Improving
Assessment
in Rehabilitation

EDITORIAL CONSULTANTS

Improving Assessment in Rehabilitation and Health

editors

Robert L. Glueckauf
Lee B. Sechrest
Gary R. Bond
Elizabeth C. McDonel

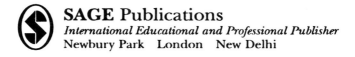

SAGE Publications
International Educational and Professional Publisher
Newbury Park   London   New Delhi

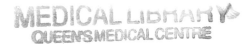

For information address:

 SAGE Publications, Inc.
2455 Teller Road
Newbury Park, California 91320

SAGE Publications Ltd.
6 Bonhill Street
London EC2A 4PU
United Kingdom

SAGE Publications India Pvt. Ltd.
M-32 Market
Greater Kailash I
New Delhi 110 048 India

Printed in the United States of America

Library of Congress Cataloging-in-Publication Data

Improving assessment in rehabilitation and health / edited by Robert
    L. Glueckauf . . . [et al.].
        p.   cm.
    Includes bibliographical references and index.
    ISBN 0-8039-5084-5 (cl).   —ISBN 0-8039-5085-3 (pb)
    1. Rehabilitation—Quality control.   2. Rehabilitation
Evaluation.   I. Glueckauf, Robert L.
    [DNLM: 1. Disability Evaluation—congresses.   2. Rehabilitation—
congresses.   3. Psychometrics—methods.   WB 320 I34 1993]
RM735.I46   1993
617.1'03'0685—dc20   93-2674

93 94 95 96 10 9 8 7 6 5 4 3 2 1

Sage Production Editor: Tara S. Mead

Contents

Introduction

Bringing the current text to fruition has been an exciting and challenging venture. During spring 1988, Rob Glueckauf and Lee Sechrest received grants from both the Ontario Ministry of Health and National Health and Welfare Canada to hold a conference, "Improving the Quality of Evaluation and Measurement in Rehabilitation," at the University of Western Ontario, London, Canada. Later that summer, however, Rob Glueckauf moved to the Psychology Department at Indiana University–Purdue University at Indianapolis (IUPUI), which necessitated the return of grant monies to the Canadian government and put the evaluation conference "on the blocks." Serendipity struck in 1989, however, when Gary Bond received a Research Scientist Development Award from the National Institute of Mental Health and suggested that a portion of his faculty release monies be used to support a working conference on assessment practices in rehabilitation. Also, around the same time, Elizabeth McDonel and John McGrew joined our rehabilitation psychology program at IUPUI, both of whom had an extensive background in assessment theory and research. Out of this fortuitous union emerged the final structure for the assessment conference and the plans for the Sage book.

Each of the book chapter contributors presented a preliminary version of his or her work at the IUPUI rehabilitation assessment conference held October 15 and 16, 1990. Most of the final papers were written subsequently, informed by lively debate and extensive editorial review. The conference planning committee—Glueckauf, Sechrest, Bond, and McDonel—decided to follow the format of the 1960 Miami Conference on research in the psychological aspects of rehabilitation (Lofquist, 1960), inviting speakers who either had expertise in rehabilitation assessment or were accomplished scientists within the broader arena of psychological assessment. Like Lofquist, we were convinced that the most productive debate would result from the juxtaposition of rehabilitation and mainstream assessment perspectives. We hope that the current text has captured the enthusiasm and rich intellectual exchange that took place at the IUPUI conference.

The primary objectives of the book are to heighten the sensitivity of practitioners and graduate students to the conceptual and methodological problems affecting the quality of assessment in rehabilitation. During the past 15 years, there has been a dramatic increase in the development and use of rehabilitation assessment techniques. Recent reports of the professional activities of rehabilitation specialists (e.g., Hickling, Sison, & Holtz, 1985; Magistro, 1989) have indicated that practitioners currently spend a substantial proportion of their time administering, scoring, and interpreting the results of assessment procedures and tests. At first glance, large investments of profession time in assessment and testing services suggest a desirable state of affairs. In this era of cost containment, few of us would be likely to argue against the need for assessment before administering expensive treatment. Unfortunately, however, there is little theory or empirical evidence supporting the widespread use of much of what is labeled "assessment" or "functional evaluation" in rehabilitation and health care (Campbell, 1987).

Although there are a few notable exceptions (see Bolton & Brookings, this volume), most widely used rehabilitation assessment procedures have not been shown to predict meaningful rehabilitation outcomes (e.g., community activity patterns, job retention) nor have they been subjected to empirical investigation. Furthermore, the findings of these assessment devices typically do not provide specific guidance for developing intervention strategies. No matter how elegant the description of physical or neuropsychological dysfunction, if assessment does not lead to specific ameliorative treatment, it offers little to the consumers of such services.

The conceptual and methodological problems facing rehabilitation today are not unique to our discipline. They pervade a number of disciplines whose primary objectives are to predict and modify human behavior, such as clinical psychology and psychiatry. There is little to be gained, however, in making assuaging comparisons between our scientific shortfalls and those of other health-related disciplines. Furthermore, our overriding goals are different: We seek to improve the quality of lives (e.g., independent living, job opportunities, and social mobility) of persons with disabilities by bringing to bear the forces of applied science and public advocacy. Other disciplines do not have as strong an interest in promoting social change.

If we are to achieve our ambitious objectives, we must go beyond minimal quality assurance standards, such as Commission on Accreditation of Rehabilitation Facilities (CARF) certification, to a full commitment to the process of scientific evaluation. Our credibility as professionals requires that we scrutinize our assumptions about the basis of practice and subject our assessment tools to scientific evaluation. But how can we make our assessment procedures more rigorous and practical? Are there basic scientific principles we can employ to increase the utility of assessment for disabled consumers? The current text addresses these and other key issues and provides concrete suggestions for improving the quality of rehabilitation assessment practice.

Each chapter addresses one of eight questions critical to the integrity and utility of rehabilitation assessment:

1. What is the role of theory in the development and evaluation of rehabilitation assessment techniques?
2. How good are current assessment methods in predicting rehabilitation treatment outcomes?
3. How adequate are the psychometric standards of current rehabilitation assessment techniques?
4. What is the role of the person with a disability in the development and evaluation of rehabilitation assessment methods?
5. To what extent are the findings of rehabilitation assessment procedures used in formulating treatment interventions?
6. How cost effective are current assessment practices in rehabilitation?

7. What are the most effective approaches for training graduate students to conceptualize and carry out rehabilitation assessment strategies?
8. How can we improve the integrity and quality of rehabilitation assessment data?

The organization of the current book revolves around these eight questions. Part I focuses on the importance of theory in the development and evaluation of rehabilitation assessment strategies. Both chapters in this part review fundamental scientific principles. The chapter by Richard McFall focuses on improving the quality of our theoretical constructs. McFall revisits some of psychology's favorite constructs with a critical eye. He persuasively argues that no amount of tinkering with the precision of the measurement model, or the psychometric properties of our instruments, will compensate for the use of fuzzy, poorly constructed, or antiquated theoretical models. The second chapter, by Robert Keith and Mark Lipsey, introduces a scheme for increasing conceptual focus on currently well-developed programs and practices in rehabilitation. Keith and Lipsey argue for a broader, more integrated theoretical formulation of health to guide the choice of constructs used for assessment. A model of health-related quality of life is presented as a potential candidate for choosing relevant assessment domains.

Part II consists of three chapters concerned with predicting rehabilitation outcomes and in judging the psychometric adequacy of standardized rehabilitation assessment instruments. Bond and Dietzen examine the array of strategies currently in use by rehabilitation professionals for making vocational training and placement decisions, asking if these practical, face-valid approaches also demonstrate predictive validity. They generally do not. Drawing on the principle that the best predictors are observations in settings that are most similar to those being predicted, Bond and Dietzen recommend assessment in real work settings, examining both worker behavior and environmental characteristics. The chapter by David Faust examines applications of neuropsychological testing, arguing that efforts to predict everyday functioning from such tests are doomed to failure—even if we incorporate actuarial decision rules that have demonstrably greater validity than clinical judgment. The problem with traditional neuropsychological batteries is not their lack of rigor but that they were not designed to predict everyday functioning. Faust suggests that we must begin again, by defining what it is that needs measuring.

The chapter by Bolton and Brookings provides optimism that excellence in rehabilitation and health assessment is possible. With their selection of exemplar instruments, Bolton and Brookings suggest that it is possible to approximate both psychometric rigor and practical utility.

Part III provides a provocative analysis of what motivates practitioners to select specific assessment instruments, who benefits most from rehabilitation assessment, and what methods should be used to teach students about rehabilitation assessment. We discover that the real-world practice of assessment departs dramatically from practices called for by the science of assessment. The chapter by Robert Glueckauf emphasizes that despite huge annual expenditures on assessment services for persons with disabilities, there is little empirical evidence supporting the clinical utility of most rehabilitation assessment practices.

Most rehabilitation assessment methods in use today have only weak conceptual and empirical linkages to intervention. Using his own Family and Disability Assessment System as a guide, Glueckauf delineates the requirements for developing utility-focused assessment methods in health and rehabilitation. The chapter by Teena Wax examines the role of the consumer with a disability in the "rehabilitation marketplace." She contends that the success of rehabilitation assessment is dependent on the assessor's ability to accommodate the needs and values of the consumer. Wax provides both a conceptual framework and illustrative examples of how assessment can be tailored to fit the functional abilities and value orientation of different disability groups. The chapter by Alfred Kazsniak and Jennifer Bortz focuses on the thorny issue of the cost-effectiveness of neuropsychological assessment. They provide a concise review of the basic theoretical issues involved in cost-effectiveness analysis and link these concepts to the practice of neuropsychological assessment. Kazsniak and Bortz emphasize the important role of neuropsychological theory in guiding the implementation of variables involved in cost-effectiveness analyses, particularly the relationship between neuropsychological assessment and theoretical explanations of functional recovery after brain damage.

The final chapter in Part III, by Timothy Elliott, addresses several important issues regarding the preparation of psychology graduate students for work in rehabilitation and health care settings. He argues that graduate training should include exposure to a variety of assessment methods as well as to didactic information about the limitations of traditional assessment methods (e.g., the Beck Depression Inventory, MMPI) with chronically disabled populations. Elliott strongly urges that students interested in working with clients in medical and health care settings should learn to integrate assessment data within theoretical models incorporating biological, social, environmental, and personality factors (e.g., Turk & Rudy, 1987; Wright, 1983).

Part IV synthesizes and integrates the key theoretical, measurement, and professional issues currently facing the field of rehabilitation and proposes new directions for improving the quality and integrity of our assessment practices. The chapter by David Cordray and Georgine Pion addresses important questions regarding the adequacy of evidence on which to base conclusions on the validity and usefulness of rehabilitation measures. They set out the points at which measurement is useful in rehabilitation work and show how that framework is related both more generally to measurement problems and to decisions about evidence. Their chapter is particularly useful in arguing that adducing evidence in favor of a proposition is almost always a matter of synthesizing a variety of findings and theoretical propositions from different sources. The chapter by Jeffrey Brookings and Brian Bolton illustrates how rehabilitation researchers can apply sophisticated statistical techniques to determine the factorial validity of assessment instruments. Their work addresses a fundamental weakness in the rehabilitation literature—the generalizability of a factor structure of tests developed in the general population to rehabilitation samples. Through LISREL, the authors demonstrate that instrument development can be much more a cumulative enterprise than the piecemeal approach that has dominated the literature.

Finally, Lee Sechrest reminds us of the enormity of the task of assessment in rehabilitation and health. He points out a number of generic measurement issues, many of them well known but still neglected. Sechrest suggests that health care scientists have lacked the will to do the hard work required to refine their assessment measures.

We have designed the book for use in graduate assessment courses across the broad spectrum of health and rehabilitation disciplines, including psychology; nursing; physical medicine and rehabilitation; and speech, recreation, occupational, and physical therapy. The material covered in each chapter may be particularly enlightening to graduate students who are preparing for fieldwork in health care and rehabilitation settings. Established practitioners and researchers may also find the current text thought provoking. It challenges a number of cherished assumptions about what constitutes reasonable and effective assessment practice and offers new approaches to increase the utility of rehabilitation assessment.

Finally, we wish to express our appreciation to Sage editor Christine Smedley for her unswerving support and guidance in publishing the current text. We wish to thank our editorial consultants, Joan Austin, Mike Eisenberg, Judy Feinberg, and Lauro Halstead, for reviewing the contents of the book and providing valuable feedback to the editors; Carolyn Farmer and Patricia Gould, for their assistance in organizing the IUPUI assessment conference and typing portions of the book; IUPUI Dean Carol Nathan for subsidizing a portion of the assessment conference; and, finally, John Hazer, former chairperson of the IUPUI psychology department, and our rehabilitation psychology graduate students for their enthusiastic support of the assessment conference.

PART I

The Role of Theory in the Development and Evaluation of Rehabilitation Assessment Strategies

CHAPTER 1

The Essential Role of Theory in Psychological Assessment

Richard M. McFall

The ideas that I will present in this chapter are neither original nor revolutionary; however, they are so fundamental to all good psychological assessment—yet so neglected in practice—that they warrant repetition, especially at the beginning of a book aimed at fostering improvement in psychological assessment. I first encountered these ideas in my graduate courses with Professors Julian B. Rotter and George A. Kelly at The Ohio State University. Soon thereafter, I encountered them again in two books published by Lee Sechrest and his colleagues in 1966. Perhaps it is not coincidental that Sechrest also studied with Rotter and Kelly at The Ohio State only a few years ahead of me.

The first of the two books was the classic *Psychotherapy and the Psychology of Behavior Change* (Goldstein, Heller, & Sechrest, 1966), which showed how productive it could be to link applied psychological interests in psychotherapy and behavior change to

AUTHOR'S NOTE: The section of this chapter dealing with the reinforcement construct is based, in part, on a symposium paper by Richard M. McFall and Richard Viken, titled *Evolving Theoretical Constructs in Behavior Therapy: From Reinforcement to Disequilibrium to Dynamic Systems,* presented at the annual convention of the Association for the Advancement of Behavior Therapy, Washington, DC, November 5, 1989.

the larger body of knowledge, research, and theory in psychology, more specifically to social psychological research on interpersonal attraction, influence, cognitive dissonance, attitude change, small group behavior, leadership, and a variety of similar topics. This was an innovative, provocative, and stimulating book.

The second book was *Unobtrusive Measures: Nonreactive Research in the Social Sciences* (Webb, Campbell, Schwartz, & Sechrest, 1966). If the average half-life of a book is somewhere in the neighborhood of 3 years, then it is remarkable, indeed, for a book to remain vital, as this one has, for more than 25 years. One of the exciting things about the book is that it frees us from the rigid restrictions of traditional ways of conceptualizing assessment tasks and encourages us to seek, instead, imaginative and nonreactive ways of solving assessment problems. Too often, psychologists think about assessment tasks only within the narrow framework of the traditional psychometrician, or "test giver." Preoccupied with administering, scoring, and interpreting established psychological tests, psychologists do not give sufficient attention to alternative approaches to psychological assessment.

The book *Unobtrusive Measures* helped broaden psychology's focus by showing us that our choice of assessment methods should depend on our theoretical preconceptions, on what we want to know, and on what information is available to us through alternative methods, at what costs. Quite often, the best way to assess something is *not* to reach for an established, off-the-shelf assessment tool, which may have been designed to assess a different theoretical construction, but instead to create a new tool, tailor-made to represent the specific construct of interest as directly and efficiently as possible. This may require more initial effort, of course, but, as Meehl (1973) has suggested, the science of psychology may be hard, if done properly.

Thus I will be stressing a pair of notions in this chapter: One is that our clinical theory and practice should be linked to the broader base of theory and knowledge in psychology; the other is that we should develop more targeted and innovative approaches to assessment problems rather than relying mindlessly on established off-the-shelf assessment instruments. I will be suggesting that both notions are central to improving the quality of our assessment practices. I will go even farther, however, by suggesting that, unless these notions are taken more seriously than they have been up to now, we cannot hope to develop a viable technology of assessment in psychology. Finally, I will suggest that rehabilitation psychology, for reasons that should become apparent, is in an excellent position to lead the way in the application of these notions to the development of an improved assessment technology.

My belief that rehabilitation psychologists are in an ideal position to lead us toward an improved assessment technology grows out of a personal experience: While a clinical psychology intern at Hines Veterans Hospital in Chicago, in 1963-1964, I was expected to do rotations on three different services. After the customary rotations on the psychiatric and neuropsychiatric units, I chose—for reasons I cannot reconstruct—to do my third rotation on the blind rehabilitation unit. In retrospect, this turned out to be the best experience of my internship and one of the more formative experiences of my career. Among other things, it gave me a high level of respect for the unique perspective of rehabilitation psychology.

Upon arriving on the blind rehab unit, I discovered that the clinical psychologists there didn't really know what to do with themselves. They couldn't administer traditional tests—Rorschachs, TATs, Bender Gestalts—to blind patients. Moreover, all of the patients on the unit were traumatically blinded veterans, so the immediate cause of their psychological problems was clear and the usual psychological interventions—talking about childhood traumas or about repressed feelings—were not particularly appropriate. No amount of such talk could change the harsh realities that had brought the patients to the hospital. Many of th ? patients had responded to their blindness with clearly diagnosable psychiatric symptoms—hallucinations, paranoid ideas, phobias, and so on. For the most part, the clinical psychologists on the unit seemed resigned to writing formal psychological reports in which they simply detailed these obvious symptoms.

Meanwhile—thank goodness—the unit also was staffed with rehabilitation specialists, who applied a very different perspective and set of approaches to the patients' problems. These specialists analyzed the problems from a competence perspective: What would the patients need to learn to live the rest of their lives at the highest level possible, despite their limited visual capacities? The specialists had identified the "problems-in-living" associated with blindness, had engineered ways for the patients to minimize or work around such problems, and had designed a treatment program specifically aimed at teaching the patients the life skills they needed to survive.

For example, the rehab specialists had determined that impaired mobility is one of the most immediate and daunting problems facing a traumatically blinded adult. Through research, they had determined the best methods of restoring the blinded veteran's mobility and had made such mobility training a cornerstone of the treatment program. As a trainee on the unit, I received mobility training and found it to be a remarkable learning experience. The mobility trainers knew their business; they went about it in an efficient, positive, and professional manner.

The rehab specialists also had determined that, if the veterans were going to support themselves, they would need new job skills and coaching in how to find a job. Thus a systematic job-skills assessment was followed by an individualized, employment-oriented training program.

The blind rehabilitation program took only 18 weeks. Typically, the veterans entered the program immobile and dependent; they would sit in their rooms, unable to get around, fend for themselves, or do many of the basic things that they had taken for granted previously. By the end of 18 weeks, however, virtually all of them were able to pass a series of stringent performance tests covering the range of independent-living skills that had been the focus of their rehabilitation treatment. The final exam in mobility training, for example, involved taking a solo trip to downtown Chicago to buy a specific item at Marshall Fields Department Store. The patients, many of whom were from rural areas, might have been intimidated by downtown Chicago even if they had been sighted, so you can imagine the sense of achievement and independence they gained from making a successful trip despite their blindness.

For each area of training, there was a corresponding final exam, or graduation test, which sampled the veterans' real-world applications of the newly acquired skills and tools. For example, the final exam in communication training tested patients' ability to solve real-life communication problems using telephones, typewriters, audiotape recorders, and other orthotic tools. These tests served both as evaluations of learning and as demonstrations of competence. As a clinical psychology intern, I was struck by how little these tests resembled traditional psychological assessments yet how well they reflected a patient's learning and how well they predicted an individual's ability to function independently.

Interestingly, as the blind veterans acquired their new skills in mobility, employment, communication, and so forth, their psychiatric symptoms tended to disappear—as if by magic. This astounded me and forced me to reconsider my theoretical assumptions about the nature of clinical problems. Subsequently, my career has been devoted primarily to research on the assessment of social skills and competencies in clinical populations, to analyzing how the fit between a person's competencies and his or her environments is related to psychological disorders, and to developing interventions aimed at improving the person-environment fit. Although I do not claim to be a rehabilitation psychologist, the perspective underlying my research has a great deal in common with the rehabilitation perspective I encountered as an intern. This perspective gives the field of rehabilitation psychology a special advantage, in my opinion, when it comes to developing new and better methods of psychological assessment.

Against the background of these personal observations, let me turn now to the central question of this chapter: How can we improve the quality of assessment in rehabilitation psychology? What I will be arguing here is that the answer to this question is grounded in the essential relationship between our theoretical models and our measurement models. Ultimately, of course, we also must be concerned with such traditional assessment issues as the reliability and validity of our measures; but, even before we can attend to such psychometric issues, we must address more fundamental questions about (a) the quality of the constructs that our measures are designed to assess and (b) the fidelity with which we have translated our theoretical constructs into specific measurement operations. Although these conceptual questions may seem "old hat," I am convinced, for reasons I will illuminate in a moment, that the sorry state of affairs in psychological assessment today is due, in large part, to psychology's preoccupation with professional practice and technique, to the relative neglect of these more basic conceptual issues. Thus these issues warrant repetition and emphasis.

Epistemology

The first step toward improving the quality of our assessments is to strengthen the scientific foundations upon which our psychological assessments are built. What do I mean by "scientific foundations"? What is "good science"? According to Karl Popper (1962), an eminent philosopher of science, the critical demarcation between science and pseudoscience is a difference in epistemology. Science can be distinguished from other approaches to "truth" by its special rules for determining whether or not we "know" something. We commonly refer to these rules as "the scientific method," although in fact there is not a single method but a general set of principles that guide how we think about "truth," how we "know truth" when we see it, and how we choose among competing claims to "truth."

To begin with, the language of science is propositional. A scientific theory says, in effect, "Suppose we impose this hypothetical order on events, or try viewing events through these artificial lenses; what, if anything, does this buy us?" Thus the scientist constructs a model of reality, then evaluates the degree to which this model does better than rival models at organizing, describing, and predicting events. To the degree that it does, then "it buys us something." Psychologists say that the model has "incremental validity" (a concept for which we are indebted, in part, to Lee Sechrest, once again).

Popper (1962) argued that scientists must go beyond merely *confirming* their pet model's theoretical predictions, however. Astrologers, shamans, soothsayers, and other nonscientists also seek to confirm their theoretical predictions. What is distinctive about the scientific approach to "truth" is its insistence on subjecting theoretical models to critical tests aimed at their *disconfirmation*.

Richard Feynman (1985), a Nobel laureate in physics, characterized the difference between science and pseudoscience in this memorable way: He equated pseudoscience with "cargo cult science," a metaphorical reference to the cargo cult culture in the South Seas. The story is that some South Sea natives had benefited from all the material that had been brought to their island during World War II, but, when the war ended and the military pulled out, these natives were thrown back to their original conditions, lacking many of the goods and materials to which they had become accustomed. In an effort to attract more material goods, the natives decided to re-create the physical conditions that had brought such goods to their island in the first place. They built runways, put torches along the sides of these, built a control tower and had a person sit in the tower with bamboo sticks, like antennae, on his head. They tried to do everything just the way they thought it had been done, and then they waited for the material to come again. Of course, nothing came. They didn't understand the essence of what had caused it to come in the first place. Cargo cult scientists, in Feynman's view, behave like these South Sea island natives; they imitate science—go through all the motions of doing science—but, because they don't understand the essence of genuine science, they don't produce anything of real scientific value.

The essence of genuine science, according to Feynman (1985), is "scientific integrity." The essential missing ingredient in cargo cult science is "a principle of scientific thought that corresponds to a kind of utter honesty—a kind of leaning over backwards."

> If you make a theory, for example, and advertise it, or put it out, then you must also put down all the facts that disagree with it, as well as those that agree with it. There is also a more subtle problem. When you have put a lot of ideas together to make an elaborate theory, you want to make sure, when explaining what it fits, that those things it fits are not just the things that gave you the idea for the theory; but that the finished theory makes something else come out right, in addition. . . . The idea is to try to give *all* of the information to help others to judge the value of your contribution; not just the information that leads to judgment in one particular direction or another. (pp. 311-312)

Thus Feynman's notion of scientific integrity is related to Popper's (1962) principle of "falsifiability." In science, a theory's status is directly proportional to its ability to survive rigorous attempts at its falsification. A good theory not only says what will happen but also prohibits other things from happening. Thus the best theories make risky predictions; the riskier the prediction, the easier it should be to falsify the theory. When a theory's risky predictions resist falsification, this is impressive to scientists. It is precisely because astrologers, shamans, and soothsayers do not make risky, falsifiable predictions that such enterprises are outside the bounds of science (see McGrew & McFall, 1990). Unfortunately, much of what goes on today under the rubric of psychology also does not meet this criterion and falls outside the bounds of science. Some psychologists—most notably Skinnerians (e.g., Bechtoldt, 1959)—have attempted to achieve scientific respectability and to distance themselves from their pseudoscientific colleagues by disavowing the use of all theoretical constructs. This is an impossible solution, however; theoretical constructs simply are unavoidable. To construe anything is to theorize at some level. Even at the most basic perceptual level, we impose order on events; we attend to some things and not to others; we chunk experience into units; we treat certain events as though they were the same, even though no two events ever are exactly the same. Our construal of events is not inductive; constructs do not arise directly from sensory ex- perience. Rather, constructs are conjectures about the order of nature; they are creative, propositional acts (Popper, 1962).

The question is not whether respectable scientists use constructs; all scientists do. The question is this: "What constructs are best, and how can we know good ones from bad ones?" Again, this is where the so-called scientific method comes in; it offers a loose set of rules by which to play the game, a system by which to choose among various competing representations of experience. The goal of science, we say, is "knowledge." Stated more formally and precisely, the goal is "information," which can be defined, in turn, as "the reduction of uncertainty" (Shannon & Weaver, 1949). Good scientific constructs reduce uncertainty by increasing our ability to predict events, to find order in events that formerly looked chaotic. Simply stated, good scientific constructs allow us to make risky predictions; poor scientific constructs don't.

Implications for Assessment: Constructs Revisited

All assessment involves the manipulation of constructs. The constructs are not manipulated directly; rather, the abstract constructs first must be translated into concrete, observable, and replicable operations. These operational definitions serve as referents, or stand-ins, for the constructs; the theory's general predictions are tested indirectly by assessing the hypothesized relationships among these referents (Cronbach & Meehl, 1955; MacCorquodale

& Meehl, 1948). To do this, we devise one or more quantitative measures of each referent and specify what mathematical relationships should be found among these quantitative measures. These operations and predicted relationships constitute our *measurement model*. When we conduct an assessment, we actually are manipulating and testing our measurement model, which is a concrete representation of our abstract *theoretical model*.

Thus there is an inevitable link between our theoretical constructs, on the one hand, and the measurement model by which we hope to capture those constructs, on the other hand. Obviously, for a measurement model to be useful, it must reflect accurately the more general theoretical model it is supposed to represent. Even the best theoretical model can be made to look bad if it is represented by a weak, poorly conceived measurement model. Conversely, if the theoretical constructs are weak to begin with, no amount of effort at careful quantification can save them; a measurement model cannot rise above the level of the theoretical model it represents. As computer scientists are fond of saying, "Garbage in, garbage out."

Now, with this brief refresher course in the philosophy of science, we are ready at last to consider the question of how best to improve the quality of assessment in rehabilitation psychology, as follows. The single most important thing rehabilitation psychologists (or any other psychologists, for that matter) can do to improve the quality of their assessment, at this point, is to begin improving the quality of the theoretical constructs that their measures are designed to assess. I am not arguing, by the way, that psychometric issues, such as sampling procedures, item selection, test reliability, or choice of statistical technique, are unimportant; rather, I am arguing that the greatest improvement in validity will come from improving our underlying theoretical constructs first. To illustrate my thesis, let's examine critically three commonly accepted theoretical constructs in use among psychologists today: "anxiety," "social skills deficit," and "reinforcement." I could have chosen any number of constructs to illustrate my point but have picked these three because they are problematic constructs that most psychologists don't stop to question, even though the research suggests that we ought to question them.

Most psychologists who routinely use these constructs probably are not aware of their shaky scientific status. These constructs have been reified; they are treated as "real," beyond question. No longer are they considered propositional; no longer must the person who uses them prove their utility by showing that they provide information, reduce uncertainty, have incremental validity. How useful are they? What, if anything, is wrong with them? Let's look briefly at the constructs of "anxiety" and "social skills deficit." Then we will look in more detail at the construct of "reinforcement."

Anxiety. The first test of any construct is this: How do you know it when you see it; can you specify its referents? The second test: How well do the different referents for the same construct hang together? The construct of anxiety has trouble satisfying these two basic criteria. I need not review all of the evidence here. Nearly a quarter of a century ago, Walter Mischel (1968), in his classic book *Personality and Assessment,* examined the evidence concerning trait constructs, including the construct of anxiety, and found them wanting. The situation has not changed much in the intervening years (McFall & McDonel, 1986), despite numerous suggestions about how to reinterpret the evidence to salvage trait constructs (e.g., Alker, 1972; Block, 1968; Epstein, 1978).

There still seems to be little consensus about the appropriate referents for the anxiety construct. Furthermore, different measures of the anxiety construct fail to show an appropriate degree of convergent and discriminant validity (Campbell & Fiske, 1959). Where there is evidence of convergence, there also tends to be a high degree of common method variance. Finally, when the construct of anxiety is invoked, it tends to be used tautologically; that is, persons observed to behave "anxiously" are said to behave that way because they *have* "anxiety" or *are* "anxious" persons. Although efforts to improve the anxiety construct have met with very limited success over the years (e.g., Kozak & Miller, 1982; Lang, 1968; Lang & Cuthbert, 1984), most psychologists blithely continue using it as though its meaning and utility have been established beyond question.

The quality of psychological assessments will not be improved until constructs such as anxiety no longer are used uncritically. Suppose, for example, that a psychologist tells us, after conducting a psychological assessment, that a patient is suffering from an anxiety disorder. Rather than accepting this conclusion as a meaningful statement, we must develop the habit of asking: What observable referents are subsumed under this diagnostic label? Is the label offered as a description of these referents or as an explanation for them? If descriptive, does the label serve as a reliable and useful shorthand for the referents; that is, given the label, could we reconstruct accurately the referents? If explanatory, was the diagnostic label arrived at independently from the very behaviors that it was designed to explain? Such questions are likely to reveal that the anxiety construct, as typically used, is vague, post hoc, and tautological, and using constructs in this way makes psychology a cargo cult science.

Social skills deficit. The construct of social skills deficit, like the construct of anxiety, also tends to be used in a vague, post hoc, and circular manner. Again, we must begin by asking, How do we know a social skills deficit when we see one? The skills concept as presented in the literature is elusive, at best (Bellack, 1979). Is shaking hands a skill? Is smiling a skill? Is blinking? What is a skill?

Typically, a social skills deficit is not observed directly but is inferred from below-average performance on some social task. If the skills deficit concept were used merely as a shorthand description of the observed performance problem, then perhaps it might be reasonable, particularly if we could reconstruct the original behavior from the information contained in the shorthand label. Unfortunately, however, the label invariably goes beyond merely saying that the performance was deficient; it is used as a putative explanation for the observed behavior. It asserts that the observed subpar performance was due to some underlying skills deficit; the person performed poorly because he or she lacked the necessary skills to perform satisfactorily. This tends to be a hollow assertion, however, because the presumed underlying skills seldom are assessed directly or independently from the performance problems that they are supposed to have caused. Moreover, no explicit theory of the underlying skills—what they are, where they come from, how they relate to performance, and how they change—is presented.

Surprisingly, the construct of social skills deficit has become popular among psychotherapists because it is so handy, so all-purpose (Hollin & Trower, 1986). Whatever problem a patient may manifest, the therapist always can explain that it is due to a skills deficit and prescribe a regimen of skills training. If the patient should improve, the therapist can declare that the patient acquired new skills; if the patient should fail to improve, the therapist can lament the patient's failure to acquire new skills. Such an analysis, of course, is circular. It has the superficial appearance of a theoretical explanation, but it is a pseudoscientific explanation. It explains every possible outcome but makes no risky predictions; thus it cannot be falsified. Used in this way, it is cargo cult science.

Reinforcement. Arguably, there is no construct with greater currency among psychologists today than the construct of reinforcement. We use it almost without thinking. Few of us bother to ask, "What do we mean by *reinforcement?*" But when we do ask that question, we discover a problem.

This is not a new problem. Meehl (1950) long ago pointed out that, for the concept of reinforcement to be useful, the effects of the reinforcing stimulus must be transituational. That is, a stimulus that serves as a reinforcer in one setting must produce reinforcement effects in other settings. If it doesn't, then the stimulus, per se, cannot be said to be "a reinforcer." The problem, stated simply, is that it is difficult to identify a priori which stimuli will serve as reinforcers, under what conditions, in which settings.

Again, we encounter the problem of post hoc, circular definitions. It isn't good science to wait to see which stimulus increases the probability of a response in a given setting, then call that stimulus a reinforcer, and finally turn around and explain that the observed increase in response probability was caused by the reinforcement value of the stimulus. This is a tautology. For the construct of reinforcement to be meaningful, we must be able to predict which consequating event will strengthen the probability of what response, in which setting; this event should strengthen the probability of the same or other responses in the same or other settings in the future. Obviously, the concept of reinforcement as it stands today does not satisfy these criteria of predictability and transituationality.

Premack offered the "probability differential hypothesis" as a solution to this classic problem. In a series of experiments (Premack, 1959, 1965), he showed that, if you pair a high probability response with a lower probability response, the former can "reinforce" the latter, but that, if you pair the very same response with an even higher probability response, it will not function as a reinforcer. This has become known as the Premack Principle. Interestingly,

Premack's experimental designs did not include some critical conditions that would have put his hypothesis at risk of being disconfirmed. He only looked at a subset of the possible combinations of conditions; he also inadvertently manipulated response rates in a way that biased the results in favor of his predictions. Other investigators who sampled the possible experimental conditions more broadly found that the Premack Principle is incorrect; that is, a higher probability response sometimes does not function as a reinforcer, and a lower probability response sometimes can function as a reinforcer (Allison & Timberlake, 1974; Eisenberger, Karpman, & Trattner, 1967; Konarski, 1985). Such disconfirming results raised the original questions: What is a reinforcer, and how can we identify reinforcers a priori?

Timberlake and Allison (1974) have taken a different approach to answering these questions. (Although there are significant differences between the perspectives taken by Timberlake and by Allison, for our current purposes we can treat them as very similar.) Timberlake and Allison reasoned that, because no single stimulus event functions as a reinforcer at all times and under all conditions, so-called reinforcement effects cannot be a function of the particular stimulus chosen as a reinforcer. Instead, Timberlake and Allison hypothesized that reinforcement effects are a function of a "disequilibrium" (Timberlake, 1980) created when a new contingency alters the relationship found in the free operant baseline levels of two responses. This is an awkward thing to explain in words alone, so let me give a graphic illustration of how this works.

Start with any organism—say, a rat—and select any two responses—say, eating and wheel running. Next, assess the baseline probabilities of these two responses in a free operant environment—that is, where there is free access to both responses and where there is not a contingent relationship between them. The relationship recorded in the stable baselines of the two behaviors typically is plotted as shown by the lines in Figure 1.1, part a, which depicts the state of dynamic equilibrium that characterizes the behaviors of eating and running at baseline. Now, when a new contingent relationship is imposed on the two behaviors, this disrupts the equilibrium by imposing a deprivation schedule on one of the behaviors, relative to its baseline. An example of such a deprivation contingency is depicted by the lines in Figure 1.1, part b.

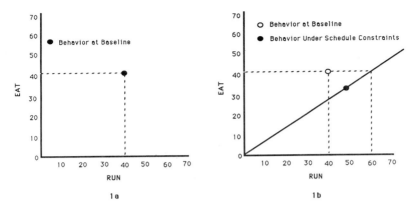

Figure 1.1. The Dynamic Relationship Between Two Responses, Eating and Wheel Running, in a Fictitious Rat

NOTE: Depicted in 1a is the initial free operant baseline levels of the two responses. Depicted in 1b are the constraining effects on behaviors of imposing a schedule contingency, represented by the diagonal line, which requires that wheel running be increased over baseline levels for eating to be maintained at baseline levels. The solid circle shows how the disequilibrium created by this schedule was resolved through a compromise; wheel running exceeded baseline levels while eating fell short of baseline levels.

Under this new contingency, the organism cannot maintain its baseline level of one behavior (eating) without exceeding its baseline level of the second behavior (wheel running). Due to the disruptive influence of the deprivation, created by this new schedule constraint, we can predict that changes will occur in both the eating and the wheel running behaviors. In effect, a new equilibrium point (sometimes called a "bliss point") is established in the paired be- haviors. This equilibrium will be a compromise (illustrated by the solid circle), in which the organism exceeds its baseline level of the operant response while falling below its baseline level of the contingent response. Given the contingent relationship imposed on the paired responses, the organism's adjusted level of responding must fall somewhere along the diagonal line that defines the contingency.

Note that the observed effects are a function of changes in the contingent relationships, relative to baseline; they are not a function of any intrinsic effects of specific stimuli. This means that we could have created a "reinforcement effect" in the opposite direction simply by reversing the contingencies, producing a disequilibrium that would have required the organism to exceed its baseline level of eating to maintain its baseline level of wheel running. Thus either response—eating or wheel running—could have served as the so-called reinforcer for the other, given the necessary contingent schedule and resulting disequilibrium in response relationships relative to their initial baseline conditions.

Timberlake and Allison's (1974) analysis of reinforcement has some intriguing implications. First, it challenges the idea that any stimulus event has intrinsic reinforcing properties. It is not the stimulus, per se, but the dynamic relationships among stimuli that produce what have been called reinforcement effects. To understand reinforcement effects, we must analyze the paired baseline probabilities of the critical responses in the relevant contexts; only then can we begin to predict the effects of imposing schedule constraints on these relationships. Only when we can predict such effects reliably can we begin to employ this knowledge with confidence in the design of interventions (see Timberlake & Farmer-Dougan, 1991, for a fuller discussion of the disequilibrium model's therapeutic implications).

Second, Timberlake and Allison's analysis indicates that we must develop a better understanding of how to classify contexts. No catalog exists that allows us to determine whether a given context should be considered as the same as, or as different than, some other context. Context categories are theoretical constructions; as such, they require the same kind of empirical validation as other theoretical constructions. What are "contexts"? What contexts go together? Such questions make the concept of reinforcement far more complex than we originally thought when at first we set out—in an atheoretical way—to shape behavior by manipulating reinforcers.

Finally, I hasten to add that Timberlake and Allison's analysis of reinforcement has raised new questions, even as it has resolved others. Allison (1983), for example, has focused on the "behavioral economics" of the disequilibrium model, searching for underlying principles by which we can predict the dynamic adjustments that the organism will make in response to different schedule constraints. What factors determine, for example, what compromise the organism will settle for under different contingencies, as illustrated by the solid circle in Figure 1.1, part b? Meanwhile, Timberlake (1980) has explored the interplay of biological constraints and schedule constraints in determining the reorganization of the organism's behavioral systems.

Cautions, Caveats, and Future Directions

My aim in this chapter has been to draw attention to the disturbing disparity between the low scientific status of the constructs underlying many of our psychological assessment methods, on the one hand, and the high level of acceptance accorded those concepts and methods by psychologists, on the other hand. Although I have illustrated my point by focusing on the constructs of anxiety, social skills deficit, and reinforcement, I could have focused just as easily on any number of other widely used psychological constructs, such as attribution, codependency, cognition, competence, compliance, empowerment, quality of life, self-efficacy, self-esteem, social support, or stress. Thus the implications of my argument are not limited to the specific constructs I have discussed but extend to the assessment enterprise in general: If the quality of our psychological assessments is limited by the quality of the constructs that our measurement models are designed to capture, then we should be concerned, given the poor quality of our current constructs, about the scientific status of our assessment enterprise.

We certainly cannot afford to be complacent or assume that the measures currently on our shelf are adequate and useful. Just because a measure has the name "anxiety scale," for example, does not mean that scores derived from it are useful indices of a meaningful construct. How can we expect useful information from a test purporting to assess anxiety when the anxiety construct itself is suspect? We need to take a skeptical look at psychological assessment in general.

For the sake of simplicity, I have taken a critical look at individual constructs and have considered these in isolation. Good psychological theories do not deal with isolated constructs, however, but with the relationships among constructs. Analyzing constructs in isolation is like planning a trip by taking scissors to the road atlas and cutting out the dots depicting the cities you plan to visit. What we most need to know about cities and constructs alike is how they are linked to the other elements in their networks.

Psychological assessment aimed at mapping the network of constructs is even more complicated and demanding than I have portrayed in my discussion of isolated constructs. Of necessity, the assessment of network relations among constructs is theory driven; it requires higher-order notions about how the elements within the network interact, how one construct can be predicted from another, how changes in one node of the system will affect other nodes. For example, when depression increases, what other changes should we expect to occur in the network?

Unfortunately, even our most successful psychological assessments have not achieved this level of complexity and precision. Our best measures, such as IQ tests, allow us to predict future behavior from past behavior only in the simplest form: A person who performs intelligently on an IQ test is likely to perform intelligently on similar tasks, such as in school. Our tests do not allow us to do much better than we could by simply using base rates at predicting whether a person with a high IQ score will become depressed, display schizophrenic symptoms, develop ulcers, be a good parent, or commit criminal acts, for example.

These sobering reflections on the weak power of our current psychological assessments should keep us humble about what psychologists can and cannot do with their tests and measures. Furthermore, they should stir us out of complacency and urge us toward improving the quality of our assessments. Next time you are tempted to pull a test off the shelf, ask yourself, "Is this really the most direct and efficient way to get quality information about the question that I'm asking?" For the reasons I've outlined here, chances are, it isn't. Unless the person who developed the instrument was asking the same question you are, the measure probably will not give you the information you need. Reaching for an off-the-shelf measure because it is convenient, or because it bears a name that comes close to what you are looking for, is like looking for your lost car keys under the street lamp because the light is better there. To get the information you need, there may be no simple and easy solution; perhaps you will have to develop a measure specifically designed for your purpose. It was in this spirit that Sechrest and his colleagues, in *Unobtrusive Measures* (Webb et al., 1966), encouraged us to develop innovative ways to use archival data and other such information to find answers to some assessment questions rather than relying exclusively on answers from psychological tests that often tend to be reactive and ill-fitted to our aims.

At the risk of overwhelming you with cautions, I want to note one more area in which we must guard against accepting uncritically the value of standard approaches to psychological assessment. When choosing statistical methods for the analysis of observed relations among various measures of different constructs, we must resist the temptation to reach automatically for off-the-shelf statistical packages, such as SPSS-X, SAS, or whatever you have in your computer. Here again, we must stop to consider whether the assumptions behind these common statistical techniques are consistent with the theoretical assumptions behind the constructs being tested. For example, most of our statistical techniques assume a linearity of relationships; yet, some promising theoretical constructs assume nonlinear relationships (e.g., the effects of arousal on performance). Statistical analyses must not violate our theoretical assumptions.

Similarly, some statistical techniques assume independence of observations; yet, some of the most interesting phenomena in the real world do not satisfy this assumption of independence (e.g., dyadic interactions across time). Before we can study the relationships among our constructs, therefore, we must think carefully about the statistical implications of our measurement model and our theory. There is no automatically correct way to analyze the relationships among variables. When we conduct an assessment, we are testing a model—our constructed representation of reality—and our choice of analyses must fit this model (see Meehl, 1971, for an extended discussion of this point).

What does all of this mean for the future of psychological assessment? One important implication concerns the approach we take toward training the psychological assessors of the future. We must teach students to think critically about assessment questions rather than simply teaching them a specific set of assessment techniques. Our current measures, which are inadequate and certain to be replaced, are doomed to obsolescence; therefore students trained in these methods, but not taught how to develop and evaluate new methods, will be trained for obsolescence.

I am not suggesting that psychological assessors should abandon standardized tests altogether and trust their clinical intuition and judgment instead. My point is quite the opposite. Psychologists must stop practicing assessment as a cargo cult science. This means that we must apply rigorous scientific standards to the skeptical evaluation of our assessment methods. We must subject our measures and their underlying theories to rigorous attempts at falsification. Clinical intuition has been a major part of the problem up to now; it cannot be a major part of the solution.

Perhaps you are asking yourself, at this point, "Is there any method available that is valid for my purposes?" It is a positive sign if this question is asked. First, by raising this question, we no longer are assuming, without evidence, that the available methods automatically will provide valid answers to our specific assessment questions. Second, we no longer are assuming that methods that are valid for other purposes will be valid for our specific purposes; we are recognizing the importance of method specificity. Third, we are beginning to evaluate the available methods by scientific criteria when we ask for evidence of their validity. The answer to this question, of course, depends on the particular assessment task.

What do psychologists working in the field do if there are no valid measures available now? What if they cannot wait 5 years for a new instrument to be developed? First, in the absence of valid measures, we gain nothing by adopting invalid or inappropriate measures just for the sake of filling the void. There are many real-life examples of circumstances in which there are no immediate answers and we simply must wait until an answer is found (e.g., AIDS, cancer, poverty); psychological assessment is no different. Second, we are more likely to find valid answers in the long run if we honestly evaluate the validity of our methods, thereby identifying the assessment tasks most urgently in need of new and better methods. Third, it need not take 5 years to develop and validate new measures for specific assessment tasks. Once again, Sechrest and his colleagues have illustrated in *Unobtrusive Measures* some imaginative ways in which we might design tailor-made assessments for specific questions.

One thing does seem clear: Psychologists who employ assessment techniques to make critical life decisions for others must be held accountable to the highest standards of "truth in advertising" (McFall, 1991). Assessors simply are not justified in using unvalidated tests in vague, unstandardized ways to guide them in making critical decisions about clients, in either a clinical or a judicial context. Recently, Matarazzo (1990) tried to defend such assessment practices, suggesting that this approach to critical decision making is better than nothing and, over time, is self-corrective; someone must make the decisions, and feedback about the accuracy of decisions should enable psychologists to home in on the truth and make increasingly accurate decisions. Matarazzo offered no evidence in support of his argument, however. At the same time, other investigators who have reviewed the evidence carefully and critically (e.g., Dawes, Faust, & Meehl, 1989) have challenged Matarazzo's conclusion. Clinical judgments seldom get checked against later data; but, even where they do, the accuracy of the judgments does not seem to improve as a consequence. We must not allow psychologists to misrepresent the validity of their clinical judgments in critical life decisions; the likelihood of errors is high and such errors can cause severe and permanent harm.

As a practical matter, psychological assessors ought to concentrate for now on making simple predictions that are relatively easy to evaluate and, if appropriate, to disconfirm. Only after achieving success with these simpler assessment problems should psychologists dare to venture into making more difficult predictions. It is amazing how willing some psychologists are to undertake assessment tasks in which events are virtually impossible to predict, where the outcomes are a function of variables that cannot be known because they themselves are unpredictable and have not yet occurred. Equally amazing is the public's apparent willingness to believe that psychologists can determine the truth about such in- credibly complex distal events, even though these same psychologists cannot determine the truth about simpler, more proximal, easily verified events.

One common argument for the perpetuation of questionable assessment practices in psychology is that market demands—most notably the demands of third-party payers—require that we provide a formal diagnosis, which calls for the use of standard tests such as the MMPI. Administering measures for these reasons alone, of course, amounts to letting the tail wag the dog. It is unethical to participate in (and accept fees for) an assessment practice that is fundamentally invalid or that is an invalid application of an otherwise valid technique.

If many of our current assessment methods lack validity, perhaps we can find shortcuts to the development of new and better methods. Are there valid methods of coming up with such assessments? Yes, but even these must be related conceptually to the underlying questions that we are asking. For example, Goldfried and D'Zurilla (1969) outlined a methodology for developing competence measures. My students and I, in turn, have used a variation of this methodology successfully with a variety of problems and populations (Fisher-Beckfield & McFall, 1982; Freedman, Rosenthal, Donahoe, Schlundt, & McFall, 1978; Gaffney & McFall, 1981; Goldsmith & McFall, 1975). It would be a mistake, however, to treat this methodology as though it were a magic road to truth. It may not provide valid information in relation to some questions or concerns, even though it has been useful in specific contexts in the past.

In a similar vein, psychologists have available in their "tool chest" a variety of methodologies that, when used appropriately, can be used successfully to generate valid assessment techniques. Some familiar examples are Likert or Guttman rating methodologies, questionnaire methods, response sampling techniques, task-analysis techniques, forced-choice rating methods, critical-incident techniques, or preference scaling. Each of these examples represents a well-studied, but relatively content-free, approach to assessment. Such tools provide extra leverage for solving novel assessment problems and eliminate the need to start from scratch with each new assessment task. Nevertheless, we still must choose and apply the tools carefully, making certain that our tools match our tasks.

I have raised a number of assessment issues in this chapter. There has been one central and underlying theme throughout, however. Let me conclude by distilling the essence of my thesis: Our measurement model and statistical methods must be faithful reflections of our underlying theoretical model—its constructs and their relations. The essential goal of psychological assessment is to provide information that illuminates the specific questions being asked about our model. If our theoretical model is inadequate, then our assessments will be of low quality, as well. Currently, our theories tend to be inadequate. Therefore the most important single thing we can do to improve the quality of our assessments is to improve the quality of our psychological theories. While there is no surefire way to do this, it is clear that we will not improve our theories if we approach the task in the manner of cargo cult scientists: merely imitating the form of science rather than understanding its essence. We must take a more careful, skeptical look at the theories, constructs, and measurement models underlying our current assessment techniques.

CHAPTER 2

The Role of Theory in Rehabilitation Assessment, Treatment, and Outcomes

ROBERT ALLEN KEITH
MARK W. LIPSEY

Rehabilitation encompasses a broad range of services and populations, including restoration for physical disabilities, psychiatric problems, developmental disabilities, substance abuse, and vocational difficulties. Even though the common theme of improving capabilities runs through all these activities, it is awkward and perhaps impossible to develop a coherent discussion that involves all rehabilitation settings and populations. The focus of this chapter is limited to medical rehabilitation: those comprehensive services that minister to the severely disabled who have had strokes, head injuries, spinal cord injuries, orthopedic disorders, and the like.

Medical rehabilitation was formed from the merging of two traditions in medicine and rehabilitation. The specialty that emerged has focused on the treatment of function: the extent to which individuals are able to perform the common activities of life. The foundations of assessment and treatment lie in many disciplines: physiology, neurology, kinesiology, and psychology, to name some of the most obvious. Other fields, such as physical therapy, occupational therapy, and speech and language therapy, have also contributed to the accumulation of applied knowledge. Because medical rehabilitation spans so many different areas of study, the development of theory has been very slow. In addition, the press of helping individuals with catastrophic problems has made theory building a low priority. The aim of this chapter is to describe some lines of inquiry that might lead to a better understanding of the relationships of assessment, treatment procedures, and outcomes. Improved theory about these relationships should result in more effective rehabilitation. Although assessment is the major theme of the volume, an examination of theory cannot isolate assessment from the other elements that make up the totality of rehabilitation. Because the conceptual problems are formidable in light of the scope of rehabilitation, the aims must be modest.

Medical Rehabilitation Services

Formulations about assessment, treatment, and outcomes first require some understanding of the nature of rehabilitation services. The trademark is the comprehensive interdisciplinary team, a group of physicians, nurses, and therapists who plan and carry out treatment (England, Glass, & Patterson, 1989; Melvin, 1989). The matching of professional talents to the problems of the patient—making the comprehensive team work effectively—challenges the most efficient organization.

There are both inpatient and outpatient programs, depending upon the severity of disability and the nature of presenting problems. Inpatients usually require close medical supervision, 24-hour nursing, and an intensive program. Outpatient programs come in a variety of forms, from comprehensive outpatient services and day treatment to single services. Residential facilities may have transitional living centers, community reentry programs, and independent living centers (National Association of Rehabilitation Facilities, 1988). Some facilities specialize in the treatment of one disorder, such as spinal cord injury, head injury, or pain.

Until recently, it was difficult to obtain statistics on patient populations, but there are now several data systems for rehabilitation. The largest, for inpatients, is the Uniform Data System. Its latest report (Granger & Hamilton, 1992), of 108 hospitals, shows that

33% of the caseload consists of people who have had strokes, with the next largest group comprising orthopedic disorders, 29%. Lesser numbers come from brain injury (8%), spinal cord injury (5%), and neurological disorders (5%). Given that geriatric patients predominate, the average age is 67 years. Patients stay an average of 28 days. The effects of cost-cutting pressures are apparent; a report of rehabilitation patients of 10 years ago showed an average length of stay of 36 days (Keith & Breckenridge, 1985).

Although medical rehabilitation is a small segment of health care, it is one of the fastest growing. The number of inpatient units more than doubled between 1980 and 1989 (American Hospital Association, 1989). There were 849 freestanding hospitals and units in 1989 with over 25,000 beds (National Association of Rehabilitation Facilities, 1991, personal communication). Hospitals with outpatient programs have increased from 27% in 1980 to nearly 40% by 1987 (American Hospital Association, 1989).

Theory in Treatment Effectiveness Research

In recent years, evaluation researchers, the individuals who do treatment effectiveness research, have become increasingly interested in developing and using theory. The writings of Chen and Rossi (1980, 1983, 1987) have been instrumental in stimulating this interest. Chen and Rossi argued that evaluation research should be "theory driven" from inception—that evaluation questions, measurement and design, and analysis and interpretation should be guided by some explicit conceptualization of the causal process through which intervention is expected to have effects. There is growing recognition that, without the use of theory, evaluators will always come up short in their efforts to explain outcome results and improve the quality of treatment (Bickman, 1987, 1990).

One might ask the relevance for rehabilitation of this preoccupation with theory by evaluators. What does it have to do with therapists, administrators, and researchers? They already have a well-developed practice tradition. Why the push for theory? A major aim of this chapter will be to demonstrate the utility of theory in the understanding of assessment-treatment-outcome relationships and, as a corollary, to show that the evaluator's views here are highly germane to the providers of care. Both, after all, are interested in maximizing the effectiveness of treatment and in being able to make rational program changes on the basis of more than intuition or trial-and-error strategies.

The Role of Theory

It is beyond the reach of the human mind to be sensitive and responsive to all the potentially relevant aspects of clinical practice. Inevitably, this complexity is abstracted, schematized, and reduced to implicit theories that summarize the most important information. It is primarily upon these implicit theories that practice is based. While formal research usually contributes, most interventions depend heavily on the accumulated clinical experience of treaters. Under such conditions, it is difficult to determine in any systematic way the most effective means of treatment. Theory can play an important role in making assumptions more explicit and in providing a coherent framework for treatment practices and innovations in those practices.

A second role of theory is in its utility as an organizing mechanism for integrating new information. As new research knowledge is developed about rehabilitation practices, it is likely to be scattered and piecemeal. Again, because of the complexities, it is difficult for researchers or practitioners to organize and synthesize this knowledge in ways that permit it to be grasped and applied without oversimplification. Without an integrating conceptual framework, its implications may not be recognized and its incorporation into common practice may be impeded.

Finally, theory has an important function in the design and methodology of treatment effectiveness research itself. It can be instrumental in implementing adequately the treatment under study, identifying potentially relevant variables, and selecting and implementing outcome measures. Only through the careful integration of theory and method can treatment effectiveness research be designed in ways that fully represent the complex causal relations under study rather than reducing them to simple input-output formulations (Lipsey, 1990).

Program Theory

Program theory has been described as "the construction of a plausible and sensible model of a how a program is supposed to work" (Bickman, 1987, p. 5). In the last several years, evaluators have been trying to formulate what such theory is and how it could be used to supply a coherent framework for analyzing the processes and effects of interventions. Chen (1990) noted that most contemporary program theory is descriptive; that is, it describes or explains facts and relationships. According to Chen, there is a second kind of theory that is prescriptive in nature—it suggests what ought to be done or how to do something better. Prescriptive theory is normative, because it provides guidance on what goals or outcomes should be pursued and how treatment should be implemented. Both kinds of theory are essential: Descriptive theory is important for explaining causal relationships, while normative theory can guide program planning and implementation and provide a rationale for program structure and activities.

Sources of program theory. Lipsey and Pollard (1989) identified three approaches to theory development in the evaluation research literature. There are, first of all, prior attempts at theory formulation that might be relevant. Some rehabilitation programs, for example, have used the principles developed in operant conditioning to modify pain behavior (Gottlieb, Alperson, Schwartz, Beck, & Kee, 1988). These principles have been well worked out with laboratory animals and later with developmentally delayed and psychiatric populations.

A second approach to the explication of program theory is exploratory research. Lipsey and Pollard noted that observational and qualitative information can provide the basis for beginning formulations, which can then be tested on a small scale. A second form of exploratory research in search of theory is the study of correlational relationships among variables characterizing patients, treatments, and outcomes. These may give some indication of causation even though the confounding of various factors precludes definite conclusions. As an example, Davidoff, Ring, and Solzi (1991) found that patients with strokes in the "middle band" of severity appeared to benefit most from treatment and hold their gains at follow-up. Because patients representing a full spectrum of severity are not admitted for treatment, it is not possible to test this assumption definitively. It does, however, furnish the beginning of a theory about level of severity in relation to rehabilitation intervention.

A third approach to theory development is to identify the implicit assumptions made by program developers, providers, and others associated with programs. This requires extracting the conceptual schemas that they hold about how the intervention works. Lipsey and Pollard described two approaches from the literature that use either *cause maps* or *concept mapping,* terms that refer to the cognitive contents and belief systems of program participants.

Treatment theory. Lipsey (1990) characterized treatment theory as "small theory" that attempts to account for the processes that occur in the transformation of inputs into outcome. It does not deal with explanations of personal or social phenomena in the larger context outside the treatment issues. There are several major components of treatment theory:

1. a problem definition that specifies what condition is treatable, for which populations, and under what circumstances; that is, a statement of the boundaries that distinguish relevant situations from irrelevant ones;
2. specification of the critical inputs, that is, what is necessary, what is sufficient, and what is optimal to produce the expected effects; inter- relationships among the inputs; the basis for judging magnitude of strength of inputs (e.g., dosage levels);
3. the important steps, links, phases, or parameters of the transformation process the treatment brings about; the intervening or mediating variables upon which the process is contingent; crucial interactions with individual differences, timing, mode of delivery, or other relevant circumstances; and
4. specification of the expected outputs, that is, the nature, range, and timing of various treatment effects and side effects; interrelationships or contingencies among the outputs. (Lipsey, 1990, p. 36)

These factors furnish a blueprint for constructing treatment theory in rehabilitation in a manner that reduces the usual trial-and-error approach of much research in this area.

Theory in Rehabilitation

The essence of theory for rehabilitation consists of identification of the distinct components of assessment and treatment, the nature of their interrelationships, and their role in treatment outcome. Though little work of this scope is available, various authors have offered guidelines for such a conceptualization.

Brook and Lohr (1985), for instance, argued: "Disease models that include comorbidity, stage, process, and outcome measures need to be built, tested, and validated so that they (or their components) can be used to evaluate quality of care" (p. 716). Fuhrer (1987a) observed that we need not only better theories of rehabilitation but better theories of the disablements to which rehabilitation responds. As a foundation for such theory, he proposed specific distinctions among the constructs of impairment, disability, and handicap taken from the formulations of Wood (World Health Organization, 1980). Equally important, in Fuhrer's assessment, are the models of the rehabilitation process (see Brown, Diller, & Gordon, 1983) and attention to the social, material, and attitudinal features of the environment that impinge upon the patient.

The WHO formulations are the most widely quoted aspects of theory in rehabilitation. They refer to the level of disablement:

Disease or Injury———▸Impairment———▸Disability———▸Handicap

A disease or injury leads to an impairment, that is, a deficit at the organ level. For example, deficiencies in vascular circulation from diabetes might require a below-the-knee amputation. When the impairment is translated into the inability to perform a task—walking in this example—the result is a disability. The deficiency in task performance—the inability to walk—results in the loss of a role performance, or a handicap, as when the individual can no longer work as a lineman for the telephone company because he is unable to walk about and climb telephone poles.

Nagi (1976) presented a similar scheme:

Pathology———▸Impairment———▸Functional Limitations———▸Disability

In this model, the first two stages are similar to those of the WHO, with functional limitations reflecting performance at the individual level. For Nagi, however, disability encompasses both role performance deficiencies and those deficiencies that result from individual characteristics. Granger (1984) has integrated these two views into a framework that stresses the importance of function as a central concern in rehabilitation. He also differentiates the emphasis on function from the usual medical model, which focuses on cure.

There has been a recent addition to the Nagi model (Institute of Medicine, 1991). Two classes of variables have been included that impinge upon the processes occurring at any stage in the disablement process. Risk factors are biological, environmental (social and physical), and life-style or behavioral characteristics that are associated with health. The second class of variables include quality of life factors, such as standard of living, life satisfaction, employment, and housing. These are obviously related to the social circumstance of the individual.

Nagi (1991) has recently reviewed the historical context in which these two models arose and has compared their utility of explanation. It is his view that the WHO concepts lack clarity and do not pay sufficient attention to social and economic formulations.

The utility of these two models has been in classifying and organizing the processes that lead to physical or mental disadvantage. They have to be viewed within a social context, because deficits in individual and role performance are social definitions with cultural values attached. The loss of a limb, for example, has different economic and personal consequences in an industrialized society than in one in which physical work is performed by nearly all its members. The models are much less helpful in the development of treatment theory, which must account for cause-and-effect relations between treatment interventions and measures of outcome.

Treatment theory in rehabilitation. Rehabilitation takes place in an organizational context that is, in turn, in a larger economic and regulatory environment. The determinants of treatment effects in rehabilitation can be organized into four components: patient characteristics, internal factors in the service organization, external or environmental factors, and the treatment regimen itself (Figure 2.1).

Patient characteristics are the first set of variables. The presenting condition or impairments, age, sex, severity, stage of recovery, and existence of comorbidities or complicating conditions are all aspects of the patient that affect treatment procedures and, ultimately, outcome. Internal organizational factors also play a part:

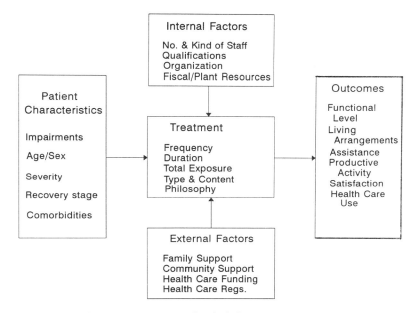

Figure 2.1. The Determinants of Rehabilitation Outcome

the numbers, type, and qualifications of staff, how they are organized, the fiscal resources at their disposal, and the physical plant in which they operate. External factors are important too: family and community support, the funding in health care, and the regulations that govern service delivery.

All of these factors impinge on the delivery of treatment itself, which can be characterized by the frequency, duration, and total exposure to treatment, its type and content, and the treatment philosophy that prevails. The totality of these factors determines what happens to patients. The outcomes can be expressed in terms of functional level, the living arrangements after discharge and how much assistance is required, the amount of health care that is needed, and, finally, the productive activities patients and family are able to engage in and their satisfaction with such activities and with the status of the patient.

Unfortunately, most rehabilitation research focuses exclusively on patient characteristics and outcomes without mention of internal or external factors or, indeed, what occurs in treatment itself.

A review of research on the prediction of function after stroke, for example, presented a table of 33 studies (Jongbloed, 1986). All of the studies concentrated on patient characteristics or patient performance during assessment; not one included a treatment variable. A second review of stroke outcomes not only looked at patient selection and outcomes but also attempted to examine the type of program and treatment intensity (Dombovy, Sandok, & Basford, 1986). The authors found generally poor description of the duration and type of therapy, if given at all. These stroke studies illustrate the incomplete nature of research when it is not guided by a larger theoretical framework.

Toward a Theoretical Framework
for Assessment-Treatment-Outcome Relations

It would be too ambitious at this point to attempt a theoretical formulation that encompasses the linkages of rehabilitation processes and their outcomes. The aim here is to identify the elements that might belong in such an exposition, to probe the assumptions behind them, and to suggest some directions that might be productive in producing a coherent theory. Because rehabilitation spans processes from a physiological and neurological level to such phenomena as social roles, it is obvious that no one set of theories will cover all of them. Explanations regarding recovery from brain injury, for example, encompass both molar and molecular theories, from issues in neural imbalance to motivation (Finger, LeVere, Almli, & Stein, 1988). The emphasis in this chapter is on the macro level, where functional skills are embedded in a social context of desirable and undesirable behavior.

Health and Health Status

Chronic disease or injury has personal, social, and economic consequences well beyond the rehabilitation setting. Restorative treatment is only an interlude in a larger struggle to overcome the effects of disability. Formulations about the nature of health and the measurement of health status in both general and clinical populations have been ongoing for many years (Bergner, 1985). Curiously, there has been very little cross-fertilization between this field and work on measurement of function in rehabilitation.

Only a couple of authors have suggested that functional assessment, as practiced in rehabilitation, should be included in the broader realm of health status (Jette, 1980; Seale & Davies, 1987). Health status indicators grew out of the need to determine more about health than just mortality and morbidity. The alleviation of infectious diseases and the saving of lives through modern methods of health care have resulted in an increase in chronic disease (Rothenberg & Koplan, 1990). Likewise, the number of lives saved in catastrophic injuries, such as brain and spinal cord injuries, has added to the numbers of disabled. Health status measures were devised to gain some understanding of the effects of both acute and chronic disease and injury on the lives of those affected.

A recent scheme by Patrick and Bergner (1990) incorporates functional status as part of the health domain, which they designate as *health quality of life.* This term has had increasing use because of the recognition that health status can have a profound impact on life-style and satisfaction with life. Table 2.1, taken from Patrick and Bergner, shows the domains involved. There is, first of all, *opportunity,* or the personal and environmental factors that encourage or restrict good health. *Health perceptions* are next, either satisfaction with health or one's perception of health status. *Functional status* encompasses social, psychological, and physical aspects, from specific physical activities to role limitations. *Impairment,* in this context, includes diagnoses, tissue alterations, evidence of disease, and subjective aspects. Last, there is *death and duration of life,* covering conventional mortality and longevity indicators.

The prominent role of functional status in this model shows the importance that function can have in formulations about health. If rehabilitation is to broaden its view to include more than the measurement of physical aspects of patient performance, it could profitably turn to formulations regarding health status.

The Nature of Recovery

If we view health as a trajectory over time that is affected by chronic and acute illness as well as the treatment applied to those conditions, we should be able to identify the factors that influence the shape of the curve. Of particular interest is the recovery curve that charts health status during and subsequent to treatment. The

TABLE 2.1
Concepts and Domains of Health-Related Quality of Life

Concepts and Domains	Definitions/Indicators
Opportunity	
Social or cultural handicap	Disadvantage because of health
Individual resilience	Capacity for health; ability to withstand stress; reserve
Health perceptions	
Satisfaction with health	Physical, psychological, social function
General health perceptions	Self-rating of health; health concern/worry
Functional status	
Social:	
Limitations in usual roles	Acute or chronic limitations in social roles of student, worker, parent, household member
Integration	Participation in the community
Contact	Interaction with others
Intimacy	Perceived feelings of closeness; sexuality
Psychological:	
Affective	Psychological attitudes and behaviors, including distress and general well-being or happiness
Cognitive	Alertness; disorientation; problems in reasoning
Physical:	
Activity restrictions	Acute or chronic limitations in activity, mobility, self-care, sleep, communication
Fitness	Performance of activity with vigor and without excessive fatigue
Impairment	
Subjective complaints	Reports of physical and psychological symptoms, sensations, pain, health problems, or feelings not directly observable
Signs	Physical examination: observable evidence of defect of abnormality
Self-reported disease	Patient listing of medical conditions or impairments

(Continued)

TABLE 2.1
Continued

Concepts and Domains	Definitions/Indicators
Physiological measures	Laboratory data, records, and their clinical interpretation
Tissue alterations	Pathological evidence
Death and duration of life	Mortality; survival; longevity

SOURCE: From Patrick and Bergner (1990); used with permission from Annual Review of Public Health Volume II, © 1990 by Annual Reviews, Inc.

generation of recovery curves assumes that there is a characteristic pattern of returning functions that is influenced by the presenting problem, spontaneous recovery, the amount and type of intervention, and the characteristics of the patient. The band of variability seen within any one impairment group would help in establishing predictability under different treatment regimens.

Recovery from physical impairment is highly complex because it spans so many levels—physiological, physical, cognitive, and social. Assessment and treatment strategies in rehabilitation are based on the assumption that there are important differences in presenting problems and the course of recovery for the impairments seen. Programs for stroke or brain injury or spinal cord injury differ and, indeed, highly specialized units are seen as the optimal mode of service delivery. Much of the clinical literature is devoted to this differentiation among diagnoses.

An important issue involves the development of recovery over time and the various phases or periods involved. Knowledge of such timing issues would allow the use of treatment interventions that could be more systematically tied to the phases of recovery. Quite a bit is known, for example, regarding the course of recovery in stroke. A number of studies have shown that the maximum physical recovery occurs within the first 3 months, whereas speech improvement is seen up to a year postonset (Andrews, Brocklehurst, Richards, & Laycock, 1981; Kelly-Hayes et al., 1989; Kotila, Waltimo, Niemi, Laaksonen, & Lempinen, 1984). A few studies, such as the long-term monitoring of individuals in the Framingham research (Kelly-Hayes et al., 1989), are community based and provide information about the course of strokes in a population that is not selected for clinical services. It is possible then to determine the progress of this condition under a variety of service conditions. Life table analysis is a promising statistical tool for studying recovery and the effect of treatment. Reding and Potes (1988) separated individuals with initial unilateral hemispheric stroke into subgroups on the basis of motor, somatic sensory, and visual field deficits. After testing patients every 2 weeks for up to 30 weeks, they were able to generate curves showing the probability of return of function over time. Of patients with motor deficit only, 90% were able to walk at least 150 feet by 14 weeks after their stroke. Only 35% of patients with motor and somatic sensory deficit and only 3% of patients with motor, somatic sensory, and visual deficits were able to attain this criterion. By this technique, the authors were able to differentiate groups on their course of recovery.

The documentation of recovery from onset through return to the community with frequent intervals of measurement is relatively rare, however. The health care system in the United States is not organized to provide care in one facility, making it difficult to maintain consistent data over the full course of a medical condition and its aftermath. The model systems programs for spinal cord injury funded by the National Institute for Disability Rehabilitation and Research were set up to remedy this discontinuity of service by dealing with this category of injury from onset to community re- turn (Thomas, 1979). Even in this program, however, many patients do not remain in one system, and records are inconsistent. Careful tracking of patients through the various stages of disability will be required if we are to understand the path of recovery and the optimal role of treatment.

The Nature of Assessment

We have taken the position that the concepts used for assessment in rehabilitation should be grounded in a broader formulation of health. Both general health measures and those used in rehabilitation currently lack an underlying theory that defines the various domains and the relationships among them. Measures of different aspects of health—for example, symptoms, psychological functioning, and patients' perceptions of health—may show low or no correlation within a patient sample (Patrick, Stein, Porta, Porter, & Ricketts, 1988). If different dimensions of health do not covary as aspects of a more global and unitary construct, then how are they related?

The assessment task. In medical care, the first step is usually diagnosis: the use of signs, symptoms, and biological indicators to determine, if possible, the cause of the ailment and to prescribe treatment that will lead to alleviation or cure. Although rehabilitation may require the same steps for treating conditions that accompany disability, such as urinary tract infections, the major task is integration of medical information with the assessment of functional performance and the nature of deficits in performance. The assessment also addresses the appropriateness of the candidate for the particular program, the treatment plan the individual requires, and an estimate of the time and resources necessary to produce an acceptable result.

All of these considerations are related to the treatment setting and the response of the patient to it. The outcomes of rehabilitation, however, must be placed within a framework of benefit external to the clinical setting. If the patient is trained to maneuver a wheelchair through hospital corridors but cannot or will not use it at home, the benefits of treatment are suspect. This dichotomy of purposes has been the source of considerable discomfort for clinicians, researchers, and evaluators. Clinicians require assessment devices that are sensitive to small increments of change in patient performance, both to guide the course of therapy and as a means of documenting progress for those who pay the bills. Outcome measures, on the other hand, must address more global issues such as the amount of assistance required or the ability of the patient to assume usual role activities.

Functional assessment measures often have been used to bridge these two aims. The Barthel Index, for example, is one of the most frequently used clinical scales (Granger, Dewis, Peters, Sherwood, & Barrett, 1979). As with most such scales, its underlying construct reflects the extent of need for a helper or for assistive devices for a series of self-care and mobility tasks. Because inpatient rehabilitation concentrates on the remediation of such deficits, the scale has considerable clinical utility. Barthel Index scores are of little interest outside such treatment, however. A total score of 80, for instance, might represent a high probability of ability to function independently at home, but such claims have to be established empirically. For those outside the rehabilitation community, such scores are meaningless and always require translation into more commonly understood competencies.

Assessment and theory. A major problem throughout rehabilitation is its ambition to influence all aspects of a patient's life: physical, cognitive, emotional, and social functioning. But there is no commonly accepted taxonomy of life activities and indeed there is not even a classification of tasks in the treatment setting (Frey, 1984). The narrow focus on activities of daily living scales in relation to the wider goals of most programs has been frequently noted (Keith, 1984; Seale & Davies, 1987). Part of the problem is the dominant emphasis on physical restoration, but it too comes from the lack of development of scales that span other areas, such as social skills. There has been a lag as well in the technical development of measures. Evidence for reliability, validity, scalability, and other measurement properties has been neglected (Johnston, Findley, DeLuca, & Katz, 1991; Keith, 1984), although there has been recent work of a more sophisticated nature that promises to strengthen scale construction in rehabilitation (e.g., Silverstein, Kilgore, Fisher, Harley, & Harvey, 1991). A task force of the American Congress of Rehabilitation Medicine is writing measurement standards for the field, which should also help.

Good assessment criteria should be conceptually connected not only to the specifics of the presenting problem but also to the more general concepts of health status already mentioned. This follows from their role in describing and defining the problems presented for treatment. Those problems represent impaired health status of some variety, hence the symptom vocabulary and other relevant assessment concepts should be part of an integrated, perhaps hierarchical, framework of health status concepts. Thus, if health status is described, at least in part, in terms of functional abilities, and assessment is described in terms of physiological or medical indicators, some further statement of the relations between the various functions and those medical states is required for full integration.

This formulation closes the circle between assessment of the initial (impaired) health status and the improvement in health-related quality of life that is the ultimate treatment goal. The problem to be remediated is specified by an assessment profile that indicates appropriate treatment. The successful attainment of treatment goals, in turn, improves health status, the magnitude of which can be assessed by comparison with initial health status. The quality of assessment in this formulation can be judged, first, by how effectively it discriminates among problems and patients requiring different treatment and, second, by how fully and accurately it indexes patients' impairments in terms meaningful to overall health status.

The Nature of Rehabilitation Treatment

Treatment delivery and research on treatment. In rehabilitation medicine, the instrument for treatment delivery is the comprehensive team, a configuration of specialists in medicine, nursing, physical therapy, occupational therapy, speech and language pathology, recreation therapy, psychology, social work, and orthotics. The team is the heart of rehabilitation and is viewed as the most appropriate means of dealing with the complex problems that patients present. Because of the broad aims of rehabilitation, a wide spectrum of professional skills are required.

The research literature on the effectiveness of rehabilitation is singularly devoid of any detailed specification of what actually constitutes the treatment delivered by the comprehensive team. Occasionally, there is a description of what the components in a treatment program were supposed to be; almost never is there an accounting of the treatment actually delivered. The assumption seems to be that a treatment protocol for stroke, for example, is fairly standard. Although there are no data on practice variations in rehabilitation, investigations in acute care have shown that large variations are common. There is no reason to assume that rehabilitation will be any different.

The use of a treatment team makes the demonstration of effectiveness very complicated. It is almost impossible to separate the influence of each individual therapy. Not only do they overlap in type of activity, they are also interactive in effect. Improvement in communication, for example, may result in faster learning of motor skills. The use of clinical trials in rehabilitation has usually involved only the molar comparison of a program of treatment with some alternative form of care. For example, Wood-Dauphinee and associates (1984) randomly assigned stroke patients to traditional and more highly coordinated team care. On outcome measures of survival, motor performance, and functional status, there was no clear-cut advantage for team care. Other studies of stroke care (Feldman et al., 1962; Garraway, Akhtar, Hockey, & Prescott, 1980; Garraway, Akhtar, Prescott, & Hockey, 1980), management of chronic illness (Halstead, 1976), and management of arthritis (Ahlmen, Sullivan, & Bjelle, 1988; Spiegel et al., 1986) have shown some apparent benefits of team care. The results are mixed, however, and do not consistently demonstrate the superiority of the comprehensive team nor differentiate the relative influences of the various disciplines on the team.

To improve understanding of what it is in the rehabilitation intervention that produces changes in the patient's performance, it is first necessary to examine closely the process of care. Though it is complicated to identify the separate components and their interconnections, it is by no means impossible. Such research requires detailed observations and is often tedious and expensive; it has had few advocates. Paradoxically, the rehabilitation hospital has been the site of some of the most detailed observations ever made in health care (Keith, 1988). As an example, Keith and Cowell (1987) observed stroke patients every 8 minutes during the working day in three rehabilitation units. They found that treatment occupied 31% of the day with passive behavior taking another 42%. Patients were in treatment most frequently in the hospital with the dedicated stroke unit. Although there were quantitative differences, the three hospitals had similar patterns of treatment activity and deployment of staff.

Even though this type of research has described the patterns of patient and staff activity and has highlighted the inefficiencies of treatment routines, it has not been connected to effectiveness and thus is incomplete. The observational methods that have been used could be employed in the search for causal linkages by placing them in a framework that addressed the specific contribution of staff members and the resultant outcomes. At a more molar level, the study of organizational effectiveness, now largely missing in rehabilitation (Keith, 1986), could provide theoretical insights regarding the most optimal program configuration.

Treatment and theory. The extensive literature on treatment in rehabilitation is primarily from a clinical perspective and is not

sufficient to establish systematically the causal connections between specific interventions and their results. Theory building
requires an alternation between formulations about treatment and
the testing of those formulations. Only a few studies have been
labeled as "controlled clinical trials" (Garraway, Akhtar, Hockey, &
Prescott, 1980; Garraway, Akhtar, Prescott, & Hockey, 1980;
Smith et al., 1981), but one could argue whether they actually fit
such a designation because of the lack of detailed specification of
treatment. Moreover, most of the research attempting to establish
the effectiveness of comprehensive rehabilitation has contrasted
treatment programs without much rationale for their differences.

The comprehensive treatment team in rehabilitation aspires to
deal with the "whole person," with all the associated deficits in
physical, psychological, social, and vocational functioning. However commendable this philosophy may be, it is quite likely that
treatment outcome depends more heavily on the remediation of
some deficits than others and, correspondingly, more on the application of some treatment elements rather than others. The increasingly selective nature of treatment funding makes more urgent the
search for these basic elements. Treatment theory will not progress until there is some identification of the essential elements
of effective treatment for a given condition—the minimal configuration and amount of treatment below which outcome is
demonstrably unsatisfactory.

The core of treatment theory, however, is some set of propositions that describe what goes on during the transformation of input
into output, that is, the actual nature of the process that transforms
received therapy into improved health. Understanding rehabilitation therapy within some conceptually coherent framework that
identifies the elements and contingencies of the causal chain that
connects provider activities with patient health will be a major
challenge.

In rehabilitation, much of what a patient is expected to accomplish involves learning, either of new skills or relearning of those
lost or diminished. Because of the attention that must be given to
patient performance, learning theory has much to recommend it
as a theoretical framework for some aspects of treatment. Motor
learning is a prominent part of therapy, although social skills and
other such nonphysical competencies are also important. A better
understanding of the conditions under which learning occurs in the

treatment setting, as well as the coordination of learning activities with phases in the curve of recovery, could further the development of theory in rehabilitation. As an example, an issue such as the use of massed versus spaced practice—a venerable topic in learning theory—has much relevance. The pioneer work of Fordyce (1971) and others in the application of operant learning principles, particularly with individuals with pain, has demonstrated the effectiveness of this orientation. In spite of such work and the large body of more general work on learning, there has been relatively little acknowledgment of its applicability to rehabilitation.

Contextual and environmental variables also must be considered in developing treatment theory because they no doubt play an important role in treatment outcome. The policy context, such as health funding and regulation, exerts great influence on the delivery of care, as do general social conditions such as the state of the economy. The nature of the rehabilitation organization—its staff, facilities, layout, social climate, and the like—also must play an important role. On the patient side, family and community support for the patient, economic resources, and other such matters may shape treatment and the patient's response to it. There is beginning to be recognition in rehabilitation of the importance of analysis of the delivery system (Batavia & DeJong, 1990). A recent conference at the National Rehabilitation Hospital in Washington, DC, addressed the issue of developing a capability for health services research in rehabilitation.

We do not want to imply that all the issues mentioned above must somehow be integrated into a single monolithic treatment theory for us to make progress in understanding and evaluating rehabilitation services. Different conceptual frames may be appropriate for different aspects of treatments and more than one may be useful and plausible for any given aspect. Nor is it necessary for treatment theory to be elaborate and detailed for it to be useful. It is far more important that the theory be explicit so that its implications for research, practice, and assessment are clear and possible to implement.

The Nature of Outcomes

The specification and understanding of the end state toward which diagnosis and treatment are directed is an essential aspect of the identification of causal linkages. The usual cliche in reha-bilitation is that the goal is to bring the patient to the highest level of independence commensurate with capabilities. But indepen-dence as a concept has had little examination. Frey (1984) observed that the field currently lacks even a rudimentary taxonomy of the minimal tasks an individual must be able to perform for self-maintenance. When it comes to the more complicated matter of self-sufficiency in the community, there are only fragments of theory. If independence is indeed one of the major criteria of rehabilita-tion outcomes, then we must have some idea of the activities and competencies involved.

The wider goal of rehabilitation, however, is to improve pa-tients' health-related quality of life. In the Patrick and Bergner (1990) scheme described earlier, the broad construct of health-related quality of life encompasses at least five concepts: duration of life, impairments, functional status, health perceptions, and opportunities. Independence is but one aspect of this construct and, moreover, is not the only aspect that rehabilitation might be expected to affect. The favored outcome measures in rehabilita-tion show good correspondence with some of these categories but they are much less complete in other areas.

Types of outcome measures in rehabilitation. Outcome measures in research on the effects of rehabilitation typically fall into four categories. First are status measures with an implied performance based on the ability to occupy that status. For example, living at home assumes the individual does not require assistance beyond that supplied by family, friends, or paid attendants. A second, re-lated group of measures involves resource use of some kind. The amount of assistance required (hours per day or week), rehospi-talization, or expenditures for medication are examples. Informa-tion about medical complications and the management of chronic disease are also included in this category.

A third category of measures describes functional perform-nces and are the favorite indicators in rehabilitation (Granger & Gresham, 1984; Halpern & Fuhrer, 1984; Keith, 1984; McDowell & Newell, 1987). They have had great utility for clinicians, particular-ly for the assessment of the basic skills in self-care and mobility that are the focus of physical medicine. The scaling of more com-plex attributes, such as social skills, has been less successful. Also included in this group are tests of speech and language, cognitive, emotional, and other sorts of functioning.

The last set of outcome measures refers to the satisfaction of patient, family, referrer, or payor with the services or their results. The subjective reaction of the benefactors of care has increasingly been seen as an appropriate outcome in health care. Even though there is a substantial literature on the topic, research in this area has just begun in rehabilitation (Winter & Keith, 1988).

Taken together, these four types of measures provide some index of overall health status but still fall short of a complete accounting. In the terms of the Patrick and Bergner (1990) scheme, they show good correspondence with the dimensions of impairment and the physical aspects of functional status. They are much less adequate in the areas of psychological and social functional status, health perception, and opportunity (see Table 2.1). If the outcome measures in rehabilitation are to represent pertinent aspects of patients' health status, they must be incorporated into a larger conceptual framework that identifies the dimensions of health and provides a rationale for the type and range of measures applied.

It is time for rehabilitation medicine to move beyond a preoccupation with scales for the rating of simple physical tasks. While such scales will continue to be important in clinical services, they do not reflect the wider goals of rehabilitation. Because the behaviors of interest in outcomes are primarily those that reflect competence in settings outside of health care, the development of measures must turn in this direction. Disablement assessment has moved beyond the boundaries of hospital and clinic to the study of general populations (Nagi, 1976; Patrick & Peach, 1989). Health status measures are likewise frequently used with general populations. A larger framework that deals with health and disablement outside of health services then is in order.

Outcomes and theory. Integrating outcome measurement into treatment effectiveness theory involves at least three important considerations. First, there must be some identification of the construct domains that are subject to change. The more complex the treatment, the more uncertainty there will be about the range and nature of outcomes. In particular, there may be adverse side effects or unintended benefits that need to be taken into account.

Improvement in independent functioning in a young patient with brain injury, for example, may produce considerable anxiety in the family about how much freedom the patient should have. The strongest basis for determining the relevant construct domains is treatment theory itself, discussed earlier. Careful formulations and testing of treatment concepts and processes will yield extensive implications for the aspects of patients' lives that may be affected by those treatments.

A second step in developing outcome measures responsive to treatment is specification of such crucial implementation details as the timing and setting of measurement. The term *outcome* is unfortunate in some ways because it implies a state of equilibrium after the cessation of services when, in fact, the patient may continue to require services the rest of his or her life. Also, gains made in the treatment setting count for little if the individual cannot function better at home or in the community afterward. Many studies measure outcome only at the termination of treatment and only in the service setting. When there is follow-up measurement, the timing is usually somewhat arbitrary. Clearly, there are a number of possible temporal patterns for treatment effects, and, indeed, different outcomes in different settings may have different patterns. The timing of outcome measurement therefore should be grounded in an understanding of recovery curves.

A last issue has to do with knowing what constitutes a meaningful outcome once adequate measurement has been operationalized. Some rehabilitation outcomes are more important than others, a matter that must be judged in the context of a broader framework of health-related quality of life and of what patients value. Closely related is the matter of judging the practical significance of the magnitude of treatment effects. Assessing practical significance requires some criterion against which effect magnitude can be compared. For example, treatment outcome might be compared with a minimal set of standards for personal functioning (e.g., Baker & Intagliata, 1982) or it might be judged in terms of the gap between the patients treated and a normative population indexed on the same measure.

Outcome measures in rehabilitation have grown without deliberate design or much thought about underlying assumptions. Although the period of practical pragmatism has been useful for clinical management, there must be a better theoretical foundation if we are to build a science of outcome measurement.

Summary and Conclusions

Quality of care in rehabilitation is not a matter that can be judged by looking at any one element or aspect of care in isolation. It ultimately refers to a configuration of assessment practices, treatment processes, and resulting health benefits that work effectively in everyday service settings to meet the needs of patients. Assessment must properly identify the optimal treatment for the presenting problem and discriminate among problems requiring different treatments. Treatments must be those that most effectively address the patients' problems and produce real benefits, benefits that would not have occurred with lesser or no treatment. The treatment benefits, in turn, must enhance patients' health-related quality of life in terms they recognize and value.

The elements and linkages of this configuration are far too manifold and complex for us to expect to attain optimal forms on the basis of trial-and-error practice. Nor can we expect the theories of practice derived from clinical experience alone to be sufficient. If we are to have the basis for evaluating, and, correspondingly, for improving quality of care in rehabilitation, we must develop explicit conceptual frameworks—that is, theory, that synthesizes knowledge and permits sophisticated understanding of the nature of the processes with which we are dealing.

In the field of rehabilitation research, theory and knowledge are at a relatively primitive level. If we fix our focus on filling in the largest gaps in our understanding, we must construct and pursue an agenda of theory-oriented treatment research. The suggestions below are advanced as part of that agenda.

1. *Treatment effectiveness.* At the center of the research agenda for rehabilitation should be differentiated, sophisticated, theory-driven experimental treatment effectiveness research and its quasi-experimental and causal modeling analogues. Such research should include both documentation and rationale for the characteristics of the patients involved, the nature of the treatment(s) implemented, and distinguishing features of the context within which treatment

is delivered, the intervening steps believed to constitute the treatment process, and the outcome variables expected to be affected by treatment. Without explicit and differentiated treatment concepts that link, on the one end, to the nature of the patients' problems and circumstances and, on the other end, to specific outcomes characteristic of effective treatment, there can be no full understanding of rehabilitation therapy, how to evaluate it, or how to make it better.

2. *Measurement.* Both assessment and outcome measurement should be integrated into some broader multidimensional, hierarchical system of indicators for health-related quality of life. Moreover, we should strive to determine the interrelations among the various domains and levels of measurement—not just the empirical intercorrelations but the reasons for those intercorrelations.

    a. Assessment instruments should be developed not just to attain conventional standards of reliability and validity but to maximally discriminate among patients needing different treatment and those responding differently to treatment. These discriminations should form the basis for assessment taxonomies that accurately classify patients into groups for which specific treatments or treatment variations are indicated.

    b. Similarly, outcome measures should be developed to respond maximally to those aspects of health-related quality of life that are at issue for patients and that are expected to be changed by effective treatment applied to appropriate patients. The conceptual framework developed for outcome measures should not only indicate how important those outcome domains are but provide a basis for assessing the practical magnitude of the change brought about by treatment.

3. *Practice variations.* As a basis for studying treatment effectiveness, in contrast to treatment efficacy, a body of descriptive data needs to be built regarding the variations in clinical practice that occur across providers, facilities, patients, and geographic regions. These variations should be used to construct normative treatment models for purposes of formal effectiveness research and as the basis for studying the factors of professional judgment, local standards, and other such matters that account for variation from the normative models.

4. *Analysis of recovery.* We need standard-setting research that describes what constitutes recovery in the various areas of rehabilitation, that is, what levels of everyday life functions and health-related quality of life constitute "normal" health. With these standards in mind, we need descriptive research that identifies the phases and pace of recovery from various impairments and the extent to which its end state attains or falls short of that standard.

While the nation's expenditures for health care have climbed to precipitous heights, only recently have major efforts been made to understand health care treatment, the basis for its effectiveness, and the costs and inefficiencies associated with its delivery. Vigorous pursuit of such a research agenda should demonstrate, if there was ever any doubt, the wisdom of Kurt Lewin's well-known dictum that "there is nothing so practical as a good theory."

PART II

Predictive Validity and Psychometric Adequacy of Rehabilitation Assessment Instruments

CHAPTER 3

Predictive Validity and Vocational Assessment: Reframing the Question

GARY R. BOND
LAURA L. DIETZEN

The point of departure for this chapter is a simple one: The adequacy of assessment approaches used in rehabilitation practice should be judged against the standard of predictive validity. We shall examine predictive validity for one type of assessment task—vocational assessment—although a similar case could be made for other types of rehabilitation assessment. *Assessment* is a broad term encompassing a range of fo mal and informal activities conducted by clinicians, researchers, clients, and others. Unfortunately, validity issues too seldom are seriously contemplated by either clinicians or researchers. When selecting vocational tools and interpreting test results, practitioners are more inclined to depend on their past experiences and intuition than on findings from research studies. Researchers also often retreat from the criterion of predictive validity to more easily attained standards of reliability, concurrent validity, and population norms, because studies of predictive validity are more difficult to conduct. Seemingly

AUTHORS' NOTE: The first author was supported by Research Scientist Development Award K02 00842 from the National Institute of Mental Health. We thank John McGrew and Michelle Salyers for their helpful comments.

far removed from rehabilitation practice is the narrow research enterprise of attempting to link a specific measure to a specific outcome in an effort to establish validity. Although we agree that it is inappropriate to fit all the functions of assessment into the procrustean bed of predictive validity, we think that the validity issues too often are postponed and neglected. Predictive validity is still the gold standard. Otherwise excellent psychometric properties do not somehow substitute for poor validity. Nor does the absence of validity coefficients excuse an instrument's use. Assessment instruments should not be presumed innocent until proven guilty.

Validity issues take on added significance in light of the importance of the decisions following from vocational assessment procedures. Assessment comes first in the prototypic sequence of assessment, training, and placement. The client's trajectory in the rehabilitation process is shaped by an initial assessment upon entry into the system. The vocational evaluator's role includes specifying the outcomes to be achieved through rehabilitation and identifying which services are needed to achieve those outcomes (Berven, 1984). By tradition, vocational evaluation is viewed as a separate "component" of the rehabilitation process, with the evaluator uninvolved with the client after the assessment is completed (Rogan & Hagner, 1990). Paradigmatically, predictive validity is measured by the correlation between a predictor variable (based on an assessment made before any intervention) and a criterion variable (a "real-world" outcome), such as job placement and retention or, even more specifically, employment in a particular occupation. Success in a training program also has been used as a criterion. Clearly, the goals of vocational assessment are congruent with the predictive validity paradigm.

Wehman (1988) has observed that "the rehabilitation service system is currently designed to give vocational evaluation a preeminent role" (p. 9). Similarly, Power (1991) has suggested that vocational assessment services must be considered among the most critical of all vocational rehabilitation (VR) services. *Vocational evaluation* (which is a term used more or less interchangeably with *vocational assessment* in the VR system) is the service most frequently purchased by state VR agencies (Bordieri & Thomas, 1986). The popularity of vocational assessment is, of course, no guarantee of its merits, any more than the use of any particular test ensures that the instrument is a good one (Glueckauf, this volume). Psychologists tend to use tests in which they have received training in internship and practicum sites (Wade & Baker, 1977). Although we have no direct evidence on this point, we speculate that a similar shaping process occurs for vocational evaluators. Exploration of the reasons for the relatively uncritical continued use of tests of dubious validity would divert us from the main focus of this chapter. Recognition of nonscientific influences on test dissemination, however, provides further fuel for our skepticism.

This chapter will not provide an exhaustive review of vocational assessment in rehabilitation, although our literature search suggests that such a review is needed. Our goal is more modest, namely, to illustrate predictive validity problems with respect to commonly used approaches. For the most part, we will not review specific instruments, although such work (e.g., Bolton & Brookings, this volume; Cook et al., 1991) is also needed. Our intent is to clarify what the issues are and should be, so that we do not simply lament the limited empirical literature but point to new ways of thinking about vocational assessment, ending with a set of principles we believe would yield more valid assessment procedures.

Four Vocational Assessment Approaches

There are various strategies for approaching the task we have set for ourselves. One strategy would be to locate "milestone studies" representing the best efforts in assessing vocational instruments. Wiggins (1973) included this strategy in his analysis of personality assessment. Unfortunately, there are few such studies that would qualify in the domain of vocational assessment in rehabilitation. Another strategy would be to identify promising instruments and to gauge their predictive validity. The piecemeal quality of this strategy is apparent, however; isolated predictive validity coefficients do not tell us much about the adequacy of the vocational assessment process. A third strategy would be to start from a theoretical framework stipulating hypotheses about predictors of successful employment and to systematically examine the components of that framework. We will have more to say about a theory-driven appraisal later.

We have chosen a fourth and familiar course for appraising the vocational assessment literature, namely, to examine generic assessment approaches, as defined by their mode of measurement. Although various reviewers have used somewhat different categories, there is general agreement that four widely used approaches are interviewing, paper-and-pencil abilities and interest tests, work samples, and situational assessment (Berven, 1984). We have made a simplifying assumption that, although predictive validity may vary among specific instruments and approaches within a specific mode of assessment, the commonalities within a particular mode outweigh their differences. Although our review strategy is vulnerable to faulty logic if we inadvertently omit important assessment domains or choose bad examples, we have attempted to be evenhanded. Our listing is not exhaustive, but we believe it to be a representative sampling of approaches in current practice.

Idiographic Specificity: Interviewing Approaches

Interviewing forms the core of the vocational eligibility and planning process (Berven, 1984). Interviewing techniques fall on a continuum from completely unstructured discussions with no prescribed focus to carefully structured interview schedules featuring closed-ended questions, with many different variations in between. Interviewing approaches of the latter type have more in common with structured paper-and-pencil tests than with the personalized exploration of vocational goals and abilities being considered in this section.

Despite their intuitive appeal, unstructured interviewing approaches have been shown repeatedly to have poor predictive validity in personnel selection studies (Eder & Ferris, 1989). Interviewers exercising clinical judgment are influenced by hidden biases. Prediction by means of job interviews is improved through the use of a structured format.

Similarly, there is some evidence that vocational evaluators, when they are asked to exercise their clinical judgment, are more heavily influenced by contextual factors than by objective test scores. For example, Murphy and Hagner (1988) found that clients were invariably recommended for training or employment in the same facility in which the assessment was conducted. The authors argued that financial, administrative, and professional factors compromised the stated goals of the assessment. In an experimental study, Cottone, Grelle, and Wilson (1988) found that vocational assessors were significantly more influenced by anecdotal observations made by workshop personnel (e.g., "Client's hair is long and unclean . . . client established little or no eye contact") than by psychometric tests or work samples. Moreover, when using anecdotal information, assessors were more likely to make recommendations for work adjustment; when using psychometric information, assessors were more likely to make recommendations for job placement. These studies dramatize the problems with "flexible" clinical decisions.

Many formal interviewing strategies have been devised. One simple improvement over the unstructured interview is a guide listing key questions and things to observe. Power (1991) has suggested that the interview can compensate for some of the deficiencies in traditional testing by providing a context for judging qualities of the client such as general appearance, communication style, mood and affect, coping resources, interpersonal skills, capacity for facing problems, energy level, and goal directedness. In a similar fashion, Marrone, Horgan, Scripture, and Grossman (1984) have offered VR counselors a practical list of positive and negative indicators of client readiness for work that can be obtained through interviews (e.g., whether the client has a course of illness that is relatively predictable, whether significant persons in the client's life support the VR involvement, and even whether the client is physically or verbally assaultive to the counselor). Neither Power (1991) nor Marrone et al. (1984), however, report validity data to back up their intuitions. Behaviors in an interview may not necessarily generalize to the work setting.

An elaborate interviewing format for assessing vocational needs and skills is the Boston University (BU) psychiatric rehabilitation approach, developed by Anthony, Cohen, and Farkas (1990). This approach involves a close collaboration between the practitioner and the client, drawing on client-centered interviewing techniques. It attempts first to establish an overall vocational goal (including a preliminary identification of an occupational objective). The next step is to identify the skills and resources needed to achieve that goal. The "behavioral requirements" for a particular job are iden- tified as well as the implicit norms in a particular work setting. In essence, the approach attempts to determine what would be necessary to achieve a good match between the client and the job so that the client not only will be successful in completing the task requirements but also will find the job satisfying.

Although widely disseminated, the BU approach is lacking in validation studies. One study employing the BU interviewing format demonstrated that clients felt highly involved in the process and well informed about the rehabilitation planning process (Wasylenki, Goering, Lancee, Ballantyne, & Farkas, 1985). Unfortunately, although this study did include a control sample, these clients were not asked parallel questions about their satisfaction with the process.

Assessment through interviewing is often based on the assumption that clients know what they want and what they can do and that the way to obtain this information is to ask questions directly. It is also sometimes assumed that interview information is more valid than objective or indirectly obtained data. The interview process does elicit a different set of reactions from clients than standardized testing, which can be perceived as dehumanizing. Client involvement in the assessment process, as enhanced through client-centered interviewing techniques, may well be a precondition for a valid vocational assessment, and one that often may be neglected in conventional vocational assessment settings. Consumer empowerment has become a major theme in the rehabilitation field and has encouraged legitimate reforms in service provision. Certainly, with regard to assessment, consumers deserve a fair hearing that includes a personalized understanding of their competencies, deficits, and compensatory coping strategies. Nonetheless, consumer-oriented interviewing techniques are not sufficient to ensure valid assessments.

Clinical judgment used in interviewing has proved to be disappointing in predicting rehabilitation outcomes. Practitioners do not combine information efficiently; they tend to formulate a small number of hypotheses early in the data-gathering process, and their opinions then become resistant to change (Berven, 1984). Such findings should not be surprising to those familiar with the broader decision-making literature (e.g., Dawes, Faust, & Meehl, 1989; Faust, this volume; Sawyer, 1966; Wiggins, 1973). It has proved virtually impossible to eradicate the conviction that informal, flexible methods of data gathering and combining information are superior to actuarial approaches, despite overwhelming evidence to the contrary.

As a method of predicting outcomes, the interview has limitations even under optimal conditions with highly articulate job applicants. Interviews require verbal clients, with skills in introspecting, describing prior experiences, and communicating effectively, all of which may be affected in some types of disability. Some clients are more capable of demonstrating skills directly rather than verbalizing them (Power, 1991). As a counseling tool, relatively unstructured interviewing has demonstrable therapeutic benefits, but, as a method of assessment, it has fundamental limitations as a primary source of information. Structured approaches are theoretically more promising, but formal studies of these are lacking.

Psychometric Excellence: Aptitude and Interest Tests

Numerous paper-and-pencil tests have been used for rehabilitation populations, some borrowed directly from the personnel selection literature and others devised or adapted either for rehabilitation settings or for specific disability groups (e.g., tests adapted for the visually impaired). These tests can be grouped into two main categories: aptitude/ability tests (e.g., the General Aptitude Test Battery [GATB], U.S. Department of Labor, 1970) and interest tests (e.g., the Wide Range Interest Opinion Test, Jastak & Jastak, 1987). Reliability studies, development of test norms, and, in some cases, validity studies have been conducted with rehabilitation samples, as reviewed by Berven (1980), Bolton (1985a, 1988b), Harmon, Sharma, and Trotter (1976), Parker and Hansen (1976), and Vandergoot (1986). Bolton and Brookings (this volume) document the care and psychometric rigor applied in the development of a number of exemplary rehabilitation assessment instruments that would fall in this category.

One general impression gleaned from these reviews is that psychometric testing has demonstrated utility for employers who wish to screen out less capable job applicants. Hunter and Hunter (1984) compiled results from a vast number of personnel selection studies, concluding that the overall validity coefficient for predicting job performance in an entry-level job from ability tests was over .50 for the general population. They further concluded that tests of cognitive abilities were typically good predictors, regardless of occupational type. The use of psychometric tests in rehabilitation settings has drawbacks, however. The first drawback is the appropriateness of the personnel selection paradigm, as discussed in a later section. Second, it appears that, even for those instruments having the rigors of psychometric development, the "fine print" often suggests that they are less useful than one might suppose for predicting vocational outcomes. Third, validity data may be available for general populations only, with the argument sometimes made that such validity coefficients can be extrapolated to persons with disabilities (Bolton, 1988b). This line of argument is debatable, especially when the tests contain items that are inappropriate for certain disabled populations. This is an issue best resolved through empirical study, not theoretical debate.

We need to ask what standardized aptitude tests are really measuring in persons with disabilities (Neff, 1980). Individuals with poor academic preparation and/or poor verbal skills will perform poorly on many of these tests. In addition, conventional tests may be anxiety producing, which could also lead to poor performance. The stamina required to complete lengthy batteries (such as the GATB) may also disadvantage clients from performing to the best of their abilities.

Most of the evidence for the validity of vocational interest inventories also comes from studies of general populations. Because experienced workers in different occupational groups show statistically significant different profiles, it can be argued that interest profiles might be used for job selection (Bolton, 1988b). In practice, however, this logic has not been entirely successful. One limitation of interest inventories is that they are dependent on client knowledge. In a study illustrating this principle, Rudrud, Wendelgass, Markve, Ferrara, and Decker (1982) showed that vocational knowledge can be increased in clients with mild to moderate retardation with a 20-minute slide show; vocational preferences also changed with the increased knowledge for half of the sample. Moreover, as Neff (1977) has suggested, paper-and-pencil tests implicitly assume that career choice is primarily a cognitive process; in fact, most career decisions are based on a process of trial and error. Without an experiential base, client preferences may be unrealistic. Bond, Bordieri, and Musgrave (1989), for example, found that clients overestimated their suitability for specific oc-cupations compared with their actual aptitudes.

It is plausible that psychometric tests would have a role in re-habilitation settings, especially for individuals whose disabilities least affect their work performance. The generalizability of such tests and their suitability for helping match clients to specific occupations, however, have not been definitively established.

Elegant Simulation: Work Samples

According to Menchetti and Flynn (1990), the work sample is probably the most popular of all vocational assessment approaches used in school programs, rehabilitation facilities, and job training programs. This approach involves simulations of tasks actually performed in specific occupations or clusters of occupations. Unlike most paper-and-pencil tests, work samples typically do not require extensive verbal abilities.

Starting in the 1970s, a number of work sample systems achieved prominence in vocational evaluation batteries (e.g., the Jewish Employment and Vocational Service System [JEVS], the Valpar System, the Singer System) (Botterbusch, 1987). A major advantage of these batteries is the frequent availability of norms for specific occupations and subscales providing guidance for job matching.

The predictive validity of work sample systems, however, has been only sparingly studied. Botterbusch's (1987) critical review of 21 vocational assessment and evaluation systems is the most extensive in the literature. He found that some of the earliest systems developed had only outdated validity information. No validity data at all were reported for many of the remaining systems; those reporting any information frequently were limited to content or concurrent validity, based on correlations with other tests. He also noted misleading validity information reported in the manual for the Microcomputer Evaluation and Screening Assessment, one of the best known systems.

Among the few published validity studies are two that are illustrative of the weak empirical foundation for the work sample approach for persons with disabilities. Berven and Maki (1979) found that only 7 of the 20 JEVS work samples predicted employment beyond chance in a mixed disability group. On the other hand,

Gannaway, Sink, and Becket (1980) found that performance on 13 of 21 Singer Vocational Evaluation System work samples was significantly correlated with job retention in "generally related jobs" for a mixed group of rehabilitation clients and economically disadvantaged participants. Based on these studies, it appears that both sampling considerations and definition of outcome influence the magnitude of the validity coefficients for work sample systems.

The almost total absence of validity studies is puzzling until one recognizes that some work sample procedures have emerged out of a different tradition than the trait approaches that underpin psychometric testing. Botterbusch (1987) has distinguished between "evaluation" and "assessment" systems, the former concerned with identifying capabilities for specific occupations, the latter concerned with traits. Work sample systems are typically evaluation systems, developed in response to the pragmatic assessment issues faced by rehabilitation programs. They assess work performance in intact tasks that may require a number of different skills. For example, the automotive work sample (from the Microcomputer Evaluation of Assessment Careers system) includes "repairing a wheel cylinder, replacing points and adjusting points" (Botterbusch, 1987). In light of their atheoretical evolution, typically in nonacademic settings, the disinterest in validity is perhaps not surprising.

By contrast, assessment systems, which share some similarities to the older work sample systems, have been more grounded in the psychometric tradition, both in their conceptualization and in their empirical underpinnings. An example of an assessment system is the McCarron-Dial System (MDS), which uses a range of tasks to assess specific traits relating to verbal and cognitive, sensory, motor, emotional, and integrative-coping factors (McCarron & Dial, 1986). Modest validity for the MDS has been found in several studies (e.g., Dial, McCarron, Freemon, & Swearingen, 1979; Fortune & Eldredge, 1982).

The primary justification for work samples is that they measure performance on skills needed for specific jobs. The commercially available systems are sometimes touted on the basis of their capacity to identify aptitudes for specific occupations or clusters of occupations; however, the meager research that is available suggests that the relationship between work sample performance and employment success is far less precise. A closer consideration of the logic of work samples suggests why this is so. It is difficult to design "pure" tests that are not confounded with contextual factors. For example, a test intended to measure dexterity may instead actually be measuring ability to understand and remember instructions (Brolin, 1976).

The laboratory-like standardization of work samples is appealing but also is the source of a major weakness, namely, the artificial conditions under which assessment is conducted. One facet of this artificiality is the brevity of the work sample. Many work samples can be completed in less than 20 minutes. How then does this speak to the individual's ability to perform during an 8-hour workday after fatigue sets in? When the disability includes attentional deficits, time-limited assessments may not adequately reflect long-term performance (Hursh, Rogers, & Anthony, 1988). A second aspect of the artificiality is the absence of natural contingencies. Pacsofar (1986) has shown how persons with mental retardation who test poorly under laboratory conditions perform much better under more realistic conditions of natural cues and reinforcers. In addition, work samples do not adequately capture the interpersonal dimension of the workplace, which is an essential component in most competitive employment situations (Neff, 1977). Getting along with others on the job may be more crucial to job retention than the technical skills required for a specific occupation (Anthony & Jansen, 1984).

Logistical Convenience: Situational Assessment

Situational assessment is an approach using staff ratings of clients' work performance and attitudes in a range of work settings, including sheltered workshops with industrial subcontracts, unpaid in-house work crews (with housekeeping, food maintenance, and clerical tasks), and temporary community jobs (Bond & Friedmeyer, 1987; Massel et al., 1990). Situational assessment is one of the most widely used tools in vocational evaluation (Hursh et al., 1988). It appears to be especially well suited for clients whose difficulties in achieving employment relate more to interpersonal issues than to the technical aspects of the job itself. Situational assessment is convenient, flexible, relatively easy to implement; provides for ongoing judgments of improvement; and makes sense to clients and staff alike. Moreover, studies have consistently found this method to yield significant predictive validity coefficients (Anthony & Jansen, 1984). Bond and Friedmeyer (1987) also have shown incremental validity for a situational assessment approach when comparing it with prior work history.

Despite its appeal, situational assessment suffers from a number of weaknesses. The first relates to lack of specificity. As it is usually practiced, situational assessment evaluates general work habits and behaviors that constitute the "work personality" (Neff, 1977) and not specific skills. Except for entry-level jobs requiring only rudimentary skills, however, most jobs also require occupation-specific skills. Thus we are led to a paradox with the use of situational assessments; if the purpose is to gauge suitability for employment, we must have already identified in advance what kind of employment a client will hold in the future before initiating the assessment. In practice, situational assessments typically involve a more primitive strategy of assessment in work settings unrelated to the ultimate employment goal.

A second issue has to do with *standardization*. Situational assessments have used a wide range of formats, with varying time frames. Without behavioral anchors, ratings are likely to suffer from a range of biases, such as "halo effects" (Borman, 1975). The psychometric work of optimizing the rating forms and duration of the situational assessments remains incomplete (Cook et al., 1991).

With work samples, we obtain clear measures of performance under carefully controlled conditions. We know with some precision how well a client can perform. The performance is disembodied from the work context, however. Situational assessments err in the opposite direction; a real work environment is approximated, but we are not always clear about which aspects of the client's performance contribute to the ratings.

General Issues in Vocational Assessment Practice

This brief review of the conventional tools used by vocational evaluators has exposed the shaky foundations for the vocational enterprise. In contrast to the development of tests within mainstream psychology, vocational assessment approaches used by rehabilitation practitioners have generally suffered from an absence of a scientific perspective. Although psychological testing has been far from perfect in its development, it has benefited from the scrutiny of careful research, critical reviews, and several high quality journals dedicated to its study. Much of the published rehabilitation research on vocational assessment is found in a single journal, the *Vocational Evaluation and Work Adjustment Bulletin*, which emphasizes practitioner-oriented studies. Moreover, a large portion of the remaining research literature consists of unpublished sources, which are relatively inaccessible and of variable quality (Fry, 1986). We believe that assessment practices discussed in this chapter would improve if they were considered to belong within the purview of psychologists. Effecting such a change in vision is no simple matter, however.

The technical capacity exists to refine and replace existing vocational tools to make them more sensitive to the target population. We have mentioned a few of these innovations in passing in the preceding review. One of the obvious suggestions would be to eliminate completely any of the approaches lacking empirical foundations. For example, currently, there is little empirical justification for the work sample approach, despite its popularity. Another suggestion is to determine the predictive validity of specific tools *for specific target disabilities* and to use these approaches selectively. Unfortunately, although it is logical to state the need for this level of precision, it is unrealistic to expect such standards to be attained soon, if ever. Other suggestions for improving validity include emphasizing the use of customized batteries of standardized instruments for each client to achieve his or her highest level of performance (for example, by ensuring that reading levels or comprehension of instructions are not interfering with test performance intended to measure some other skill), reducing test anxiety, and eliminating items that are biased against persons with disabilities.

Still another technological improvement that is attainable is more stringent enforcement of standards of assessment practices derived from the psychometric literature. Systematic application of decision rules based on objective information is a more promising strategy for improving predictive validity than is clinical prediction (Dawes et al., 1989; Faust, this volume).

Admirable as these technological refinements might be, we believe that this energy would be misdirected. There are larger problems with the vocational assessment process, suggesting a need for a complete reconceptualization. These problems include (a) the exclusionary bias in assessment when it is focused on individual traits and abilities, (b) the failure of the vocational assessment process to improve future employment, and (c) the theoretical sterility of conventional vocational assessment.

Exclusionary Bias

Wehman (1988) has been one of many commentators to note that vocational assessment procedures often have the effect of screening clients out from the opportunity to receive services. From a commonsense standpoint, it is not surprising that persons with disabilities would be found deficient on traditional vocational measures. By definition, the presence of a disability means that an individual has difficulty performing one or more functions in major life roles (Wood & Badley, 1980). Because vocational assessment approaches identify those who are least capable of working, this process should logically lead to the determination that a sizable proportion of clients with disabilities are either ineligible for services altogether or unlikely candidates for competitive employment. This, in fact, is very much what has happened in the field of rehabilitation. The exclusion can occur at very basic levels. Menchetti and Flynn (1990) have noted that "IQ scores remain an almost impenetrable screen for persons with mental retardation seeking community employment" (p. 117). Similarly, cursory information about psychiatric diagnosis and symptomatology sometimes has been used to reach judgments about the unemployability of an individual (Anthony & Jansen, 1984). Such program decisions are not inherently illogical, even though the professionals making these judgments have presumed greater predictive validity than is warranted from the existing literature. After all, assessment of individuals is based on the premise that there are individual differences. This selection process is appropriate for personnel selection tasks, in which employers are seeking to maximize the capabilities of their businesses by hiring those who have the best chance to succeed. In the rehabilitation field, the personnel selection paradigm is inappropriate. The goals of rehabilitation services are quite different; they include the goal of maximizing the vocational outcomes of the consumers of these services.

Ironically, some tests may have excellent predictive validity, *but only if clients do not receive training*! Exclusionary criteria become self-fulfilling prophesies. Conversely, Rudrud, Ziarnik, Bernstein, and Ferrara (1984) found that clients trained in their rehabilitation program achieved far greater success than would be predicted by vocational testing. The paradox in traditional rehabilitation practice is the exclusion of those who are judged least capable of working and who therefore need services most. Over the past two decades, rehabilitation legislation has attempted to redress this bias. Starting with the Rehabilitation Act of 1973, this legislation has given high priority to persons with severe disabilities. The theory and practice of vocational assessment, however, have not yet changed perceptibly in response to the intent of this legislation.

Unhelpfulness of Current Vocational Assessment Practice

Another way to think about the validity of vocational assessment is to ask about the validity of the process itself. Simply put, is a client better off having received vocational assessment services? Although this question has not been examined thoroughly in the literature, the available evidence is not encouraging.

Vandergoot (1986) has reasoned that, if assessment does facilitate the rehabilitation process, then clients receiving more extensive vocational assessment services should have better vocational outcomes. From his review of the literature, he concluded that the amount of time spent in vocational evaluation has little obvious value for job placement. He found that "only services provided in close proximity to the job search appear to impact placement rates" (p. 2).

If vocational evaluation is accomplishing what it is intended to do, then we would also expect recommendations made by vocational evaluators to show some correspondence to eventual placements. Vandergoot's (1986) review of the rehabilitation literature suggests that the relationship is at best tenuous. Taking into consideration that recommendations are typically made for specific forms of training (which then lead to placement), recommendations and eventual placement are two steps removed in the causal chain. Several studies suggest that both links in the chain (assessment to training and training to placement) are suspect (Caston & Watson, 1990; Cook, 1983; Cook & Brookings, 1980).

Several studies have suggested that reception of vocational assessment services may be associated with poorer vocational outcomes, especially when the assessment involves observation in a sheltered or prevocational setting. In a correlational study, Caston and Watson (1990) found that, among clients who received a successful closure (i.e., were judged as having a positive vocational outcome), only 15% had received a formal vocational evaluation. By contrast, 47% of those with an unsuccessful closure had undergone vocational evaluation. The authors speculated that only when counselors felt they had "difficult" cases (typically clients with severe disabilities) were they inclined to recommend an evaluation. If the authors' interpretation is correct, then referral to vocational evaluation was used as a de facto screening process.

In another study, Roessler and Boone (1982) examined the validity of a screening decision after 2 weeks of interviews, psychological testing, and a series of work samples in a rehabilitation center. Clients assigned to long-term evaluation had no different training program outcomes than those placed directly into training. The authors speculated that early screening was not only uninformative but also may have resulted in stigmatizing clients referred to long-term evaluation. They recommended discontinuing this early screening procedure.

In an experimental study examining the impact of placement in a prevocational setting for the purposes of assessment and training, Bond and Dincin (1986) found that clients with severe psychiatric disabilities had significantly better employment outcomes if randomly assigned to transitional employment (TE)–that is, temporary paid positions in community businesses, without *any* prior vocational assessment–than if they were initially assigned to unpaid prevocational work crews. A recent experimental replication yielded similar results (Bond & Dietzen, 1992).

In a separate analysis of the Bond and Dincin (1986) study, Bond and Friedmeyer (1987) examined situational assessment ratings made by rehabilitation staff supervising the prevocational work crews and the TE positions. Staff ratings were examined for 77 clients who were not early dropouts (of the 131 initially entering the study). Clients observed in prevocational work crews received significantly lower ratings than those observed in TE. The authors speculated that clients in unpaid work settings were less motivated to do their best, because less was expected of them and because they were not paid for their work. In a related study, Moryl (1991) found that clients observed in both prevocational work crews and TE positions received significantly lower ratings in the prevocational setting.

Other investigators have also concluded that the setting in which a client is observed influences staff evaluations. Laird and Krown (1991) noted that sheltered workshop staff were more severe judges of client performance than were community employers or the clients themselves. They speculated that "the work manager's first impression of a client, who is usually unskilled at work, and may be disorganized or acting out, is so paramount that later improvement and stabilization goes relatively unnoticed" (p. 8).

Only one study was located that directly supported the view that vocational assessment can have beneficial effects on employment outcomes. Using an experimental design, Potsubay and Fredrickson (1985) examined the hypothesis that systematic vocational assessment procedures enhance vocational outcomes. Fifty clients with a range of disabilities (66% with physical disabilities, 28% with mental disabilities, and 6% with both) were randomly assigned to one of two groups. The control group received an eligibility determination by interview, whereas the experimental group received a systematic assessment battery, including aptitude and interests tests, a labor market analysis, and choice of a work goal. Neither the clients nor the rehabilitation counselors were told beforehand of the experimental manipulation. The difference between groups in the percentage placed, stabilized for a 2-month period, and matched to a job consistent with their vocational choice was significant, with 76% of the experimental group successfully placed compared with 32% of controls. Unfortunately, the authors combined placement, retention, and matching into a single index without also reporting the results in separate outcome categories, precluding more fine-grained interpretations. Their findings, however, do suggest that systematic assessment is preferable to an unstructured approach.

Although this last study is encouraging, by suggesting that rigorously implemented vocational assessment procedures have the potential for improving outcomes, it is the only study found that supports this conclusion. One recurring theme is that extended evaluations in artificial settings, whether they are conceived as "assessment" or "training," appear to take on a life of their own, with sometimes tenuous connections to their stated purpose. The criticism in this section is directed more to this form of assessment than to brief, focused assessments. Nonetheless, we wonder if the standard in medical practice, "First, do no harm," could be met by current vocational rehabilitation assessment practice.

Lack of an Adequate Theoretical Framework

To understand the underlying weaknesses of conventional vocational assessment approaches, we need to examine the implicit and explicit models on which they are based. As a field, rehabilitation does not have a unified theory, nor is such consensus realistic for a domain spanning such a wide range of disabling conditions and interventions. Certainly, however, rehabilitation principles have been historically rooted in the assumption of the interaction between the person and the environment and the need to assess, and make adaptations to, both factors (Eisenberg & Glueckauf, 1991). The approaches reviewed above, however, have focused exclusively on the *person* side of the prediction equation. This bias is apparent in the vocational assessment field, despite the lip service given to environmental factors.

Current vocational assessment practice is also limited by its implicit dependence on a model of rehabilitation services that has proved to be unworkable for a large segment of the disabled population. More than two decades ago, Newman (1970) questioned the appropriateness of the traditional VR assessment-training-placement sequence for clients with mental illness. More recently, Wehman and his colleagues have generalized these arguments to all clients with severe disabilities, suggesting that assessment that occurs prior to training and placement has little validity (Revell, Wehman, & Arnold, 1984; Wehman, 1986). These investigators subsequently demonstrated the viability of an alternative rehabilitation model that has become known as supported employment (SE). In their formulation, assessment is not a "program" or "service" that is provided before a client begins training but it is an ongoing process that occurs intensively *after* the placement is made. Although a preliminary assessment step is needed to ensure that the client is matched to an appropriate job, much of the traditional ability determination occurs on the job rather than being predicted beforehand.

The SE model helps clarify several misguided factors in traditional vocational assessment services. Both the *context*—occurring in artificial settings under artificial conditions—and the *timing*—occurring before the client has begun real work—make the conventional prediction task a virtual impossibility. We have asked too much of our vocational assessment procedures.

Reframing the Question: What Do We Really Want to Know?

At this juncture, it is appropriate to repeat the platitude that it is easier to criticize traditional approaches than it is to suggest alternatives. Current vocational assessment practice needs rethinking, precipitated by the need for changes in rehabilitation training and placement models. The needed reframing of the vocational assessment question is put concisely by Rogan and Hagner (1990):

> Within a supported employment context, the question is not, "which people belong in community settings?" Nor is it correct to ask "in which of a series of continuum options should this person be placed?" . . . The appropriate questions are, "in which community settings is this person likely to be successful?", "what adaptations are required?", and "what support services should be provided?" (p. 50)

Our reframing of the question is based on the assumption that no vocational assessment approach that stops prior to job placement will ever achieve adequate validity. We hypothesize that a substantial proportion of the assessment process should occur at the workplace in which the client expects to be employed, either in the short term or permanently. This does not mean that no assessment is needed prior to placement, although preplacement assessment procedures need to be rethought as well.

For many clients, we hypothesize that the optimal assessment approach includes only minimal prevocational training and assessment. The "place-train" paradigm is especially suited for entry-level jobs, which we assume will continue to be realistic job options for some clients, especially many of those excluded by traditional VR services. There are other clients for whom careers requiring educational preparation (e.g., college preparation) are appropriate. The assessment paradigm is no doubt different for this latter group and may include aptitude and interest testing as is often currently used in industry. Focusing on clients with severe disabilities, we hypothesize the following guidelines for vocational assessments to be maximally valid:

1. Vocational assessment should occur in real work settings.
2. Assessments should be made repeatedly over time. Adequacy of assessment instruments should include sensitivity to measuring change in client behavior.
3. The opportunity for job tryouts in more than one job will increase the likelihood of a job match.
4. Vocational assessment measures should include the following:
   a. supervisor ratings of worker performance and attitudes,
   b. client ratings of job satisfaction and perceptions of the workplace, and
   c. objective ratings of the work environment.

Community-based assessment. Although assessment through on-the-job evaluation (OJE) was a familiar strategy even two decades ago, it has never been widely used by rehabilitation programs. Genskow (1980) found that only 21% of 106 facilities surveyed reported using OJEs. Illustrative recent examples of community-based assessment are provided by demonstration projects in Virginia and Washington states.

In Virginia, a series of demonstration projects conducted by Wehman and his colleagues have shown that the community assessment model is viable. Revell et al. (1984) have argued that the proper context for vocational assessment is in the community work site and that assessment should focus on the specific skills needed in a specific work environment. Prior to placement, clients go through an orientation, which does not entail assessment for the purposes of determining readiness but assessment to gauge client-employment fit with respect to coworkers, employer, job requirements, and travel to and from the job. This process concretizes rehabilitation efforts and reduces irrelevant preparation.

Ruddy (1987) has described a related approach, the "community-based, time-limited assessment," which was developed by the state VR agency in Washington state. This pilot project allowed a client and the rehabilitation counselor to determine the fit between the client and an occupation with up to 120 hours of exposure to a specific job. The philosophy of this program was that, because the process was an assessment, the client did not "fail" at a placement even if a particular job proved to be a poor fit. Instead, the client and counselor had an opportunity to learn concretely how a client might function in a particular job. Over a 5-year period, 1,500 clients participated in this pilot project, including 40% with mental retardation, 18% with mental disorders, 8% with spinal cord injuries, 7% with hearing impairments, and 27% with other disabilities. Altogether, 44% of the sample went into competitive employment directly from assessment without additional services from the state VR agency.

Formal instrumentation. The feasibility of community-based assessment, however, is only the first step in demonstrating the predictive validity of these approaches. Formal instrumentation also must be developed.

As noted above, situational assessment is a general approach for assessing adjustment to the work situation. Although the technology for defining target skill areas and for anchoring ratings is needed before the community-based situational assessment approach is considered to be scientifically rigorous, it remains a promising approach. Depending on the level of precision desired, such assessments are likely to be labor intensive.

Another essential ingredient of any complete vocational assessment is an analysis of the environmental context. The Minnesota Theory of Work Adjustment (Dawis, 1976) has proved to be one productive theoretical framework for assessing not only objective characteristics of the worker and the environment but also outcomes relating to both satisfactory work performance and job satisfaction. Instruments measuring aspects of this model have been developed in general populations and used with rehabilitation populations (Bolton & Brookings, this volume).

Menchetti and Flynn (1990) have also argued for assessing the environment in their description of the "ecological alternative" to traditional vocational assessment. They propose measuring characteristics of the job site such as the physical environment, the social climate, and organizational variables.

There is an extensive research literature examining employee ratings of the work environment, in particular, using job satisfaction ratings (e.g., the Minnesota Satisfaction Questionnaire; Weiss, Dawis, England, & Lofquist, 1967) and, to a lesser extent, work environment scales (Moos, 1974). Application of these instruments with rehabilitation populations has just begun. Regarding objective measures of the work environment, Bond and Dietzen (1992) developed a 10-item Quality of Employment Scale (QOES) from the criteria identified by Schalock (1988) for an SE program evaluation. Ratings of the work site were made by employment specialists at the point each client began a job. The QOES was correlated .49 with client ratings of job satisfaction approximately 3 months later.

A further justification for an environmental analysis is related to the recognition that person-environment fit can be enhanced not only by changes in the individual (e.g., through skill training) but also through environmental changes. The Americans with Disabilities Act, with its concept of "reasonable accommodation," provides legislative encouragement for making modest environmental adjustments that may eliminate or reduce barriers to employment in specific jobs. The task of identifying instances of "reasonable accommodation" will require practitioners to become accustomed to divergent thinking if we are to extend the concept beyond stereotypical examples (e.g., removal of architectural barriers; use of large print). For clients with psychiatric disabilities, reasonable accommodation might include: wearing a Walkman to filter out auditory hallucinations, allowing time off to go to psychiatrist appointments, allowing drinking water at one's desk if dryness of mouth is a medication side effect, working reduced hours if stamina is a problem or if prodromal symptoms arise, allowing time off when medications are adjusted, or providing written rather than verbal instructions for clients who have attention problems (Selleck, 1991).

These rudimentary examples suggest that environmental assessment is a promising avenue for increasing successful and satisfying employment outcomes for rehabilitation clients. In the rush to embrace this perspective, however, the point should not be lost that the work of developing psychometric instruments has only begun. Although it is plausible to expect reasonable predictive validity for measures obtained directly from employment settings, such studies have yet to be done. One encouraging finding from the personnel selection literature is a composite validity coefficient (based on various employment criterion measures) of .44 for job tryouts among applicants for entry-level jobs (Hunter & Hunter, 1984).

Complications. One crucial issue in community-based assessments is how they are conceptualized. Are these assessments actually thought of as assessments per se, as they are in the Washington project? Or are assessments thought of as job tryouts intended to lead to permanent employment if the fit is adequate? A third alternative is the transitional employment model (Bond & Dincin, 1986), in which the community placements are conceived primarily as temporary training opportunities for clients to gain confidence as workers without regard to the job fit and where they also are assessed on their work habits and attitudes. There is virtually no empirical literature to indicate which of these approaches might be more fruitful, or for whom, or under what circumstances.

If vocational assessment has as its primary focus client adjustment to community jobs, then a host of other new issues emerge. How readily will community employers participate in such activities? How do we choose the first community assessment site for each client? How long in duration must a community-based assessment be before it is valid? How do we decide on subsequent assessment sites if a given site does not work out? How many different assessment sites are necessary to determine the best fit? These are but a few of the host of logistical and technical questions that emerge once the focus of assessment is shifted from the rehabilitation setting to the community. We shall focus on but a couple of these.

Regarding the choice of the initial assessment, we are thrown back to the point of departure for this chapter: how to conduct a vocational assessment prior to any training or placement. One possible solution would be placement literally without any prior assessment, as has been the strategy in accelerated placement programs (e.g., Bond & Dincin, 1986). A doctrinaire rejection of vocational assessment, however, is unrealistic, not only because of the federal statute requiring VR counselors to determine eligibility and to develop a rehabilitation plan but also because implicit assessment processes will inevitably evolve in the absence of a formal structure. Rogan and Hagner's (1990) suggestion that VR counselors "get to know" clients by interacting with them in natural environments is a start toward a more ecological approach. Their suggested context for evaluation is consistent with SE principles, but, as we have seen, informal judgment processes are vulnerable to subjective biases.

Some SE proponents have suggested measuring client preferences and their general work and social skills (Menchetti & Rusch, 1988), falling back on methodologies that do not depart drastically from conventional thinking (Rogan & Hagner, 1990). One difference in the SE preplacement assessment approaches is that their intended use is for choosing among placement alternatives and not as a basis for screening out clients.

In terms of recommendations of specific instruments, Menchetti and Rusch (1988) have suggested that preplacement assessment should include "identification and measurement of actual skills required for employment" (p. 85). One such instrument is the Job Skills Inventory (Belmore & Brown, 1978), which involves three steps: identifying the general vocational and social skill requirements, observing workers in the target job and breaking down their actions into specific steps, and identifying factors such as transportation and independent living skills needed to succeed.

Once the initial community-based placement is made, a key question is how many job tryouts are required (or permitted) before a client is matched to a job. Some degree of exposure to alternative work settings and occupations can be healthy in widening the individual's life experiences. Clearly, however, a completely unguided trial-and-error process is inefficient and might ultimately tax the goodwill of employers. Yet we have no known technology for helping clients "converge" on the appropriate job. In theory, one could envision a decision tree in which the assessment information obtained on a particular job could be used to decide the type of site desired for a subsequent evaluation. A perhaps farfetched analogy is the adaptive testing technology used in well-defined fields such as mathematics (e.g., Hsu & Shermis, 1989). In adaptive testing, students are not asked a full battery of test items, as is the custom in traditional psychometric testing. Instead, the results from a student's answer to each question are used to select the next question to be asked, until the computerized decision tree converges on the exact level of that student's competence. One major advantage of adaptive testing is that the number of questions needed to determine competence is far smaller than in traditional testing. One disadvantage is that the bank of items needed is far greater.

A modification of the multiple job tryout approach might be to mix and match it with "researching" job options through observation, visits to job site, and other activities that stop short of the client's actually working in the setting. The assumption is that some jobs may be ruled out quickly based on cursory information.

In practice, community assessment placement decisions are typically made intuitively and on the basis of site availability. If we are committed to a vocational assessment technology centering on community-based assessments, however, then these are the kinds of questions worth raising.

Conclusion

We agree with proponents of SE, who have argued that the traditional view of vocational rehabilitation—as a linear process starting with assessment, leading to training, and culminating in placement—is inadequate. The SE model suggests a fundamental change in the role of assessment, to view it as an ongoing process incorporating client preferences. In the reformulated approach, the work environment becomes the "vocational instrument."

The role of vocational assessment in the SE paradigm is in transition. It would be a mistake to assume that, because the old paradigm is flawed, the new paradigm is better. We need a more comprehensive theory to link together the various elements of assessment described above. We must move beyond the shotgun approaches to community-based assessment currently available in the literature.

The hard work of developing and validating new assessment procedures remains to be done. Some of the SE literature reflects the perennial tension between intuitive judgments based on "knowing my client" and hard-nosed assessment procedures. Our reading of the assessment literature is that it would be a mistake to regress into purely qualitative methodologies.

Ironically, the reformulated assessment model does not eliminate the desirability of assessment approaches outside the workplace. If community-based assessments are to be employed efficiently, we need preplacement assessment tools to guide decision making. Instruments tailored to specific work settings may be more valid than off-the-shelf instruments.

In this ideal formulation of vocational assessment, the role of the assessor has been expanded dramatically. The role requirements are more labor intensive, more interactive with employers, and more involved in the creation of new tools than are those in the traditional role. Most important, the assessor's job does not end when the initial assessment is completed but continues as long as the client is involved in the employment process.

CHAPTER 4

The Use of Traditional Neuropsychological Tests to Describe and Prescribe: Why Polishing the Crystal Ball Won't Help

DAVID FAUST

When Dr. Thomas J. Guilmette asked a national sample of neuropsychologists to indicate the areas of research they considered of greatest priority, the assessment of everyday functioning and its relation to rehabilitative planning topped the list (Guilmette, Faust, Hart, & Arkes, 1990). These practitioners would likely suggest that the editors of the current text chose their topic wisely. In their everyday practices, neuropsychologists—psychologists specializing in brain-behavior relationships—are frequently involved in the design and implementation of rehabilitative programs for the brain injured and cognitively impaired.

Although new methods are being devised to assess functioning in everyday life (see Tupper & Cicerone, 1990b), I would conjecture that many or most neuropsychologists pursuing this assessment task still place primary reliance on "traditional" neuropsychological tests and methods (with some mix of behavioral observations, historical data, and interview data from collateral sources sometimes thrown in). To my knowledge, no formal survey has specifically examined the methods neuropsychologists use to appraise everyday functioning, but general surveys of test usage among practitioners, discussions with colleagues, and the opportunity to review the work of many neuropsychologists lead me to this conjecture. My use of *traditional* here refers solely to the tests used and not to the strategy of application—that is, whether they are employed in a set or flexible manner—although I will have a good deal to say about assessment strategies later. I am referring to tests of the type that generally have been in use for many years, such as the Wechsler Intelligence Scales (e.g., Wechsler, 1981), the Wechsler Memory Scale or its revised version (Wechsler, 1945, 1987), and the components of the Halstead-Reitan Neuropsychological Battery (H-R) (Reitan & Wolfson, 1985).

I will argue that the use of traditional tests to describe everyday functioning or to prescribe rehabilitative strategies is, as currently practiced, likely to be ineffectual and that efforts to apply them in new ways to fulfill these aims are unlikely to succeed. Rather, we typically would be better off limiting their application to other and more appropriate purposes and getting (or continuing) on with the task of developing new methods and approaches to description and prescription. In setting forth this argument, I will first review the role of diagnosis, then examine major approaches to neuro-psychological assessment and their application to the assessment of everyday functioning, and finally suggest some possible approaches to description and prescription.

"I don't care about diagnosis. I just treat individuals." We have not yet fully shaken the antinosologic malady that gripped psychology in the 1960s. Many psychologists still seem to believe (pragmatically and even theoretically!) that diagnosis and prediction are of little importance. Instead, so the argument goes, down in the trenches, one is too busy treating the sick to be concerned with diagnosis or prediction.

Of course, treatment choice is *sometimes* arbitrary. For example, one may be down to two options, and the knowledge that is available may not help at all in selecting one over the other. There obviously are instances, however, in which we know enough to prefer one intervention over another or can select in a way that improves the chances of success. For example, if a patient with a long history of extreme mood swings presents in a hypomanic state, and has responded positively to lithium in the past but stopped taking his medication 3 weeks ago, resuming lithium is a better choice then putting him on the couch and initiating a Freudian analysis. Further, the extent to which we currently possess knowledge that helps to guide treatment choice is separate from the potential value of such information or the worth of attempts to obtain it. Unless one contends that perfect knowledge would show that all current and future treatment approaches are equally effective in treating all conditions (and who would hold this absurd notion?), then assessment/appraisal/diagnosis is a desirable objective. As long as there are possible choices, and as long as all of these choices are not equally likely to succeed, there is an assessment task that needs to be done. If I cannot currently cure an infectious disease, I would not conclude there is no point in conducting further research on antibiotics. Thus one can maintain that many assessment efforts, given the current state of knowledge, do not help matters very much, and concomitantly maintain with perfect consistency that assessment should be pursued where feasible and should be further developed.

For one who argues that she does not diagnose but just treats individuals, it would seem fairly clear that the treater typically (or one would hope) sets out with some assumptions or guesses about what will result from the intervention or strategy selected. Thus one treats based on implicit or explicit predictions. In addition, as an increased range of treatment options become available, and as practitioners increasingly face constraints on expenditures in the helping fields, assessment will take on greater and greater importance. Diagnosis and description also, of course, ultimately inform intervention, as intervention ultimately informs diagnosis.

One sometimes wonders whether those who voice general opposition to diagnosis and prediction would maintain their position were the tables turned. Would they say to their neurosurgeon, "I don't care whether it's a brain tumor or a spinal cord tumor; and, yes, I understand you think a CT scan would clarify things, but I prefer a trial-and-error approach, so get out that scalpel and just start somewhere." Although it is difficult to anticipate the form that diagnostic entities or categories will eventually take in a system that encompasses everyday functioning and its failures, or the extent to which future assessment methods will resemble current ones, these are matters separate from whether assessment, diagnosis, and prediction are relevant clinical endeavors. Where there is the potential for a complexity of disorders representing as heterogeneous a mix as failures in meeting everyday life demands, I would conjecture that it simply impossible to optimize treatment effectiveness without an adequate diagnostic system.

Methods of Assessment

Currently, there are two major orientations to neuropsychological assessment: set approaches and flexible approaches. A clinician may place sole or primary emphasis on one or the other approach or may combine the two approaches. Initially, I will deal with each approach in its relatively pure or unmixed form.

Set or Structured Batteries

The most commonly used standard or set battery is the H-R (Guilmette et al., 1990), although the term *set* is something of a misnomer as H-R users may differ in the precise stimulus materials, instructions, and scoring procedures they apply (Snow, 1987). At the time the H-R was developed, neurological investigative techniques were far less sophisticated, and more dangerous, than they are today, and thus a central intent was to aid in the identification of brain damage. The H-R was a monumental achievement, one that did much to lay the groundwork for the emergence and growth of neuropsychology. I fear that many current neuropsychologists fail to accord Halstead and Reitan the credit they deserve or recognize the intellectual powers that were required.

If one's primary objective is to identify brain damage, then, obviously, one selects tests that are maximally sensitive to brain damage. Maximizing sensitivity in the detection of brain damage *and* specificity in the description of everyday functioning are, however, in no small part, incompatible aims. In general, as sensitivity increases, specificity decreases, and vice versa.

For the purposes of this discussion, I will assume that specificity is a key objective in the description of cognitive and everyday func- tioning, as it provides the information needed to design individually tailored rehabilitative strategies and programs. (I realize that opposing arguments are possible and that this could appear to be an oversimplification.) Although certain placement decisions are well served by general or global information, such as a client's standing on an index of overall cognitive abilities, such coarse information is usually of limited value in making specific treatment decisions (especially as treatment options are further developed and refined). In contrast, tests generally become more sensitive to brain dysfunction as they become less specific.

The hypothetical perfect test for identifying brain damage simultaneously demands intact functioning in all areas. As such, brain damage of any type that creates functional impairment will be detected by the test. For example, the Bender-Gestalt Test (Bender, 1938), which, despite its critics, shows a reasonable sensitivity to brain damage as a single measure, simultaneously requires such capacities as motor coordination, spatial analysis, the integration of these two functions, planning, and other abilities. At the other end of the continuum, a (hypothetical) test that requires only a single function will be failed only by those select individuals who have brain damage of a type that affects that function. Of course, the requirement to perform multiple functions simultaneously and integratively is not the sole factor that increases sensitivity; various other factors also affect this parameter, such as the frequency with which functions are affected, the distribution of the measured ability in the healthy versus disabled population, and sensitivity to extraneous factors as opposed to primary ones. Still, all other things being equal, the greater the number of functions required, the greater the likelihood of detecting brain dysfunction. As the number of functions required increases, the specificity of the test decreases, however, and hence the greater the difficulty determining the particular factors leading to task failure and the what and how of rehabilitation.

One can "eyeball" the results of tests requiring multiple functions and attempt to determine which particular abilities have been affected. For example, if the patient reproduces each of the Bender figures with reasonable exactness but spaces them erratically across the page such that many of the figures collide, one can reasonably postulate that the motor components of this task have been handled adequately and that the problem lies elsewhere. Having eliminated one factor, however, numerous other possibilities remain. Further, one often lacks specifically related or relevant observables for evaluating various functions tapped by the test (beyond the general correlation between task success and the integrity of the various functions underlying performance, and task failure and problems with one or more of these functions). For example, the failure to solve orally presented mathematical problems may provide little or no information about the underlying processes related to task failure. Opponents of structured batteries have long pointed out their lack of specificity and weakness in identifying the factors underlying impaired performance (see, for example, Milberg, Hebben, & Kaplan, 1986).

A supporter of structured batteries may agree that performance on a limited number of items or tasks might not help much in identifying specific impairments but argue that examination of performance across a series of tests often allows for such distinctions or permits one to identify common threads underlying task failures. The problem is that this approach requires the evaluator to comprehend a series of comparisons in which, in each case, multiple variables are changing simultaneously. One might label this the "multiple confounded comparisons problem." Suppose someone performs poorly when I ask them to repeat digit series in the forward order. I am not sure whether this difficulty is due to limitations in short-term memory or inattention. I notice, however, that this individual performs reasonably well on a passage recall task. I might hypothesize that short-term memory is intact, given normal performance on this latter task, and, further, as passage recall tasks place less demand on attentional capacities than digit recall tasks (for reasons that need not be gone into here), that attention is the compromised function. The problem with all this is that digit recall tasks and passage recall tasks do not differ in just their attentional demands but in multiple ways. For example, with passage recall tasks, one is dealing with meaningful versus rote material, which allows for different ways of organizing or chunking information for purposes of recall. Further, word knowledge and other factors related to verbal comprehension are now relevant, and more material must be placed in temporary storage: One can often perform active rote rehearsal of most or all of the material as digits are being presented but cannot do so with passages as the amount of material is so much greater. Given simultaneous alterations in multiple variables, it is difficult to determine which one accounts for the change in performance. Additional tasks that require short-term memory are also likely to differ from these first two tasks in multiple ways. Thus the data base from the evaluation, in large part or entirely, violates logically necessary requirements for isolating variables and determining their operation. Whatever the correctness of this theoretical analysis, studies examining the relation between H-R performance and everyday functioning generally show modest or weak associations between the two, especially when one analyzes specific or more delineated activities (see Chapter 4 of Faust, Ziskin, & Hiers, 1991). Dunn, Searight, Grisso, Margolis, and Gibbons's (1990) study provides an example. Dunn et al. obtained modest relations between H-R scores and results on a measure designed to assess everyday functioning among geriatric patients (the difficulties and paradoxes relating to criterion measures in studies of this type are evident). The authors indicated that cross-validation of their results is needed and that even the modest relations they obtained may have been inflated. Even disregarding this possibility, they noted that, given such modest relations, individuals who perform poorly on neuropsychological tests may show adequate everyday living skills, and vice versa. They further noted that the relations obtained between test performance and various facets of everyday functioning did not necessarily align with previously described, clinically based guides (or what might be considered clinical lore). Dunn et al. also indicated that the neuropsychological test results, although globally related to overall functioning, did not demonstrate more specific relations with particular functional capacities. They stated, "A clear pattern of specific neuropsychological functions meaningfully associated with specific daily living skills did not emerge in this study. Therefore, while the two domains appear to be moderately related, prediction of a patient's daily functioning in a particular area from neuropsychological test data is not supported by the results of this study" (Dunn et al., 1990, p. 115). Of interest, Dunn et al. observed that many neuropsychologists seem willing to address questions about everyday functioning, despite the lack of necessary or supportive scientific data. They noted that such predictions are based on the assumption that individuals who have difficulties on neuropsychological tests will also have problems in everyday living but stated that "at present the validity of the relationships between the two domains has not been established empirically" (Dunn et al., 1990, p. 104).

The intent here is not to single out the H-R, and I have focused on it because it is the most widely used structured battery and has been the subject of most studies examining neuropsychological test performance and everyday functioning. For other structured batteries, such as the Luria-Nebraska Neuropsychological Battery (Golden, Purisch, & Hammeke, 1985), the same theoretical limitations described previously would seem to apply, and there has been little or no research examining the relation between performance on such batteries and everyday functioning.

In conclusion, given the format and approach used in the H-R and other structured batteries of this type, it is difficult to imagine a circumstance in which they would prove very useful in determining everyday functioning in specific areas, particularly given the current state of knowledge about brain-behavior relations. If we had a more highly developed theory of brain structure as it relates to higher order behavioral/cognitive functions (and if that theory turned out to be of a certain type), then determining the presence, location, and severity of brain damage might help considerably in designing specifically tailored rehabilitative interventions. To the extent these conditions hold, however, it will most likely follow that neuroimaging and related techniques will gain ascendancy over neuropsychological methods for purposes of rehabilitative planning, for the capacity of neuropsychological tests to identify, locate, and delineate brain damage will probably never catch up to imaging techniques and rather will continue to fall further and further behind. I would thus suggest that, for structured batteries of the traditional type, tinkering with, or polishing, the crystal ball will not help much in achieving the descriptive or prescriptive objectives associated with rehabilitative planning.

Descriptive, Flexible, and Process/Qualitative Approaches

According to surveys of the field, many neuropsychologists alter the tests or methods they use based on the questions of clinical interest and, often, the data that come in as testing proceeds (Guilmette et al., 1990; McCaffrey, Malloy, & Brief, 1985). Many neuropsychologists who use these tailored and flexible approaches also emphasize the manner in which the examinee approaches or solves (or fails to solve) tasks. Some such practitioners also change the format of standardized tests at their discretion. For example, the examiner might extend time limits on items, provide extra presentations of the to-be-memorized material, or alter the test stimuli. Some of this simply represents the testing of limits following normal administration of the test, but in other cases the standard procedures themselves are altered. Muriel Lezak (Lezak, 1983) and Edith Kaplan (see Milberg et al., 1986) are among the leading spokespersons for these approaches.

Limits of FLX and P/Q approaches. One fundamental limit of flexible (FLX) and process/qualitative (P/Q) approaches is the nearly complete absence of formal scientific research examining or backing proponents' claims. From one perspective, research on these methods is extraordinarily difficult to conduct. The same practitioner may alter her procedures considerably across examinees, and different practitioners using the same general strategy may differ completely in the specific methods or test items employed. It would be relatively simple, however, to determine the accuracy that clinicians using such approaches achieve. For example, one could examine initial judgments and outcome in such areas as occupational functioning to determine predictive success.

The accuracy of FLX and P/Q approaches is commonly taken for granted, probably in part because leading advocates are persuasive individuals and *some* of the underlying theoretical premises are fundamentally sound. For example, for reasons described earlier, structured neuropsychological batteries often provide little help in determining the specific problems or dysfunctions underlying task failure. FLX and P/Q approaches detail methods for attempting to pinpoint specific underlying causes, as perhaps best described by the great A. R. Luria (1980). For example, one can readminister a task that was failed while altering only one variable, such as requirements for the processing of orally presented information (e.g., one might readminister the test in a visual format). The variable that is eliminated is usually the one hypothesized to account for task failure. If performance normalizes once this variable has been eliminated, one has initial evidence that it is a specific cause for task failure. There clearly are major advantages gained in manipulating a single variable at a time, as opposed to the situation with structured batteries in which multiple variables are changing simultaneously. (Whether one really is altering only one variable when redesigning tasks with this aim in mind is another matter.)

Despite the intuitive appeal of FLX and P/Q methods in their current form, their seeming verification in practice, the importance and legitimacy of the problems they are designed to address, and their meritorious elements, there are strong reasons to believe that, when research on their accuracy is finally undertaken, they will be found to be far from optimal. A large body of research supports this supposition.

Fixed Versus Flexible and Clinical Versus Actuarial Methods

Considerable research has examined fixed versus variable methods of data collection. In the "fixed" method, one follows a set or prespecified procedure for data collection; in the "variable" method, the data collector alters procedures at his discretion. Structured versus unstructured interviews serve to illustrate the distinction. Over the years, numerous studies have compared fixed versus flexible methods, and even in 1966 Sawyer was able to conduct an extensive literature review. Sawyer found that, in *every* comparison in which the method of data interpretation was held constant, fixed methods of data collection were as or more accurate than variable methods. In general, fixed methods of data collection increase reliability or reduce error variance, which, so long as the data have potential predictive power, increases accuracy. Such methods also protect against certain frailties of the human mind, in particular, biases stemming from preconception or initial hypothesis formation (see Faust, 1984), because the order and type of information sought is not altered in accord with the examiner's developing impressions.

In addition, there is a large body of research on approaches to data interpretation, in particular, clinical and actuarial methods. As originally described by Meehl (1954), the major contributor in this area, *clinical judgment* refers to decisions reached in the "head," using whatever type of knowledge and information the practitioner has at her disposal. Actuarial methods are defined by two features: (a) Data combination is routinized or prespecified, and (b) it is based on empirically derived relations or frequencies. A method is *not* actuarial unless *both* requirements are met. The *source* of data is *irrelevant* in distinguishing clinical and actuarial approaches. Rather, the relevant dimension is how data, of whatever kind, are combined. If they are combined in the head, the method is clinical, and, if they are combined following a predetermined method that is based on observed relations, it is actuarial. Virtually any form of information can be made amenable to actuarial analysis. For example, if the clinician's qualitative observations are coded (e.g., 0 equals absent; 1 equals present), they can be entered into the actuarial mill.

Many studies have examined the accuracy of the two methods in an equal horse race, that is, when both start with the same information. In virtually every one of these studies in the social sciences, the accuracy of the actuarial method has equaled or exceeded that of the clinical method (Dawes, Faust, & Meehl, 1989). The same holds even when the actuarial method is placed at an informational disadvantage, for example, when those using the clinical method have access to test and interview data and the latter data are not available for actuarial analysis. Studies in neuropsychology also demonstrate the superiority of the actuarial method (see Wedding & Faust, 1989). A study by Heaton, Grant, Anthony, and Lehman (1981), which is sometimes cited as an exception to the actuarial advantage, is not correctly viewed as such because it compared clinical judgment with judgments that were routinized but were not founded on empirically established frequencies. Therefore the latter judgment method was not actuarial.

Many clinicians resist the outcome of these studies, not uncommonly on the basis of counterfactual or conceptually questionable positions. For example, it has been argued that the studies forced clinicians to engage in less familiar predictive tasks, did not include experts, or denied practitioners access to crucial information. All of these objections have been met in various studies, which failed to yield contrary results (see Dawes et al., 1989). It has also been argued that group statistics do not apply to individual cases, but tallied observations obviously can have predictive power. If the argument were literally correct, the clinicians in these studies, who made judgments based on individual case analysis, would have beaten the actuarial method (which depends on generalities), but they did not. More conceptually interesting possibilities include, for example, the identification of rare events not included in actuarial formulas or shifts in cost-benefit ratios that actuarial formulas may not be designed to evaluate. Studies on these possible exceptions (e.g., Goldberg, 1968; Leli & Filskov, 1984) have not been supportive, although insufficient research is currently available to draw firm conclusions (Dawes et al., 1989).

It is thus clear that the practitioner who uses a flexible approach to gather data and clinical judgment to integrate that data is depending, in both cases, on generically inferior methods. Contrary to common belief, the complexity of the data or the judgment task does not reverse these advantages but tends to extend them (see Faust, 1984). The problem is made more serious by the paucity of formal scientific evidence examining or supporting the FLX and P/Q approaches. In the context of neuropsychological assessment, it is conceivable that good comes from the use of generally inferior strategies, but the prior odds clearly go against the possibility.

A sophisticated proponent of FLX or P/Q approaches might cite Meehl (1954) in arguing that the clinician can exceed the actuary when complex pattern recognition or analysis is required. They might further argue that complex pattern analysis is exactly what is required in deciphering data generated through a comprehensive neuropsychological evaluation. When Meehl initially proposed this possible exception to the actuarial advantage, it was stated as just this—a possibility—not as a scientifically demonstrated outcome. In fact, this possibility has not panned out, as Meehl himself has noted (1986). One can develop actuarial procedures that incorporate configural or complex patterned relationships, and thus, as Goldberg (1968) indicated, such capacities are not the clinician's "ace in the hole." Additionally, the potential advantages of configural analysis or optimal weighting of variables are often far overestimated (see Dawes, 1979). Also, many studies show that individuals have considerable difficulty deciphering complex cue configurations or analyzing complex data (see Faust, 1989). Finally, even simple actuarial methods equal or exceed the accuracy of clinicians who claim to have employed complex configural strategies (see Faust, 1984).

To my knowledge, only one study has directly examined neuropsychologists' capacity to analyze or integrate configural patterns.

Arkes and Faust (1987) had practitioners review a series of cases in which the presence, area, severity, and pattern of impairment varied. Although the first three variables influenced judgments, in no instance did pattern or configuration alter conclusions. Not much can be determined from a single study of this type, but it does align with a large body of literature suggesting that individuals, clinicians included, have a surprisingly limited capacity to integrate complex data.

These restrictions in human cognitive ability aside, there is good reason to argue that the FLX and P/Q approaches tend to obscure, rather than clarify, patterns in nature. For example, if the approaches increase error variance, patterns will be (more) distorted. Russell, one of the major developers of formal decision aids in neuropsychology, has stated: "Accurate pattern analysis is only possible when a set rather than a flexible battery of tests is utilized" (1984, p. 50). He stated further, "If the tests are changed each time a different patient is tested, a pattern cannot be observed and established" (p. 57), a statement that may be too extreme but at least suggests something about the difficulties involved.

The Weakness of "Supportive" Arguments for FLX and P/Q Methods

Lacking formal research support, advocates of the FLX and P/Q approaches rely on subjective impressions about the effectiveness of their methods and often cite the power of judgment that is developed and refined through extensive experience. Such forms of evidence or support are weak and illustrate the need for scientific evaluation. Across various studies analyzing the subjective appraisal of judgment accuracy, the pervasive finding is overconfidence; that is, individuals are more confident in their judgments than is warranted by their true level of accuracy (Lichtenstein, Fischhoff, & Phillips, 1982). Clinicians tend to hold inflated beliefs in their diagnostic and predictive abilities, and personal experience may be accorded evidentiary superiority over well-conducted studies. I am not mindlessly arguing that research findings should *always* be accorded superiority over personal impressions. When subjective experience leads to one belief and a large and consistent body of literature suggests another, however, it is the research that is most often correct. One who is placing rational bets should be guided accordingly.

Hyman (1977), a palm reader (turned psychologist), reports that his initial personal experiences led him to believe in the method. He was convinced, however, to perform a number of readings in which he gave the opposite interpretations to those "indicated." For example, if the sign indicated introversion, he reported extroversion. To his surprise, the subjects of the inverted readings agreed with his statements at a similar rate. Hyman began to look at things much differently, and he has subsequently spent much time analyzing the ill-founded faith that others develop in personality readers of various sorts. He points out that the high rate of agreement with interpretations often leads the readers themselves, whether palmists or psychologists, to develop false or exaggerated beliefs in their judgment powers.

There are many instances in which conclusions based on experience are found to be wrong when put to scientific test, such as the notion that bleeding individuals with leeches was a medical panacea. False impressions or "illusory correlations" (Chapman & Chapman, 1967, 1969) are not uncommon in neuropsychology. For example, at one point or another, it has been purported that the tendency to draw circles in a clockwise direction is indicative of learning disability and that rotations or reversals on visual-motor tasks strongly suggest brain dysfunction (for a review of these and other possible illusory correlations in neuropsychology, see Chapter 5 of Faust et al., 1991).

Considerable research examining mental health professionals' experience and judgment accuracy shows little or no relation between the two (see Dawes, 1989). Studies conducted on this topic in neuropsychology have yielded similar outcomes (see Wedding & Faust, 1989). For example, Faust et al. (1988) obtained no significant relations between neuropsychologists' training, education, or experience and their accuracy in determining the presence, cause, and location of brain damage. The same negative findings were obtained even when professionals were divided into highly contrasting groups, such as those with a mode of approximately 500 versus 12,000 hours of clinical experience.

There are numerous obstacles to learning through experience (see Dawes, 1989; Faust, 1991). For example, as noted, interpreters' erroneous conclusions are often accepted as correct (Hyman,

1977; Snyder, Handelsman, & Endelman, 1978). Stated differently, the frequency of feedback that seems confirmatory exceeds the clinician's true rate of accuracy. It is not surprising that clinicians develop inflated confidence under such circumstances and have difficulties benefiting from feedback. Feedback is useful only to the extent it is accurate, and, as the error component in feedback increases, learning from experience can become extremely difficult (Dawes, 1989), particularly when judgments are founded on a shaky knowledge base.

Human judgment biases can further impede the accurate interpretation of feedback that is received. For example, individuals tend to remember their initial judgments as more consistent with outcomes than is actually the case (Fischhoff, 1980). Again, this leads to inflated confidence and to difficulties identifying, and hence learning from, mistakes. Also, in the context of clinical activities, practical and ethical grounds usually prohibit one from systematically manipulating variables. As such, one does not know what would have happened had one done otherwise. For example, the clinician does not know how the patient would have fared had he initially selected a different intervention. Finally, judgments can lead to self-fulfilling prophecies. When one rejects a certain intervention approach with a particular patient, one's conclusion that the option was inferior cannot be overturned if the approach is never enacted.

These problems with clinical judgment, including our limited capacity to integrate complex data and the ease with which we develop illusory beliefs, highlight certain restrictions of the human mind. This is not, however, an argument for eliminating human judgment from evaluative processes. For example, human judges have unique observational abilities, and computer technology cannot yet match human capacity for language interpretation or the invention of deep structure theories. In addition, human judgment and experience are essential in identifying possible predictive variables, developing assessment technologies, and generating hypotheses. Thus, for example, there are certain important data that could not be observed or recorded without human involvement. Arguments for human observational abilities should not, however, be confused with arguments for integrative abilities. The evidence suggests that, in the context of psychological and neuropsychological evaluations, once the data are gathered, they are best integrated by the actuarial method, not the human judge.

The unique abilities and contributions of the human judge notwithstanding, given the current status of FLX and P/Q approaches, polishing the crystal ball will only further perpetuate the appearance of remarkable vision that might characterize a few adherents of exceptional talent but not the many that remain. Even were the crystal ball polished, the odds are high it would not show us what we need to see or greatly alter the current limitations of our vision.

False Synthesis and False Dichotomy

Some argue that the division into clinical and actuarial camps is artificial and needless and, instead, that the two methods can easily be combined. As Meehl (1986) noted, certain versions of this argument are nonsensical. In a considerable percentage of cases, clinical and actuarial methods lead to different conclusions, and one is faced with a dichotomous choice. For example, if actuarial judgment suggests that antidepressant medication is needed and clinical judgment suggests it is not, one cannot "integrate" the two conclusions and decide that one will and will not medicate the patient. Further, many proposals for so-called clinical-actuarial approaches essentially dictate that one follows actuarial conclusions at one's discretion (in effect, when it agrees with one's clinical judgment), which is not much different than simply depending on one's clinical judgment. The available research on the topic, although limited in scope and coverage, thus far consistently suggests that the "clinical-actuarial" approach leads to less accurate judgments than the strict actuarial approach.

There is a related, although not parallel, argument in neuropsychology about the relative merits of quantitative versus qualitative data. One should not confuse source of data with method of judgment, although this mistake is common, probably due to the way these dimensions are perceived to covary; that is, those with a quantitative bent are believed to prefer actuarial judgment and those with a qualitative orientation to prefer clinical judgment. (My wager would be that most practitioners in *both* camps depend on clinical judgment in reaching final conclusions, with actuarial judgment used somewhat more often, but still infrequently, in the quantitative camp.) Despite these notions, qualitative data can be interpreted actuarially and quantitative data clinically. For example, a clinician eyeballing results on the H-R and integrating this data in his head is exercising clinical judgment, no matter the level of reliance on numbers.

Arguments about combining clinical and actuarial data, which often involve a false synthesis, are opposite in kind to arguments about quantitative and qualitative data, which often create a false dichotomy. Virtually any form of qualitative data can easily be quantified. Take, for example, the tendency to break gestalt on the Block Design subtest of the Wechsler Intelligence Scales. One can code such occurrences as 1 and nonoccurrences as 0. Even highly subjective, impressionistic judgments about the patient can be similarly coded. The argument that one who attends to numbers cannot take qualitative information into account or give it its just due is highly questionable. One irony here is that, although Reitan has frequently been criticized as unduly emphasizing quantitative data, his suggested use of pattern and pathognomonic signs fits within the rubric of most qualitative strategies.

A similar type of confusion is to view flexible assessment procedures as incompatible with an emphasis on quantitative data or set decision rules. No matter the particular slant the clinician takes toward assessment, it seems virtually unimaginable that one would advocate following *exactly* the same procedures with all patients. When one looks closely, it is apparent that we almost *never* do this, even across any two patients. For example, one stops administration of items on the Wechsler Intelligence Scale subtests, which are arranged in order of difficulty, after a certain number of consecutive errors. Across the subtests, different patients often reach discontinuation points on different items. As such, one has a flexible but structured procedure in which decisions to continue or stop a subtest are governed by systematic and empirically based rules. These rules relate to the probability of passing subsequent items once a certain number of consecutive items have been failed.

These types of hybrid assessment methods are so widespread and taken for granted that those who argue that structured and flexible approaches are incompatible may not realize that they commonly use what they believe cannot exist! The hybrid methods in current use are extremely rudimentary and could be much further refined. For example, decision rules could be used to determine the starting point of assessment and, based on the results obtained at each point in the process, the subsequent steps to take. In a separate piece (Faust, 1991), I have described what a procedure of this type might look like in the future. Some beginnings have been made along these lines (e.g., adaptive testing), but the approach can be expanded greatly and can combine the flexibility needed to conduct optimal evaluations with the rigor and consistency needed to minimize measurement error and compensate for human judgment limitations. Qualitative and quantitative approaches, and standardized and flexible approaches, can be combined in a way that eliminates these false dichotomies and that is likely to maximize evaluative accuracy and efficiency. For purposes of subsequent discussion, I will refer to the combined quantitative-qualitative/flexible-structured approach as "flexibly structured."

Toward a Neuropsychology
of Everyday Functioning

I suspect that neuropsychological methods for assessing everyday functioning will take the flexibly structured approach, using a combination of traditional (or derivatives or parts of traditional) cognitive measures and methods that sample everyday activities more directly. The latter type of tasks seem necessary because the probabilistic links between fundamental cognitive capacities and everyday life functioning are modest to weak in many areas. For example, in some areas, once skills surpass a certain minimal threshold, more advanced skills do not create additional performance advantages. Alternatively, motivational or affective factors may determine whether competencies are realized in task performance. Although simulations and direct observation are obvious choices for assessing everyday functioning, the role of self-reports and relatives' reports seems less clear. For example, if a patient's condition did not affect self-appraisal, and if that patient generally had excellent insight, self-report might sometimes serve as an incredibly efficient method for appraising everyday functioning. Of course, certain things are difficult to self-appraise, especially when prediction is involved; for example, the patient might have trouble determining how likely she is to succeed upon returning to work. This immediately leads one to think of hierarchically arranged choice points or branching procedures, in which assessment begins at different points with different individuals. Based on the individual's standing on background variables, empirical knowledge, and set decision procedures, one determines what information to seek initially. For example, one might first evaluate the accuracy of self-insight (using cross-checks that are easily ascertainable). If the results are positive, self-reports might serve as the initial focal point in evaluating certain functions. If we eventually develop a large compilation of assessment devices or methods, and if the selection of method is properly guided, then even components that are generally unrevealing, but sometimes tremendously informative, can combine to form a powerful assessment technology.

The predictive power of simulations and observations of everyday functioning follows from the principle that the more direct the measurement and the more closely one mimics the relevant conditions, then (with certain important exceptions), all other things being equal, the greater the degree of accuracy or generalization to real-life situations. This is another variant of the tenet that the best predictor of future behavior is past behavior. If this is so, then performance in an earlier situation (i.e., the evaluative context) should best predict performance in later, parallel situations. Simulations can be most effective when one wishes to evaluate limited and discrete skills. For example, if I want to know whether someone can dial a number, I simply ought to hand them the phone and let them give it a try rather than have them free associate to ink blots.

One limitation of simulations is the almost endless number of activities and situations one confronts in life. One certainly cannot run the patient through a simulation for each such possibility. Further, to the extent one views everyday life activities as consisting of many discrete tasks, it is difficult even to think about how one might pursue representative sampling. How does one obtain a representative sample of a heap? It is easy to overlook the extent to which representative sampling increases efficiency, thereby making otherwise prohibitive assessment tasks manageable. Imagine trying to assess a patient's vocabulary by starting at the beginning of the dictionary and proceeding through, or following the patient around for a week and seeing what words he utters, rather than using 30 or 40 appropriately selected and scaled items.

In addition, as studies on artificial intelligence have shown, to perform many human activities at anything approaching an optimal level, an underlying framework, or basic competencies, are required. If one were to design an everyday functioning machine, one's programming should surely include overreaching conceptualizations or mental abilities, such as the capacity to remember, reason, and abstract. Human competence is not a collection of discrete, unrelated skills and behaviors but is built around more general functions and capacities.

Unlike a heap of discrete entities, these broader intellectual skills and capacities are far more amenable to representative sampling. Further, determining the status of overreaching capacities often allows for prediction across a variety of domains. For example, a Full Scale IQ score provides some predictive power across many situations. I am reminded of a former secretary, whom I once asked to save postcards from reprint requests so that I might maintain a file for purposes of correspondence. In sending out reprints, she clipped the return addresses off the postcards and used them as mailing labels, making no record of them, and then gave me what remained, believing she had satisfied my request. When I relayed this story to a psychologist friend of mine, he commented, "Well, it goes to show that g bears on performance in just about any type of job." The problem, however, is that, across most domains, the level of predictive power one gains by assessing these more general capacities is modest or worse.

Thus, on the one hand, there is assessment of more general capacities, which tends to be efficient and provides predictive breadth but lacks precision in most specific domains. On the other hand, there are simulations and direct observations of life behaviors, which allow for greater predictive power but lack efficiency and breadth. Stated in another way, we can predict a little about a lot and a lot about a little. If our assessment task is to determine everyday functioning in all relevant areas of life, then we need some way of combining approaches to achieve the aims of accuracy, efficiency, and breadth of sampling.

Under certain conditions, the appraisal of core cognitive abilities may allow one to form relatively powerful generalizations about performance in multiple realms. The fundamental methodological or epistemological problem is that our current knowledge of such abilities generally fails to meet the conditions necessary for a high level of predictive accuracy. If we had better developed theoretical constructs and networks, and better measuring devices, then the assessment of such capacities might provide considerable predictive and descriptive power. Efforts to develop such knowledge certainly should continue.

I can think of a number of approaches that might increase the efficiency of assessment efforts, including those that incorporate simulations and direct observation. One is to use more complex or advanced tasks that require competence in a number of less complex or advanced areas. One can thus rapidly establish competence in multiple component activities by assessing more complex activities (assuming the latter are completed successfully). As a simple example, if a patient can spontaneously recall orally presented instructions under conditions of interference after a 30-minute delay, it is a good bet that similar types of materials can be recognized and recalled on an immediate basis, on a recent basis, and under noninterfering conditions. If an individual can recall material spontaneously, she should be able to recognize it. If she can recall material later, she (usually) should have been able to recall it earlier. If she can recall it under interfering conditions, she should be able to recall it under easier circumstances or in the absence of interference.

A related approach, which might serve as a supplemental assessment device, is to examine performance on laboratory tests that require all or more of the skills needed to perform classes of everyday tasks. For example, if one is concerned with the patient's ability to discriminate sounds when listening to conversations, crossing the street, or whatever, one might design a relatively difficult task that, if successfully completed, allows for confident predictions about the capacity to handle certain activities in the natural environment. There are some frightening complications with such an approach, including the possibility that a laboratory task permitting highly accurate predictions about competence in the natural environment will need to be so hard that most normal individuals will fail it. As a component in a hierarchical branching procedure, however, such tasks might serve as initial screening procedures, in which one can eliminate the need to conduct more detailed as- sessment in certain areas. Thus, for example, if one had 40 areas each requiring, say, a 5- to 10-minute assessment procedure, and one could eliminate the need to conduct more fine-grained evaluation in 10 or 15, or perhaps 20, areas, these screening procedures might greatly increase efficiency. A critic might object that this is too much time spent on evaluative activities, but one should consider the magnitude of rehabilitative efforts with some patients and the wasted time, expense, and heartache resulting from false starts and misdirected efforts.

As another approach, assume we begin to construct an adequate taxonomy of everyday abilities, and of cognitive capabilities and behavioral competencies, and gradually develop knowledge about the covariation between the two classes. One might then first assess cognitive abilities/behavioral competencies and then use actuarial methods to form tentative conclusions about functioning in everyday areas. One would check, or calibrate, the accuracy of these actuarial judgments by selecting a representative sample and determining how well they predict related simulations or samples of everyday performance.

Many other variations of flexibly structured approaches are possible. Whatever the specific forms, I believe we will increasingly move toward methods that combine the assessment of basic or overriding competencies with simulations and direct observations aimed at more specific functional capacities, and that representative sampling, breadth of coverage, and efficiency will be key organizing concepts. None of these approaches is easy, but, then again, who would argue that the development of methods for assessing every-day functioning is anything less than an incredible undertaking.

CHAPTER 5

Appraising the Psychometric Adequacy of Rehabilitation Assessment Instruments

BRIAN BOLTON
JEFFREY B. BROOKINGS

The purpose of this chapter is to provide an appraisal of the psychometric adequacy of eight exemplary assessment instruments currently used in rehabilitation. Following an introductory overview, a taxonomy of functional areas of rehabilitation measurement is presented. Capsule reviews of eight selected instruments establish the basis for appraising the psychometric status of rehabilitation assessment.

The Scope of Rehabilitation Assessment

If we define rehabilitation assessment as the specialized application of measurement principles to the unique problems of people with disabilities, then the earliest assessment efforts in rehabilitation would be the development of activities of daily living scales. In their comprehensive literature search, Donaldson, Wagner, and Gresham (1973) located 25 instruments published between 1950 and 1970 that satisfied two of the following three criteria: (a) a mechanism for scoring, (b) use in a survey or other type of research, and (c) applicability to a general rehabilitation population. Activities of daily living scales, also referred to as *independent living* or *adaptive behavior scales,* measure a variety of self-care, communication, and mobility variables.

As rehabilitation psychology developed into an independent professional and academic discipline in the 1950s and 1960s, the separate measurement specialty of rehabilitation assessment emerged. The Handicap Problems Inventory (HPI; Wright & Remmers, 1960) illustrates an initial attempt to measure the psychosocial impact of disability, as perceived by the person with a handicap. The HPI is a checklist of 280 problems representing four life areas (personal, family, social, and vocational) that may be attributable to physical disablement. Respondents mark those problems that they believe are caused or aggravated by the handicapping condition. In contrast to the HPI, the vocational assessment instruments developed in conjunction with the Minnesota Theory of Work Adjustment (Dawis, 1987) between 1957 and 1972 are psychometrically sophisticated measures. One of the instruments, the Minnesota Satisfactoriness Scales (MSS), is described below.

Because of the rapid expansion of rehabilitation assessment methodology in the 1970s and 1980s, a comprehensive review and evaluation of rehabilitation assessment instruments is beyond the scope of this chapter. Persons interested in examining the population of rehabilitation instruments available for use are referred to the following volumes: Bolton (1987a), Bolton (1988a), Bolton and Cook (1980), Fuhrer (1987b), and Halpern and Fuhrer (1984). Rather than identifying a random or representative sample of instruments, we decided to select a set of exemplary rehabilitation instruments that span the full range of assessment procedures in rehabilitation, although our choices emphasize instruments that assess vocationally relevant traits and capabilities. For these selected instruments, we provide capsule summaries and then evaluate their psychometric adequacy against explicit criteria.

To place our selected exemplary instruments in the broader perspective of rehabilitation assessment methodology, we present a taxonomy of instruments based on functional areas of rehabilitation measurement applications.

1. *Vocational assessment instruments.* Because occupational considerations are central to the goals of the rehabilitation enterprise,

the assessment of work-relevant attitudes, behaviors, values, and preferences assumes special importance. Examples of vocational instruments are the Functional Assessment Inventory (Crewe & Athelstan, 1984), the Minnesota Importance Questionnaire (Gay, Weiss, Hendel, Dawis, & Lofquist, 1971), the Preliminary Diagnostic Questionnaire (Moriarty, 1981), and the United States Employment Service Interest Inventory (U.S. Department of Labor, 1982b).

2. *Work behavior rating scales.* Observational ratings of persons with handicaps in workshop evaluation settings are fundamental to assessment for vocational evaluation. Examples of instruments are the Becker Work Adjustment Profile (Becker, 1989), the Work Adjustment Rating Form (Bitter & Bolanovich, 1970), the Work Personality Profile (Bolton & Roessler, 1986), and the Workshop Scale of Employability (Gellman, Stern, & Soloff, 1963).

3. *Independent living scales.* Referred to in physical medicine settings as *activities of daily living scales*, and with school-age youth as *adaptive behavior scales,* these instruments measure the extent of independent functioning in the areas of self-help, mobility, and communication. Examples of independent living scales are the Rehabilitation Indicators (Brown, Diller, Fordyce, Jacobs, & Gordon, 1980), the National Independent Living Skills Assessment Instruments (Dunlap & Iceman, 1985), the Social and Prevocational Information Battery (Halpern, Irwin, & Mundres, 1986), and the Independent Living Behavior Checklist (Walls, Zane, & Thvedt, 1979).

4. *Psychosocial assessment instruments.* The range of psychosocial characteristics that may be relevant in rehabilitation assessment include temperamental traits, needs, motives, and adjustment to disability. Examples of instruments are the Sixteen Personality Factor Questionnaire-Form E (Institute for Personality and Ability Testing, 1985), the Human Service Scale (Kravetz, Florian, & Wright, 1985), and the Acceptance of Disability Scale (Linkowski, 1987). Of course, standard clinical instruments, such as the Minnesota Multiphasic Personality Inventory (Hathaway & McKinley, 1989), may be appropriately administered in some situations.

5. *Tests of intellectual abilities.* Two intelligence tests have been developed expressly for use with examinees with handicaps. The Hiskey-Nebraska Test of Learning Ability (Hiskey, 1966) is an

individually administered instrument for persons with severe hearing impairment. The Haptic Intelligence Scale (Shurrager, 1961) is a performance intelligence test for clients with visual impairments. Standard clinical instruments, such as the Wechsler Adult Intelligence Scale-Revised (Wechsler, 1981) and group-administered general ability tests, such as the General Aptitude Test Battery (U.S. Department of Labor, 1982a), however, are widely used in the assessment of persons with handicaps.

6. *Rehabilitation outcome measurement.* Instruments have been developed to evaluate client outcomes that result from the provision of rehabilitation services, both for the general population of persons with disabilities and for specific disabling conditions (see Fuhrer, 1987b). Examples are the Minnesota Satisfactoriness Scales (Gibson, Weiss, Hendel, Dawis, & Lofquist, 1970), the Levels of Cognitive Function Scale (Hagen, Malkmus, & Durham, 1979), the Arthritis Impact Measurement Scales (Meenan, Gertman, Mason, & Dunaif, 1982), and the Service Outcome Measurement Form (Westerheide, Lenhart, & Miller, 1975).

7. *Attitudes toward disability scales.* A recently published compendium of scales that measure attitudes toward people with disabilities describes 22 instruments (Antonak & Livneh, 1988). The most popular of these are the Disability Factor Scales-General (Siller, 1969b) and the Attitudes Toward Disabled Persons Scale (Yuker, Block, & Young, 1970).

8. *Work sample systems.* Standardized assessment of vocational aptitudes and skills using work samples has a long history of application in vocational rehabilitation, beginning with the well-known TOWER system. Botterbusch (1987) has provided a descriptive review and comparative evaluation of 21 commercial work sample systems. In general, work sample systems are deficient when evaluated by basic psychometric criteria.

Evaluating Rehabilitation Instruments

After reviewing the principles and guidelines presented in *Standards for Educational and Psychological Testing* (American Educational Research Association, American Psychological Association, National Council on Measurement in Education, 1985) and the *Handbook of Measurement and Evaluation in Rehabilitation* (Bolton, 1987a), we decided that the evaluation scheme developed by Hammill, Brown, and Bryant (1989) constitutes a useful distillation of the major issues that pertain to the psychometric adequacy of assessment instruments (see Table 5.1). We reject as too rigid, however, the absolute standards that Hammill et al. (1989) stipulated in their criteria. For example, although reliability coefficients of .80 and above are certainly desirable, scales with lower reliabilities may be useful in situations where no other decision-relevant data are available. Also, validity must be considered simultaneously with reliability; lower reliability may be offset by good validity evidence. Knowledgeable professionals take the unreliability of scores into account when interpreting test results, usually by calculating the standard error of measurement and reporting interval rather than point estimates.

Because we do not believe that the application of absolute test evaluation standards is appropriate, instead preferring a global assessment of instrument characteristics and features, our evaluations of the psychometric adequacy of eight selected rehabilitation instruments consist of capsule summaries followed by brief comments. The chapter concludes with an overall summary of the psychometric status of rehabilitation assessment instruments. We also recognize the importance of nonpsychometric features of assessment devices, which may actually be the critical factors that influence test adoption (see Sigafoos, Cole, & McQuarter, 1987). The nontechnical test characteristics listed in Table 5.1 were also modified from Hammill et al. (1989).

The eight "exemplary" instruments reviewed below satisfy one or more of the following criteria: (a) The instrument is widely used in rehabilitation assessment practice; (b) the instrument represents a unique contribution to assessment methodology in rehabilitation; and/or (c) the instrument possesses outstanding psychometric characteristics for the population of persons with disabilities. In addition, the final choices reflect the authors' experience with the instruments: using them in research studies, investigating their psychometric properties, and writing reviews for test evaluation volumes. Of course, the ultimate criterion for selecting an instrument for inclusion in this review was a matter of the authors' judgment.

TABLE 5.1

Characteristics of Assessment Instruments

Technical Characteristics:

I. Norms
   A. Representativeness
      1. How selected/sampling plan (evidence of representativeness)
      2. Demographic description: thoroughness and relevance
   B. Subgroup partitions (sex, disability, employment status, and so on)
   C. Size of norm group(s)
   D. Recency of norm data (year of collection)
   E. Type of normative scores (raw, percentile, standard scores)

II. Reliability
   A. Internal consistency (single administration)
      1. Split-half
      2. Coefficient alpha, KR-20, and so on
   B. Experimental (two administrations)
      1. Retest
      2. Parallel forms
      3. Short term (1-2 weeks): instrument reliability
      4. Long term (6 months+): trait stability

III. Validity
   A. Content
      1. Sampling plan for items
      2. Framework for subscales (rational)
      3. Factorial derivation of subscales
   B. Concurrent
      1. Correlates with measures in expected way
      2. Convergent versus divergent predictions
   C. Predictive
      1. Intermediate
      2. Long-term outcomes
   D. Construct (subsumes above categories)
      1. Differentiation between groups identified by independent assessment
      2. Theoretical relationships confirmed
      3. Treatments modify/change scores in expected ways
      4. Confirmatory analysis of structure

Nontechnical Characteristics:

I. Administration
   A. Individual versus group
   B. Level of qualification
   C. Special training required
   D. Time to administer

II. Response Format
   A. Respondent reads items (or listens to audiotape)
   B. Examiner observes and rates examinee

    C. Respondent marks answer sheet
    D. Examiner records answers from interview
    E. Third-party respondent (parent/supervisor)
III. Scoring
    A. Clerical task
    B. Judgment required
    C. Computer-generated report
    D. "Clinical" data recorded
IV. Utility: relevance and usefulness of data (scores) in rehabilitation diagnosis and service planning

---

SOURCE: Adapted from Hammill, Brown, and Bryant (1989).

The eight instruments do not represent all eight functional areas that compose our taxonomy. We selected three instruments from the vocational assessment domain and none from the intellectual and work sample areas. We omitted intelligence tests because instruments for the nondisabled population are commonly used in rehabilitation assessment practice; regarding the work sample systems, it is our judgment that none qualifies as an exemplary instrument.

Five of the eight instruments were developed specifically for use with persons with disabilities, whereas three (the USES Interest Inventory, the Sixteen Personality Factor Questionnaire-Form E, and the Minnesota Satisfactoriness Scales) were constructed for application to the general population. These latter three instruments, however, have been used extensively in research and practice with individuals with disabilities. All eight instruments are multiscale measures, with each scale (or area of functioning) composed of multiple items. Seven of the eight instruments rely on norm-referenced score interpretation, with only the Rehabilitation Indicators reporting skills mastered rather than standard derived scores.

Functional Assessment Inventory

The Functional Assessment Inventory (FAI; Crewe & Athelstan, 1984) is a 42-item rating instrument designed for use by vocational rehabilitation counselors. All FAI items are focused on vocationally relevant behaviors and capabilities and provide data essential in rehabilitation service planning.

Construction of the FAI began with a review of 150 client case files for the purpose of identifying potential barriers to work. This initial inventory of vocational barriers was extended through discussions with experienced counselors and subsequently organized into a preliminary checklist. After several revisions, the checklist was converted to a series of behavioral rating items.

The current version of the FAI consists of 30 behaviorally anchored rating items that assess the client's vocational capabilities and deficiencies, 10 items that identify unusual assets, and 2 global items judging severity of disability and probability of vocational success.

Factor analytic studies of the FAI with diverse samples of vocational rehabilitation clients spanning the spectrum of physical, intellectual, and emotional disabilities have identified a consistent dimensional structure underlying the 30 behavioral items. These seven subscales are the primary organizing scheme for reporting FAI results: Adaptive Behavior, Motor Functioning, Physical Condition, Communication, Cognition, Vocational Qualification, and Environmental Orientation.

The FAI can be hand scored easily. Percentile equivalents for three categories of disability (physical, behavioral, and blind) are available for items, subscale scores, and the total Functional Limitation score. The Functional Assessment Rating System (FARS) computer program generates the best score report, however, because it incorporates the largest and most representative normative samples.

The FARS is a comprehensive eligibility determination and case planning program that enables the counselor to complete a functional assessment using the FAI, from which a series of normative functional profiles are provided, and guides him or her in designing a service plan that links functional deficits to needed services.

Two interrater reliability studies found that (a) 75% of the behavioral ratings made by pairs of counselors were identical, and another 23% differed by only one position on the four anchors, and (b) the average item reliability (alpha) coefficient was .80.

The available validity evidence strongly supports the objective of the FAI, which is to assess vocationally relevant functional capabilities of applicants for VR services. Scores on FAI items, subscales, and total limitations and strengths distinguish between disability groups in logically expected ways, identify applicants for services who are judged to have substantial vocational handicaps, correlate with global evaluations of severity of disability and probability of employment, and predict rehabilitation outcome criteria such as work status, earnings, and service costs. Readers interested in statistical details and references are referred to Bolton (1990).

Comments on the FAI. The Functional Assessment Inventory was developed and validated for use in vocational rehabilitation counseling settings. The instrument spans the full range of work behaviors, is applicable to all disability groups, and does not require extensive client observation. The FARS computer program incorporates extensive normative data in its report; the interrater reliability of the FAI items is very good; and the validity evidence for the FAI scores is excellent. Furthermore, the FAI is unique in its focus on behavioral capabilities with specific vocational relevance.

Preliminary Diagnostic Questionnaire

The Preliminary Diagnostic Questionnaire (PDQ; Moriarty, 1981) was developed to assess the functional capacities of persons with disabilities in the context of employability. Implicit in the construction of the PDQ was the assumption that a preliminary assessment of work-relevant characteristics should be possible without special tools and equipment and should take about an hour to administer.

The PDQ was designed to assess four broad areas of functioning relevant to the employability of persons with disabilities: *cognitive* (measured by Work Information, Preliminary Estimate of Learning, Psychomotor Skills, and Reading Retention subtests); *motivation or disposition to work* (measured by Work Importance and Internality subtests); *physical* (measured by the Personal Independence subtest); and *emotional* (measured by the Emotional Functioning subtest).

The 148 PDQ items are administered in a structured interview format using a self-contained, consumable 12-page booklet. All examinee responses and examiner notes are recorded in the booklet. Item scoring is accomplished simultaneously with test administration by the experienced examiner and the profile of standard scores can be calculated in a few minutes. A computerized PDQ report is available on floppy disk and a computer-based decision support system for rehabilitation counselors incorporates PDQ results as client data base elements.

The normative sample that constitutes the basis for converting raw scores on the eight PDQ subtests to stanine scores consists of 2,972 vocational rehabilitation clients from 30 state agencies. Comparisons on demographic variables demonstrated that the PDQ normative sample is representative of the population of disabled persons who receive services through the state/federal vocational rehabilitation system.

Internal consistency reliabilities for the eight PDQ subtests average .81, with a range from .69 to .90. Retest reliabilities calculated for six of the subscales with an interval of 30 days average .78, with a range from .47 to .97. The subtest with the lowest retest reliability has adequate internal consistency reliability, as do the two subscales for which retest data are not available.

Because the PDQ purports to assess the employment potential of persons with disabilities, evaluation of its validity should be based on the prediction of employment outcomes. Two subtests were significant predictors of earnings after case closure for a sample of former clients, whereas three subscales were predictive of minimum wage attainment. Although only some of the relationships were statistically significant, all eight PDQ subscales were positively correlated with the two employment criteria.

A discriminant analysis of the PDQ was carried out for the purpose of developing a global Feasibility Index. Of the minimum wage earners, 95% scored in the top third on the Feasibility Index. Additional evidence supportive of the validity of the PDQ includes the careful scale construction procedures and expected convergent and divergent relationships with standard aptitude, intelligence, and achievement tests. Readers interested in statistical details and references are referred to Bolton (1991a).

Comments on the PDQ. The PDQ represents a truly innovative approach to the psychosocial evaluation of applicants for vocational services. Three features of the PDQ are noteworthy: (a) It measures comprehensively the functional capacities that are considered essential in preparation for competitive employment; (b) it is administered in a structured interview format and therefore provides both clinical and psychometric information of value to the counselor; and (c) it has been demonstrated to be adequately reliable and valid for the purpose of assessing the employment potential of rehabilitation clients.

United States Employment Service Interest Inventory

The United States Employment Service Interest Inventory (USES-II; U.S. Department of Labor, 1982b) is a self-report instrument that measures the respondent's relative strength of interests in 12 broad categories of occupational activity. The 12 occupation interest areas constitute the primary organizing theme of the U.S. Department of Labor's (1979) *Guide for Occupational Exploration*.

The USES-II consists of 162 items of three types: job activity statements, occupational titles, and life experiences. Twelve interest areas are measured: Artistic, Scientific, Plants & Animals, Protective, Mechanical, Industrial, Business Detail, Selling, Accommodating, Humanitarian, Leading-Influencing, and Physical Performing.

The USES-II can be appropriately used with the general adult population aged 16 years and above. The reading level required is about third grade, but an audiotape version for administration to poor readers is easily prepared.

After a profile of 12 raw scores is obtained by counting the number of "liked" items for each of the 12 interest areas, the raw scores are translated into standard T-scores using a geographically and racially representative normative sample consisting of 6,530 students, job applicants, and employed workers.

The USES-II is the product of a careful program of developmental research. A series of preliminary factor analyses and item analyses eventually reduced a pool of almost 1,000 interest items to the final set of 162 items. Although the inventory was not developed specifically for use with persons with handicaps, several psychometric studies of the instrument have been carried out with rehabilitation client samples.

Internal consistency reliabilities for the 12 scales averaged .82, with a range from .75 to .87; retest reliabilities with a 1-week interval averaged .83, ranging from .73 to .88. A confirmatory factor analysis provided strong support for the 12-scale interest structure in the rehabilitation client population. Finally, the USES-II predicted with substantial accuracy graduation from various vocational training curricula at a comprehensive rehabilitation center. The USES-II is the only interest inventory designed to be used with the most thoroughly occupationally validated multiaptitude test available, the General Aptitude Test Battery (U.S. Department of Labor, 1982a), and is directly linked with an occupational exploration system that encompasses all jobs in the U.S. economy. Clearly, the USES-II is preferable to pictorial interest inventories sometimes used with rehabilitation clients, such as the Reading-Free Interest Inventory and the Vocational Interest and Sophistication Assessment. Readers interested in statistical details and references are referred to Bolton (1985b).

Comments on the USES-II. The psychometric foundation of the USES-II is outstanding and the excellent normative sample is representative of the nonprofessional U.S. labor force. The reliability and validity of the USES-II for the population of rehabilitation clients can be regarded as definitively established.

Becker Work Adjustment Profile

The Becker Work Adjustment Profile (BWAP; Becker, 1989) is an observer rating instrument designed for use with persons with physical, intellectual, and emotional disabilities who are clients in vocational rehabilitation programs. The primary purpose of the BWAP is to identify deficits in clients' work behavior that can be remediated in vocational training facilities. Use of the BWAP assumes that the evaluator has had ample opportunity to observe the client in a simulated or real work setting.

The conceptual domain measured by the BWAP includes work skills, habits, attitudes, and personal traits that constitute "vocational competency," a construct of central importance in vocational rehabilitation. The BWAP consists of 63 items that are allocated to four subscales: Work Habits/Attitudes, Interpersonal Relations, Cognitive Skills, and Work Performance Skills. A total score, called Broad Work Adjustment, is also calculated.

Scoring the four subscales is accomplished by summing the raw item ratings. The total score is the sum of the four subscale scores.

Raw scale scores are translated into percentile equivalents, normalized T-scores, and stanines using standardization samples representing four populations of vocational rehabilitation clients: mental retardation, medical disabilities, emotional disturbance, and learning disabilities. All clients in the normative samples had participated in vocational adjustment programs conducted in workshop facilities.

Potential BWAP items were located by reviewing existing work behavior scales and the professional literature on work evaluation of persons with disabilities, supplemented by suggestions given by experienced work evaluators during interviews. The four subscales were constructed by factor analysis of preliminary item pools (principal factor condensation and varimax rotation of four factors retained by the scree criterion).

Three types of reliability evidence are given for the BWAP subscales: internal consistency, rerating by the same evaluator after 2 weeks, and interrater agreement by independent evaluators. The median coefficients for the three kinds of reliability are .87, .86, and .82.

Several kinds of evidence support the validity of the BWAP. The multiple item sources and developmental factor analysis that pertain to content sampling have already been mentioned. The pattern of relationships obtained with the concurrently administered Adaptive Behavior Scale includes high positive correlations with social and vocational competencies and negative correlations with maladaptive behavior indices.

Average BWAP scores for four diagnostic categories of mentally retarded clients (profound, severe, moderate, mild) correspond to the degree of intellectual handicap present. Emotionally disturbed clients scored lower on Interpersonal Relations, a result consistent with the central feature of the disabling condition, that is, difficulty with social and emotional adjustment.

Measured intelligence is highly correlated with the Cognitive Skills subscale. The correlation of .81 approaches the theoretical maximum, reflecting the nature of the Cognitive Skills items (e.g., memory, reading level, problem solving, and job task learning). Hence the Cognitive Skills subscale may be regarded as an index of intellectual functioning. Although the correlations of IQ with Work Performance Skills (.57), Habits/Attitudes (.39), and Interpersonal Relations (.30) are somewhat lower, it is apparent that the BWAP is, in part, measuring intelligence. Readers interested in statistical details and references are referred to Bolton (1991b).

Comments on the BWAP. The BWAP is a comprehensive and easily administered behavior rating instrument. The norm groups are relevant to the purpose of the instrument; the subscale reliabilities are excellent for a rating procedure; and the validity evidence supports the interpretation of the BWAP as a measure of vocational competency. One important type of validity evidence missing is data relating BWAP scores to successful completion of different types of vocational placements.

Rehabilitation Indicators

The Rehabilitation Indicators (RIs; Brown et al., 1980) constitute a comprehensive assessment system for describing the functional capabilities of rehabilitation clients. RIs focus on observable elements of client behavior, using lay terminology to characterize a broad range of content (e.g., vocational, educational, self-care, communication, mobility, household, recreation, and transportation) at varying levels of detail from specific to general.

There are three types of RIs. Status Indicators (SIs) describe categorical statuses or roles that are crucial to clients' functioning. Activity Pattern Indicators (APIs) describe clients' daily living activities in terms of frequency, duration, social interaction, and assistance needed. Skill Indicators (SKIs) describe the behavioral tools that clients need to attain their rehabilitation goals.

The RIs form a standardized procedure for quantifying rehabilitation clients' activities of daily living and their independent living skills. The RIs assessment materials include instrument forms, training manuals, and various supplementary resources. All materials are printed, with "pencil-and-paper" formats; no apparatus or hardware are required.

The RI materials were devised to provide maximum flexibility for users with each component (SIs, APIs, and SKIs) being administrable by interview, by independent observation, or by self-report. Furthermore, the user selects only those items from the SIs and SKIs that are relevant to the purpose for which the RIs are being used. The SIs consist of 48 indicators that represent six role categories; the APIs include 106 items organized into 15 categories of activities; and the SKIs consist of more than 700 skills that represent 78 skill areas organized under 14 categories of functioning.

RIs were developed for the explicit purpose of describing rehabilitation clients' statuses or life roles, daily living activities, and behavioral competencies or skills in ways that are especially helpful in the provision and evaluation of rehabilitation services. Depending on the mode of administration (interview, observation, or self-report), the RIs can be administered in almost any setting, ranging from the examiner's office to the client's home.

Assessment data for the SIs and SKIs are typically reported in a behavioral format, while APIs are usually summarized in a profile. The nature of the SIs virtually precludes any type of data aggregation. The most common application of the SKIs is to diagnose specific skill deficits so that remedial training can be initiated. In contrast, API data are meaningless without the provision of comparative scores across the spectrum of daily activities. Computer programs have been developed for scoring and reporting the SIs, APIs, and SKIs.

Reliability evidence for the RIs is of several types. For example, each of the SIs was refined until across-recorder and test-retest consistency was obtained in 10 out of 10 respondents. Based on a thorough literature review, it was determined that under optimal conditions the reliability of activity clusters and summary scores can be quite high. And, when a data collector interviewed 10 resident staff members, each of whom reported on one client's functioning twice (with a 2-week interval between reports) with respect to 269 SKIs in 18 skill areas, the average test-retest correlation for the 18 skill area scores was .92.

The validity of the SIs was assessed by comparing 100 clients' self-reported SIs with data obtained from available records and significant others: Agreement for all items exceeded 95%. Statistical analyses of API inventory data for 75 spinal cord injured individuals who used wheelchairs as their principal mode of ambulation located numerous within-sample differences that were consistent with clinical experience or commonsense expectations. Likewise, an SKIs validity study that involved comparisons of groups of paraplegic and quadriplegic patients found that paraplegic individuals performed better on all motor skills, whereas there were no differences in skills involving predominantly social judgment and cognitive abilities. Readers interested in statistical details and references are referred to Bolton (1992).

Comments on the RIs. The conceptual foundation of the RIs is excellent and their technical development is outstanding. The RIs provide rehabilitation professionals with a standardized common-language system for assessing clients' daily living activities and independent living skills. The instruments were carefully designed to ensure maximum user flexibility and application in a wide range of settings. The reliability and validity data supporting the RIs are fairly extensive and generally good. Despite the substantial investment of time and resources in the development of the RIs, however, use by practitioners is not commensurate with the instrument's potential to assist service providers in their work with clients with severe disabilities.

Sixteen Personality Factor Questionnaire-Form E

The Sixteen Personality Factor Questionnaire-Form E (16 PF-E; Institute for Personality and Ability Testing, 1985) is a special-purpose personality inventory that was designed for use with persons with limited educational and cultural backgrounds. In particular, it is appropriate for individuals whose reading level is no more than third grade.

As its name indicates, the 16 PF-E measures 16 primary characteristics of the normal personality sphere, such as Outgoing, Assertive, Conscientious, Imaginative, Apprehensive, Self-Sufficient, and Controlled. In addition, five second-order dimensions are also scored: Extraverted, Adjusted, Tough-Minded, Independent, and Disciplined.

Two simplifying features of 16 PF-E are as follows: (a) A forced-choice format is used rather than allowing an "in-between" or "uncertain" response to each item, and (b) all 128 items are phrased as simple questions consisting of two options separated by the conjunction *or.*

Each of the 16 primary scales is represented by eight items. The five secondary scales are scored according to formulas derived from the results of a factor analysis of the protocols of more than 10,000 respondents. Norms are available for a heterogeneous sample of almost 1,000 rehabilitation clients, subdivided by sex and age.

The 16 PF-E rehabilitation client norms are incorporated into a computer-generated report, the Vocational Personality Report (Bolton, 1987b), that provides scores on the five second-order personality scales, two psychopathology dimensions, three vocational interest scales, and Holland's six occupational types.

The 16 PF has been used in at least 20 investigations designed to identify the unique personality traits associated with various types of disability, thus to better understand reactions to disablement (Roessler & Bolton, 1978). Furthermore, several basic psychometric studies of 16 PF-E have been conducted on samples of rehabilitation clients.

Test-retest reliabilities with a 1-week interval averaged .66 (with a range from .43 to .78) for the 16 primary scales and averaged .77 (with a range from .73 to .86) for the five secondary scales (Bolton, in press). Stability coefficients with a 6-year retest interval averaged .45 (with a range from .14 to .80) for the primary scales and averaged .58 (with a range from .40 to .75) for the secondary scales.

Traditional and confirmatory factor analyses at the item, parcel, and scale levels have consistently supported the factorial structure of 16 PF-E with rehabilitation clients (Brookings & Bolton, 1988). In longitudinal follow-up studies, several 16 PF-E scales were predictive of self-evaluated physical and mental health as well as salary level of employed former clients. The 16 PF-E did not, however, predict job satisfaction, job satisfactoriness, or persistence in looking for work (Bolton, 1983). Finally, the 16 PF-E is essentially independent of both self-reported and objective measures of psychopathology (Bolton & Dana, 1988).

Comments on the 16 PF-E. The 16 PF-E measures personality constructs isolated and validated in programmatic research carried out over more than 25 years by Raymond B. Cattell and his colleagues. Hence the validity of the inventory relies on theory and evidence that extend beyond studies with rehabilitation clients. The reliability of the primary scales is lower than desirable but raises the legitimate bandwidth/fidelity dilemma. (This dilemma refers to the measurement in a fixed period of time of either many variables with modest reliability or few variables with high reliability.) With the 16 PF-E, the easiest solution is to focus interpretation on the five secondary scales.

Minnesota Satisfactoriness Scales

The Minnesota Satisfactoriness Scales (MSS; Gibson et al., 1970) is an observer rating instrument that summarizes an employee's level of job performance, as judged by the employer. Use of the MSS presumes a work environment composed of a series of tasks that must be performed and a set of rules that must be followed.

The MSS consists of 28 items that can be completed by the employee's supervisor in about 5 minutes. It is scored on four factor analytically derived subscales (Performance, Conformance, Personal Adjustment, and Dependability) in addition to a total score for general satisfactoriness.

Raw scores for each of the four subscales and general satisfactoriness may be converted to percentile equivalents using normative tables for four occupational groups and a workers-in-general group that is representative of the entire U.S. labor force. Extensive descriptive data for each of the normative samples are provided in the manual.

An especially commendable feature of the MSS scoring procedure is the recommendation that scores be reported as percentile bands rather than point estimates. Standard errors of measurement for each of the five scales are given in the normative tables.

The development of the MSS began with a thorough literature review that suggested several types of information that employers might use to evaluate employee satisfactoriness. The third and current edition of the MSS refined the items, identified the fourth subscale, revised the scoring weights, and expanded the normative groups.

Internal consistency reliabilities for the four subscales and general satisfactoriness for the workers-in-general norm group were .90, .85, .85, .74, and .94, respectively. Corresponding values calculated for 174 former rehabilitation clients were .91, .91, .86, .78, and .95. Test-retest stability coefficients (with a 2-year interval) for a sample of 725 workers were .59, .50, .45, .49, and .59, respectively.

A confirmatory factor analysis of the MSS for the sample of former rehabilitation clients established that the four subscales and the total score are generalizable to the population of workers with severe handicaps to employment. Additional data suggest that the MSS is a valid measure of job satisfactoriness: Satisfactory workers are less likely to leave their jobs than unsatisfactory workers; employee age is meaningfully related to MSS scores; and rated satisfactoriness is virtually independent of measured job satisfaction. Readers interested in statistical details and references are referred to Bolton (1986).

Comments on the MSS. The MSS is a carefully constructed measure of the job satisfactoriness of former rehabilitation clients. The advantage of an occupationally representative norm group is mitigated by its age (more than 20 years). The reliability data, including long-term stability, support the use of the MSS as an outcome assessment. The initial literature search and developmental factor analyses support the content validity, whereas the confirmatory factor analysis and the results of other studies indicate that the MSS measures the construct of job satisfactoriness.

Disability Factor Scales-General

The Disability Factor Scales-General (DFS-G; Siller, 1969b) is a self-report instrument that measures seven replicated components of attitudes toward people with physical disabilities. The DFS-G was developed in conjunction with a research program undertaken for the purpose of investigating the implications of psychoanalytic theory for understanding the nature and origins of attitudinal reactions to people with disabling conditions.

The DFS-G consists of 69 statements that express reactions, describe assumed attributes, or advocate policies toward nine types of disabling conditions: amputation, blindness, deafness, facial scars, epilepsy, cancer, paralysis, spinal deformity, and heart trouble. The disabilities were chosen to represent a wide variety of conditions varying in visibility and seriousness. Respondents indicate their opinions about each statement using a 6-point Likert format ranging from "Strongly Agree" to "Strongly Disagree."

The DFS-G can be appropriately administered in small groups to most adolescents and adults. The instrument is scored objectively by summing the scores for the items composing each attitude component. The seven attitude scales are Interaction

Strain, Rejection of Intimacy, Generalized Rejection, Authoritarian Virtuousness, Inferred Emotional Consequences, Distressed Identification, and Imputed Functional Limitations.

The DFS-G has been used primarily as a research instrument in projects designed to investigate the nature and causes of prejudicial attitudes toward people with physical disabilities. The inventory also has been used in psychoanalytically oriented counseling with clients for whom physical disablement is a threatening issue and as a sensitization device for rehabilitation personnel in training. In addition to assessing prejudicial attitudes held by people without disabilities, the DFS-G can be used in counseling and research applications with persons who have disabilities, serving as a measure of self-esteem or disability acceptance for this population.

All clinical applications have to rely substantially on the analysis of item content, however, because the DFS-G normative data are more than 20 years old. Milestone events in the Disability Rights Movement, including the Rehabilitation Act of 1973 and subsequent reauthorizations culminating in the Americans with Disabilities Act of 1990, as well as renewed activity by disability rights organizations, have most certainly produced significant changes in attitudes toward people with disabilities.

Internal consistency reliabilities for the seven DFS-G scales average .82, with a range from .69 to .89. There are no published retest reliability data for the DFS-G, but retest coefficients for earlier versions of the DFS-G with a 2-week interval averaged .84, with a range from .76 to .89, and, with a 3-month interval averaged .78, with a range from .68 to .87.

The DFS-G was developed through a series of factor analytic studies that initially focused on one disability for each investigation. After a consistent set of attitudinal dimensions emerged repeatedly, the research effort shifted to construction of a general measure of attitudes toward persons with physical disabilities. The final result was the current 69-item DFS-G.

Three independent factor analyses of the DFS-G replicated the seven attitude scales, including an analysis of a Hebrew translation administered to a sample of Israeli students. Other studies have provided support for the theoretical rationale and construct validity of the DFS-G. Readers interested in statistical details and references are referred to Bolton (1991c).

Comments on the DFS-G. The DFS-G is the product of a sophisticated program of research on the nature and determinants of attitudes toward persons with physical disabilities. Unlike many rehabilitation instruments, the development of the DFS-G was embedded in a theoretical framework, in this case, a traditional psychoanalytic perspective. Thus the research produced a meaningful taxonomy of components of attitudinal reactions to disablement as well as a general-purpose instrument for reliably and validly measuring the attitude components identified.

Conclusions About Rehabilitation Instruments

Because the eight instruments reviewed do not constitute a representative sample of rehabilitation assessment measures, it is not possible to frame any conclusions about the psychometric status of the population of rehabilitation instruments. It is, however, entirely reasonable and appropriate to draw conclusions about the "better" assessment instruments—as "better" or "superior" is reflected in the three selection criteria cited earlier. Our evaluation of the psychometric adequacy of the eight instruments follows the characteristics outlined in Table 5.1.

Norms. Although there occasionally is some question concerning the choice of proper norms for interpreting the test performance of examinees with disabilities, the general rule is to use rehabilitation client norms for diagnostic applications and general population norms for decisions about employment in the competitive labor market. The type of normative data available for seven of the eight selected instruments (the RIs do not have norms) conform to the principle that rehabilitation diagnostic instruments should have rehabilitation client norms, with only two instruments, the USES-II and the MSS, having general population norms. The norms for the seven instruments typically are representative of the target population, with demographic descriptions provided, often partitioned on sex, age, disability, and/or employment status, usually sizable and current, and providing one or more types of derived scores.

Reliability. The two basic approaches to estimating instrument reliability involve either a single test administration (internal consistency reliability) or two test administrations (test-retest reliability). Additionally, interrater agreement should be calculated for observer rating instruments. For seven of the eight exemplary rehabilitation instruments, the median internal consistency coefficient was in the low to middle .80s. (The one exception, the 16 PF-E, was designed to have scales with only moderate internal consistency.) The median retest reliabilities for the five instruments with data available range from the high .70s to the low .90s (the 16 PF-E primary scales are excluded). Interrater agreement is very good for the three measures with this form of reliability information. Considering the nature of the subject population, the reliability evidence for these instruments should be regarded as fully satisfactory.

Validity. Four classes of validity evidence may be considered in evaluating assessment instruments: content, concurrent, predictive, and construct evidence. The items constituting the eight rehabilitation instruments were typically derived from multiple sources, including client case files, interviews with practitioners, literature reviews, systematic examination of other instruments, and (in one case) psychoanalytic theory. Concerning the development of subscales, six of the eight instruments are based on factor analyses, whereas the scales of the PDQ and RIs resulted from rational analyses. Concurrent validity data presented include correlations with other tests and analyses of convergent and divergent relationships with aptitude, intelligence, and adaptive behavior measures. Predictive evidence includes correlations with rehabilitation outcomes, such as work status and earnings, and the prediction of graduation from different vocational training areas. Several instruments distinguished between disability groups in expected ways, or were related to independently measured severity of handicap, or identified workers who left their jobs, whereas one instrument correlated with other variables in ways predicted by theory. Finally, the subscale structure of three instruments was verified by confirmatory factor analysis, and another was supported by three independent (traditional) factor analyses. In conclusion, the eight instruments are strongest in the areas of content and construct validity but somewhat weaker in the areas of concurrent and predictive evidence.

Utility. The fourth category for evaluating assessment instruments is the nontechnical characteristic of utility, which refers to the usefulness of assessment data in making decisions about rehabilitation diagnosis and service planning. Six of the eight instruments were developed for the purpose of helping counselors and other rehabilitation practitioners (e.g, vocational evaluators and independent living specialists) to provide optimal services to persons with disabilities. The other two instruments also serve important functions: the MSS generates information about the job performance of former clients and the DFS-G provides a conceptual framework for understanding attitudes toward persons with disabilities. Examples of utility-oriented features of rehabilitation assessment instruments are the comprehensive case planning program based on the FAI that relates functional deficits to needed services, the structured interview administration of the PDQ, which generates both clinical and psychometric data valuable in service planning, and the computer report that translates the 16 PF-E protocols into a series of vocational scales. This review suggests that rehabilitation assessment instruments are designed to benefit persons with disabilities by enhancing the service delivery process.

Summary

In the 40 years since rehabilitation psychology emerged as a recognized specialization in the field of psychology, enormous progress has been made in establishing the theoretical and empirical foundations of the discipline. It is generally acknowledged by authorities in psychology that measurement is the foundation of science and that assessment is the foundation of clinical diagnosis and service planning. Because assessment is the application of measuring instruments to the individual case, it can be argued that a good barometer of progress toward full professional status is the existence of a sophisticated armamentarium of assessment instruments.

In this chapter, we defined rehabilitation assessment instruments as those instruments that measure variables relevant to the unique concerns of people with disabilities. Rehabilitation assessment instruments measure the functional status of people with disabilities in three major areas: vocational, psychosocial, and independent living. Because of the impracticality and limited generalizability of a comprehensive review of all assessment instruments in rehabilitation psychology, we selected eight exemplary instruments, which we described and evaluated according to stipulated criteria.

Our evaluation of the eight exemplary instruments suggested that the following conclusions are warranted: (a) Norms are typically representative of the target population, fully described, usually sizable and current, and providing one or more types of derived scores; (b) internal consistency data, retest reliabilities, and interrater agreement statistics are all satisfactory indicators of the dependability of the scores; (c) validity evidence, including multiple item sources and factor analysis, is strongest in the areas of content and construct validity and somewhat weaker in the areas of concurrent and predictive data; and (d) assessment information generated by the instruments is clearly useful in rehabilitation diagnosis and service planning, thus benefiting persons with disabilities by enhancing the service delivery process.

PART III

Utility and Cost-Effectiveness of Rehabilitation Assessment

CHAPTER 6

Use and Misuse of Assessment in Rehabilitation: Getting Back to the Basics

ROBERT L. GLUECKAUF[1]

During the past two decades, there has been a dramatic increase in the popularity and use of assessment devices in rehabilitation and health. Recent reports of the professional activities of health care specialists (e.g., Hickling, Sison, & Holtz, 1985; Jansen & Fulcher, 1982; Magistro, 1989) have indicated that practitioners currently spend a substantial proportion of their time administering, scoring, and interpreting the results of assessment procedures and tests. At first glance, large investments of professional time and effort in assessment and testing services may suggest a desirable state of affairs. In this era of cost containment, few of us are likely to argue against the need for assessment prior to the administration of expensive treatment. Unfortunately, however, there is little empirical evidence supporting the widespread use of much of what is labeled "assessment" or "functional evaluation" in rehabilitation (Campbell, 1987).

The primary drawback with the majority of these instruments is their failure to meet fundamental scientific standards for utility in clinical practice. To be effective in guiding rehabilitation intervention, assessment techniques should (a) provide an adequate

135

description of "target" behaviors, abilities, and so on of the client and/or significant others; (b) propose an explanation of the factors that influence or control the behaviors of interest; (c) correlate with external criteria that are linked conceptually or empirically to the behaviors of interest; and (d) lead to a specific plan of treatment (see Kanfer & Saslow, 1967; Mischel, 1968; Peterson, 1987). A substantial number of assessment procedures currently employed in rehabilitation do not meet these standards; most do not meet more than one criterion (see Bond & Dietzen, this volume; Campbell, 1987). The most troublesome of these deficiencies is that most rehabilitation assessment procedures do not provide specific guidance in formulating intervention strategies. Despite the high cost to the consumer with a disability and the public at large, we continue to lack basic information about how and under what conditions rehabilitation assessment influences the success of intervention.

The primary objectives of the chapter are to raise several concerns regarding the current use of assessment devices in rehabilitation and to propose new directions for research. The specific issues to be examined are as follows: (a) What are the typical assessment practices of rehabilitation professionals? (b) For what reasons do rehabilitation professionals conduct evaluations? (c) Do rehabilitation professionals know more about assessment than they currently put into practice? In other words, is there a disparity between practitioners' knowledge of appropriate rehabilitation assessment methods and what they currently practice? In examining each of these issues, special emphasis will be given to the identification of barriers that limit the optimal use of assessment methods. Finally, new directions for research on rehabilitation assessment will be suggested, in particular, the author's work on problem-specific family assessment.

Assessment Utilization Patterns in Rehabilitation and Health Care

Although it is standard practice to perform evaluations upon admission to a "rehab" program, during the course of treatment, and at discharge, there is surprisingly little information about the actual assessment utilization patterns of rehabilitation professionals.

What we do know about assessment in rehabilitation comes from a handful of survey studies on practitioners affiliated with large professional organizations and from anecdotal observations. Survey studies typically ask respondents to provide information about the types of assessments and interventions they perform and their reasons for using these procedures. These reports, of course, are prone to a number of biases, particularly social desirability and recency effects. In the absence of more rigorous observational or self-report data (e.g., diary accounts), however, survey studies provide, at least, a "first cut" in depicting the assessment practices of rehabilitation professionals.

In a recent study of the assessment activities of health psychologists (N = 271), Piotrowski and Lubin (1990) found that the MMPI ranked first in popularity among frequently used assessment instruments. Among the 89% of the sample who employed the MMPI, 64%, or 125, incorporated the MMPI 50% or more of the time into routine assessments combined with an unstructured clinical interview. Although the Symptom Checklist-90-R (Derogatis & Cleary, 1977) and the Millon Behavioral Health Inventory (Millon, Green, & Meagher, 1982) were ranked second and third in usage, respectively, both fell far short of the use rates of the MMPI. These findings were consistent with other recent studies of psychological assessment practices in pain clinics (Hickling et al., 1985), Veterans Administration medical centers (Lubin, Larsen, & Matarrazzo, 1984), and pediatric hospitals (Tuma & Pratt, 1982). Thus it appears that psychologists in health care settings predominately use the MMPI and unstructured clinical interviews to assess the psychosocial functioning of clients with physical and mental disabilities.

The popularity of an assessment instrument, however, may not be a good indicator of its appropriateness and utility for clinical practice. A number of studies (e.g., Pincus, Callahan, Bradley, Vaughn, & Wolfe, 1986; Williams, Thompson, Haber, & Raczynski, 1986) have shown that the MMPI yields *false positive* results in chronically disabled populations because it incorrectly identifies disability-related symptoms (e.g., fatigue, irritability) as signs of psychological distress. The low reliability and validity of unstructured clinical interviews are also well known to professional psychologists (Dawes, Faust, & Meehl, 1989; Meehl, 1954). Nonetheless, health and rehabilitation psychologists persist in their use of these assessment procedures.

Unfortunately, research showing low validity and utility has had little impact on assessment practice throughout most quarters of rehabilitation. Physiatrists, nurses, physical therapists (PTs), and occupational therapists (OTs) routinely employ interview procedures and structured tests with limited or unknown predictive validity. For example, physiatrists typically perform mental status exams to assess intellectual functions, such as memory, affect, insight, and numerical ability (Stolov, 1982). Although the protocol for conducting mental status exams has been well established, there is little empirical evidence that the results are either reliable (stable across time) or valid (correlate with other indices of neuropsychological dysfunction). OTs working with individuals who have neurological disabilities (e.g., stroke, multiple sclerosis) are also frequently called upon to assess functional and orientation difficulties. Although, over the past decade, OTs have become routine users of standardized tests, such as the Benton Visual Retention Test (Benton, 1974), it is unclear whether the results of these procedures have increased the validity of their traditional functional assessments or have simply provided the "trappings of scientific rigor" (Haworth & Hollings, 1979).

Reasons for Choosing Assessment Devices

Given that most assessment in rehabilitation rests on shaky scientific grounds, on what basis do practitioners select the tests and procedures they use in daily practice? We will need to rely once again on surveys of the assessment activities of professional psychologists to answer this question. Fee, Elkins, and Boyd (1982) surveyed a random sample of Division 17 (Counseling Psychology) members of the American Psychological Association. Respondents were asked to rate the importance of 10 factors or reasons counseling psychology students should learn testing techniques. The most highly rated reason was the "capacity of psychological tests to reveal information about the personality structure" of clients (p. 110). Other highly rated reasons were these: enhances employability or income, satisfies legal requirements, provides a specialty, saves therapist time, and satisfies institutional demands.

Although counseling psychologists strongly felt that personality tests yielded insights about the personality makeup of clients, the most "highly rated" reasons for encouraging students to learn psychological tests focused on the expectations and demands of the workplace. In essence, respondents indicated that new counseling psychology graduates were less "marketable" if they had limited or no preparation in administering and interpreting standard psychological tests. Increases in behavioral prediction and treatment efficacy were clearly secondary reasons (rated in the bottom third of 10 reasons) for encouraging students to learn psychological tests.

In a recent survey of the Association for Advancement of Behavior Therapy (AABT), Piotrowski and Keller (1984) offered compelling evidence of the preemptive influence of marketplace factors in guiding the assessment practices of psychologists. Despite their familiarity with research showing low predictive validity and clinical utility, 70% of the AABT respondents felt quite favorable toward the use of the MMPI in clinical practice. The authors proposed several reasons so-called objective personality tests were popular among "card-carrying" behavioral therapists: (a) Behavioral clinicians are cognizant of agency and third-party payers (who do not reimburse for the extra time involved in conducting intensive, community-based behavioral assessments); (b) objective personality tests, such as the MMPI and the Millon Clinical Multiaxial Inventory (Millon, 1982), can be used as a quick means of making a diagnosis required by insurance companies for reimbursement; and (c) the recent trend toward computer scoring and interpretation has made the use of personality inventories more appealing despite their numerous shortcomings. Thus factors operating in the psychological marketplace appear to influence assessment practices substantially more than scientific merit and clinical usefulness.

Although the generalizability of psychology-based studies is questionable, it is my opinion that professional identity and "guild" issues largely control the kinds of assessment practices conducted by workers in the field of rehabilitation. There are a number of reasons to support this contention: First, most rehabilitation professionals are not actively encouraged to question the validity and utility of their assessment practices. They are generally not given time to seriously critique their assumptions and to rethink the basis for their clinical measurements. Employers, clinical supervisors, and frontline staff are likely to share a common belief that they are paid to provide a service, not to scrutinize the benefits of assessment and intervention. The latter role is typically assigned to rehabilitation educators and scientists.

Unfortunately, rehabilitation educators and researchers have perpetuated this cycle of ignorance by employing a double standard in training graduate students. On the one hand, we encourage students to critically evaluate rehabilitation principles and concepts in the classroom and laboratory but, on the other hand, we either implicitly or explicitly ask them to suspend their critical thinking skills when they perform assessment and intervention procedures at community practicum or internship sites (see McFall, 1991). To my knowledge, most rehabilitation training programs do not systematically instruct students in how to incorporate theory and research into routine rehabilitation practice. Students are generally left on their own to resolve contradictions in what they have been taught in the classroom and what procedures they are encouraged to perform in practicum and internship settings. In some cases, they may be explicitly told that conformity to the tenets and practices of community-based supervisors is an expectation of the training program. Students quickly learn that disagreements with community supervisors about the usefulness and validity of clinical procedures may reflect negatively on their perceived competence as therapists and jeopardize their status in the program. If these conditions prevail early in the careers of rehabilitation professionals, it is not surprising that passive acceptance of unproven assessment and treatment methods may be the final result.

Second, a substantial proportion of rehabilitation practitioners lack the research skills to adequately evaluate the adequacy and utility of their assessment procedures. Most rehabilitation disciplines (e.g., physical medicine and rehabilitation, OT, and PT) emerged in response to the necessities of treating victims of war and thus did not have a rich research tradition to guide their assessment and treatment practices (Keith, in press). It is only over the past decade or so that research in the allied health disciplines has begun to flourish (Campbell, 1987). Most allied health practitioners currently in the field have not had extensive course work in measurement and research design or conducted independent research. Magistro (1989) indicated that only 50% of physical therapists "claim to have sufficient working knowledge of research design and methods of statistical analysis to critically read and evaluate reports of research . . . published in professional and scientific journals" (p. 525). Thus it would be unrealistic to assume that most rehabilitation therapists would be able to evaluate the adequacy and efficacy of their assessment procedures; nor would they necessarily feel a compelling need to do so. If Ph.D. psychologists who have undergone extensive training in research methods show greater concern for meeting employment expectations than examining the validity and utility of their assessment methods, we cannot reasonably expect rehabilitation nurses, physical therapists, and physiatrists, who have fewer research training requirements, to rigorously uphold the cause of science.

Finally, the mounting drive among rehabilitation disciplines for professional autonomy and independent practice status may further shift attention away from key scientific matters, such as the accuracy and utility of clinical measures, to entrepreneurial concerns, such as market saturation and adequate liability coverage (see Hayes, 1987). As Magistro (1989) has asserted, with direct access to patients (i.e., independent practice), physical therapists will be "infinitely more responsible and accountable for the outcomes of their intervention" (p. 526). The referring physician will no longer be culpable for a client's failure to respond to treatment. This issue would not pose a major dilemma for physical therapists if there were a significant body of scientific knowledge to support the use of common clinical tools such as goniometry, manual muscle testing, and observational gait analysis (Campbell, 1987). Recent studies, however, have found serious problems with the reliability and validity of these procedures (see Rothstein, 1985).

Although we can only make educated guesses about the assessment utilization patterns of most rehabilitation professionals, there is good reason to believe that much of what is being done under the rubric of assessment lacks scientific support. Lister (1987) noted that we cannot take for granted the efficacy of PT measures (e.g., goniometer readings) and assessment forms just because they are used routinely in rehabilitation practice or because their results are documented in medical records. He asserts that our "credibility as professionals mandates that we constantly critique our assumptions" (p. 1829) about the basis of practice and subject our assessment tools to scientific investigation. But how can we make our assessment procedures more rigorous and practical? Are there basic scientific principles we can use to increase the utility of assessment for consumers?

Increasing the Utility of
Rehabilitation Assessment Methods

These and other pertinent assessment questions have been the focus of considerable debate and research in the psychological sciences over the past two decades (Goldfried & Kent, 1972; Kanfer & Saslow, 1967; McFall & McDonel, 1986; Mischel, 1968; Peterson, 1968, 1987). A broad set of standards for improving the quality and rigor of assessment procedures have emerged from this literature and have been summarized recently by the American Psychological Association's Task Force on Standards for Educational and Psychological Tests (1985, 1986). Although questions regarding clinical utility are more circumscribed, they nevertheless have been discussed at considerable length by investigators, such as Mischel (1968), Glaser, Abelson, and Garrison (1983), and Patton (1986). Instead of conducting a cursory review of the main points of these authors, I have opted to intensively examine three key strategies that have been shown to increase clinical utility in previous research. Following this discussion, an example of rehabilitation research linking assessment and treatment will be presented.

In their classic chapter on behavioral diagnosis, Kanfer and Saslow (1967) described two essential requirements of an adequate assessment system. First, they argued that *the constructs of an assessment system should be closely tied to the basic concepts of treatment.* This requirement is particularly important because it suggests that assessment and intervention form a theoretical and empirical whole. The implications of this recommendation are profound: For assessment to be clinically useful, it should have direct theoretical ties to the primary constructs guiding rehabilitation intervention, and, conversely, the utility of intervention depends on the extent to which assessment results are conceptually linked to treatment.

Most rehabilitation assessment practices have only weak theoretical links to intervention. A compelling example of the theoretical schism between assessment and intervention can be found in the domain of neuropsychological rehabilitation. Clinical neuropsychologists typically administer a battery (or a portion of a battery) of structured neuropsychological tests (see Osmon, 1983, for a review) to assess the cognitive impairment of persons with recent traumatic brain injuries (TBI). The results of these tests are then used to formulate recommendations for treatment. As Faust (e.g., Faust, this volume; Faust & Ziskin, 1988) has noted, however, the cognitive and behavioral processes assessed by neuropsychological tests may bear only a weak relationship to the daily activity and community living skills employed by persons with TBI. The memory, organizational, and social judgment problems faced by persons with TBI in the community tend to be more complex and more anxiety provoking and include more interpersonal contact than the cognitive tasks measured in the neuropsychological laboratory. Furthermore, social and architectural barriers (e.g., limited peer support, steep staircases) that may significantly influence performance in work and educational settings are not routinely accounted for in neuropsychological evaluations and therefore limit the utility of treatment recommendations. Thus the lack of formal theory taking into account the impact of situational variables, such as peer support and physical characteristics of the work site, on the implementation of treatment, has severely limited the utility of neuropsychological assessment. A similar theoretical gap between assessment and intervention has been reported in the occupational therapy literature. Bear-Lehman and Abreu (1989) found that increased use of sophisticated technological equipment (e.g., Valpar Work Samples) to measure dexterity and range of motion has had little impact on the treatment interventions selected by occupational therapists. The latter's treatment decisions tend to be guided by clinical intuition and situational factors (e.g., the value coworkers place on the benefits of technology) rather than the increased precision and accuracy afforded by advanced technology.

A second requirement for improving the quality of assessment (Kanfer & Saslow, 1967) is that an *assessment scheme should lead logically to a specific program of treatment.* In other words, the ultimate goal of assessment is to produce specific intervention plans for specific client problems. Note that this conception differs substantially from traditional views of assessment as a systematic collection of information about individual differences in personality, aptitudes, or abilities. As Peterson (1987) and Wax (this volume) have suggested, the nomothetic or individual differences approach to assessment serves the aims of researchers and assessors interested in ordering subjects along a continuum of a particular trait or ability but does not lead to the development of intervention strategies tailored to the specific needs of the consumers. Although professional psychologists have asserted that the results of nomothetic assessment devices, such as the MMPI and Millon Behavioral Health Inventory (Fee et al., 1982; Hickling et al., 1985), are helpful in providing insights into personality dynamics, there is little evidence that clinicians can translate information about personality characteristics into specific and effective programs of behavior change (Peterson, 1987). The schism between assessment and treatment intervention is not only a problem for psychologists, it pervades the practices of many occupational therapists and vocational rehabilitation specialists who rely on test batteries to assess the cognitive skills of neurologically and psychiatrically disabled clients, despite their lack of real-world significance (see Bond & Dietzen, this volume).

Although influential rehabilitation researchers, such as Wilburt Fordyce (e.g., Fordyce, 1976) and Leonard Diller (e.g., Diller, 1987), have spoken to the need to use assessment systems whose results are tied to treatment, the impact of their work has been felt primarily in the areas of psychiatric rehabilitation and special education. Bond and Friedmeyer (1987), for example, have reported that work assessments of persons with severe mental illness performed in conditions closely resembling the actual job environment not only improve prediction of future work performance but also provide useful data on previously unwitnessed social strengths and problem behaviors. Furthermore, once the conditions associated with specific strengths and problem behaviors have been identified, work supervisors can directly test their assessment hypotheses by altering working conditions or prompting effective interpersonal skills and subsequently measuring their effects across time and/or situations.

Finally, one of the most effective methods for ensuring the utility and relevance of rehabilitation assessment is to *involve expert consumers* (e.g., professionals and consumer advocates with disabilities) in the instrument development and evaluation process (see Glueckauf, 1990; Patton, 1986). One of the basic philosophical assumptions of modern rehabilitation practice is that clients or consumers form the "hub of the clinical intervention wheel" (Wright, 1983). All intervention decisions are ideally carried out in consultation with the consumer and tailored to his or her personal needs and characteristics. Consumers, in turn, are responsible for selecting and carrying out rehabilitation goals, providing feedback on the strengths and weaknesses of professional intervention, and, ultimately, judging the efficacy of treatment (Anthony, 1979; Wright, 1983).

Unfortunately, this principle tends to be significantly underutilized by professional staff working in rehabilitation facilities and even more rarely applied in the development and evaluation of rehabilitation assessment instruments. Assessment content and objectives guided by the priorities of expert disabled consumers are not only more likely to be relevant to the concerns of the target population but also more closely associated with pertinent treatment outcomes (see Glueckauf, 1990, for a description of the use of expert consumer panels in rehabilitation research).

Illustrative Example of
Utility-Focused Assessment Research

Despite the promise of utility-focused assessment, there are few examples of rehabilitation research that have been guided by clinical utility principles (e.g., Koren, DeChillo, & Friesen, in press). The majority of these studies are either in the planning or in the early implementation phases and have gathered only initial data. Although it is premature to draw definitive conclusions about the benefits of utility-focused assessment research, a case example will serve to illustrate the distinguishing features of this approach.

Family and Disability Assessment System

Objectives and assumptions. Over the past 3 years, Glueckauf and colleagues (e.g., Glueckauf, 1990; Glueckauf et al., in press) have initiated a series of studies on the Family and Disability Assessment System (FDAS). The specific objectives of the first phase of this ongoing research program were (a) to assess the psychometric adequacy (i.e., intercoder agreement) of the FDAS and (b) to determine whether therapists can systematically use the FDAS in matching specific family problems to specific family interventions. The long-term goal of our research is to develop an assessment system that links the *specific* problems of at-risk adolescents and adults with chronic disabilities and their families to *specific* ameliorative intervention strategies.[2]

Three basic assumptions have guided the development of the FDAS. First, family interactions are reciprocal in nature and are amenable to change by multiple factors both within and outside the family system. We eschew the notion that the problems of persons with chronic disabilities, particularly children and adolescents, are "caused" by poor family upbringing, or, conversely, that the problems of parents (e.g., marital distress) are the result of misbehavior or poor functioning of the person with a disability. Previous research has failed to take into account the reciprocal influences of parenting roles, the actions of community professionals (teachers, physicians), and the behavior problems of children with disabilities (Quittner, Glueckauf, & Jackson, 1990).

Our second major assumption is that the individual with a disability and family members are the "experts" in identifying their own concerns and treatment goals and in setting priorities for intervention (i.e., the order in which specific goals should be addressed). This assumption differentiates the FDAS from other family assessment approaches, which rely heavily on therapist judgment to "decipher" family concerns and to establish therapeutic objectives (e.g., Minuchin's [1978] Structural Family Therapy).

Finally, the FDAS emphasizes the importance of having explicit theoretical linkages between assessment and intervention. Each of the major dimensions of the FDAS (i.e., repetitive behavior patterns, roles, and beliefs and values) represents a major organizing principle "driving" family systems interventions in the field of rehabilitation (see Efron & Glueckauf, 1989).

The FDAS appears to be particularly sensitive to the alterations in roles, beliefs, and behavior patterns that persons with disabilities and their families typically confront. Examples of common disability-related *role* problems assessed by the FDAS include not being able to obtain a driver's license, difficulties finding employment, and lack of available marital partners; examples of common *belief* conflicts include discrepant perceptions about the dangers of sports and differing beliefs about the importance of regularly

TABLE 6.1

Brief Version of Categories of Family Issues

Category	Example
Relationship Issues: Family and Significant Others	1. Lack of closeness among family members or partner, such as family members spending little time together, brothers and sisters ignoring identified client, and concerns about emotional closeness with partner or spouse 2. Concerns about intrusiveness of a family member 3. Sibling problems
Intrapersonal Issues	1. Emotional difficulties (not related to symptoms of illness) such as depression, paranoia, or fear of losing control over life 2. Concerns about self-esteem and body image 3. Lack of direction in life
Psychosocial, Vocational, and Educational Issues	1. Job-related concerns, such as employment concerns or concerns about volunteer work 2. Transportation problems 3. School or educational issues
Issues of Disability, Symptoms, and Medical Concerns for Identified Client	1. Concerns about cause(s) of symptoms or seizures (medical and psychological) 2. Concerns about medical treatment such as medication ineffectiveness, doubts about the effectiveness of medical treatment, or complaints about inconsistency or lack of medical treatment 3. Interactions with health care professionals

taking medications; examples of common *repeating behavior patterns* include dealing with frequent "put-downs" from peers and arguing over restrictions about drinking alcohol (see Table 6.1 for a brief version of the FDAS Categories of Family Issues).

The FDAS not only identifies specific disability-related issues or problems but, more important, matches the specific problems of specific family members to specific intervention strategies. This is a distinct and important feature of the FDAS because therapy has been shown to be more effective when tailored to the specific concerns of individual clients (see Paul, 1987). A description of the "problem-specific matching approach" of the FDAS follows.

Key features of the model. As shown in Table 6.2, the FDAS links the specific problems and concerns of individuals with disabilities and their families to seven categories of family and community functioning. The three primary dimensions of the FDAS and their theoretical origins are (a) *repetitive behaviors* (sequences of behaviors, thoughts, or feelings that occur repeatedly over time) representing the major theoretical focus of brief interactionist therapy and behavioral marital therapy (e.g., Jacobsen & Margolin, 1979; Watzlawick, Weakland, & Fisch, 1974); (b) *roles* (a prescribed set of behaviors that family members are expected to carry out with other persons in the family or in the community) forming the key conceptual focus of structural therapy and family psychoeducational treatment (e.g., McFarlane, 1991; Minuchin, 1978); and (c) *beliefs and values* (beliefs are expectations about how people, interactions, things, or events actually are; values are ideals about how people, interactions, things, or events should or should not be) representing the primary theoretical focus of the systemic school of family therapy (Selvini Palazzoli, Boscolo, Cecchin, & Prata, 1978). The rationale for selecting this combination of dimensions derives from the earlier theoretical work of Efron and Glueckauf (1989), who categorized family systems interactions into three fundamental patterns: habits, structures, and understandings. In the FDAS, these patterns have been relabeled *repetitive behaviors, roles,* and *beliefs and values*.

Assessment using the FDAS is based on an analysis of issues presented by the at-risk person with chronic disability and family members during the course of an initial evaluation interview. The semistructured family interview consists of a series of open-ended questions regarding the nature of each family member's issues. At the beginning of the interview, each family member is asked, in turn, to describe his or her current concerns or problems. The interviewer then pursues a line of questioning focusing on (a) what family members believe "causes" the problem(s), (b) who in the family is most concerned about the

TABLE 6.2
Categories of Family and Community Interaction Patterns

FCIP Categories	*Definitions*
Single category	
1. Repetitive behavior pattern	Sequences of behaviors, thoughts, or feelings occurring repeatedly over time
2. Roles	A prescribed set of behaviors that family members are expected to carry out with other persons in the family or in the community
3. Beliefs/values	Beliefs about the cause and maintenance of family problems; family values (expectations about how family members ideally should behave, feel, or think)
Two categories	
4. Roles-repetitive behaviors	Repeating behaviors that affect family roles
5. Roles-beliefs/values	Individual's beliefs or values about roles
6. Repetitive behaviors-beliefs/values	Evaluation or a judgment about the cause or consequences of a repeating behavior pattern
Three categories	
7. Roles-repetitive behaviors-beliefs/values	Refers to a belief about the way in which repetitive behaviors influence family roles

NOTE: FCIP = family and community interaction patterns.

problem(s), (c) how often the problem occurs, (d) what each family member does when the problem occurs, (e) who is responsible in the family for trying to solve the problem, (f) how the family would change if the problem were resolved, and (g) what the family has already done to try solve the problem.[3]

Family assessment interviews are videotaped and transcribed verbatim. All family issues are content analyzed using a set of coding instructions developed by Glueckauf et al. (in press) and placed into one of seven categories (see Table 6.2). Family issues can convey information linking specific problems to a single category of family and/or community functioning (either roles, repetitive behaviors, or belief/values), two categories (roles-repetitive

behaviors, roles-beliefs/values, or repetitive behaviors-beliefs/
values), or to three categories of family and community functioning (roles-repetitive behaviors-beliefs/values).

For example, the assessment system identifies simple family
processes, such as a *repeating behavior pattern* characterized by
a father "putting down" his daughter when she forgets to take her
antiepilepsy medication. It also identifies more complex combinations of problems (e.g., values-repetitive behaviors), such as a family
value's conflict about a 15-year-old's "right" to choose the person
she is going to date "even if he is uses marijuana" (*repetitive
behaviors*).

As noted previously, a major advantage of the FDAS is its capacity to guide treatment intervention. Table 6.3 provides a brief representation of how the model links assessment to treatment. If the
problem is judged to be a role issue (e.g., loss of a job due to prejudice against multiple sclerosis), then the counselor can suggest
a strategy from an array of interventions proposed by role-oriented,
psychoeducational, or structural family therapy (e.g., taking a
proactive role in educating prospective employers about multiple
sclerosis). If the problem is located in a repetitive behavior pattern
(e.g., frequent arguments between parents and their teenage son
with epilepsy about medication routines), a "pattern-breaking" intervention (e.g., encouraging the teenager to "take charge" of designing a more effective medication schedule acceptable to both
him and his parents) proposed by brief interactionist or cognitive-
behavioral therapy might be suggested. If the issue is judged a belief/
value conflict (e.g., negative self-perceptions due to the slowness
of speech), then the counselor can suggest a belief-oriented intervention proposed by Milan systemic or psychoeducational therapy
(e.g., reframing slowness of speech as a sign of careful delibera-
tion or thoughtfulness).

Of course, this form of matching represents the simplest case.
Matching also can be made between problems located in two or
three categories of family/community functioning (e.g., beliefs-
associated repetitive behavior problems) and combinations of two
or three intervention strategies (e.g., reframing a belief about a
problem combined with prescribing a new behavior pattern).

Preliminary findings. The findings of two early studies on the psychometric adequacy of the FDAS have been promising. The objec-

TABLE 6.3
Brief Overview of Intervention Strategies Linked to Specific Family and
Community Interaction Patterns

Family/Community Interaction Patterns	*Intervention Strategies*
Beliefs/Values	Providing education to introduce new information
	Considering pros and cons of actions
	Positively reframing situations that can be changed
	Embedding new ideas during interview
Roles	Altering existing role patterns during counseling sessions
	Assigning homework in taking on new roles
	Providing new vocational roles
Repetitive Behavior Patterns	Altering ineffective behavior patterns through skills training
	Disrupting ineffective behavior patterns by adding new steps
	Restraining change when benefits of change are unclear

tive of our first study (Glueckauf et al., in press) was to assess intercoder agreement on three primary measures included in the FDAS: (a) the content of family problems (see Table 6.1), (b) the family system or community interaction patterns (FCIP) associated with each issue or problem (see Table 6.2), and (c) the specific family members most concerned about each identified problem.

Thirty persons with neurological disabilities and their families participated in this ongoing reliability investigation. Twenty subjects were diagnosed with epileptic seizure disorders; four had traumatic brain injuries, and six persons were diagnosed with multiple sclerosis.

The overall consistency of FDAS judgments among trained *undergraduate* coders was in the acceptable range for a newly developed assessment instrument. The average proportion of agreement (i.e., number of agreements divided by total agreements and disagreements) for the content of family problems and the family/community interaction patterns was .75 and .51 (average Cohen's kappa = .61 and .23), respectively. The average proportion of agreement and Cohen's kappa for the family members most concerned about specific problems/issues were .82 and .73, respectively. Thus agreement among undergraduate coders was generally high across the FDAS measures. The overall pattern of results suggests that advanced training in family systems therapy may not be necessary for consistent application of FDAS-guided counseling judgments.

Our second investigation is ongoing and focuses on the question of the accuracy in using a brief, "therapist version" of the FDAS. The primary objective of the study is to assess the accuracy (i.e., agreement with criterion) of therapist judgment in "matching" specific family problems to specific family interventions. Graduate student volunteers receive 15 hours of preparatory instruction in the theory and application of the FDAS. Each student views 10 videotaped family assessment sessions, previously conducted by Glueckauf et al. (in press). After viewing each videotape, students are asked to analyze five specific family issues (selected a priori by the investigators) on three dimensions: (a) the degree of disruptiveness of the issue, (b) members in the family/community most concerned about the issue, and (c) the family and community interaction patterns associated with each problem (e.g., role, repetitive behavior pattern). Finally, each student is instructed to formulate specific intervention strategies for each of the five presenting problems. Although the results are only preliminary (n = 3), the average proportion of agreement with criteria (i.e., the investigators' judgments) in matching family systems interventions (e.g., behavioral family therapy, psychoeducation, strategic family therapy) to specific family problems was .83. After only 15 hours of training, students showed a high degree of accuracy in matching theoretically relevant treatment strategies to specific family problems.

In summary, the results of early investigations of the psychometric adequacy of the FDAS have been promising. We believe that the careful construction and strong theoretical foundation of the FDAS bodes well for this measure. Nonetheless, until the appropriate predictive validity and utility studies have been performed, the efficacy of the FDAS remains in question. In the near future, we plan to conduct our first intervention outcome study comparing FDAS "issue-specific" family counseling with a broad-based family psychoeducation approach for at-risk adolescents with epilepsy and their parents.

Conclusions and Recommendations

Although the field of rehabilitation has recently enjoyed unchallenged growth and prosperity, it is essential that we do not become complacent and neglect the painstaking work of scientifically evaluating our assessment methods. We are at a turning point in our evolution, one that may set the stage for further advancement or one that foreshadows the emergence of an entrepreneurial pseudoscience.

There are a number of reasons at this time to be particularly concerned about the status of assessment in rehabilitation. First, despite huge annual expenditures on assessment services for persons with disabilities, there is little empirical evidence supporting the clinical utility of most rehabilitation assessment instruments. As noted previously, rehabilitation researchers have largely neglected to examine the impact of assessment on the selection and outcome of rehabilitation interventions. To be fair, this shortcoming is not unique to our discipline; older and more established disciplines (e.g., public health and clinical psychology) continue to struggle with the same problems. Nonetheless, if our goal is to become an applied science, we must go beyond minimal quality assurance standards (e.g., CARF accreditation) to a full commitment to the spirit and process of scientific evaluation. One simple step in the right direction, for example, would be to routinely give rehabilitation consumers an "assessment report card," that is, a status report on the strengths and limitations of our current assessment practices. This might temporarily diminish our "expert image" but in the long run may engender greater respect for knowledge and scientific integrity among both rehabilitation professionals and consumers.

A second reason for concern lies in the lack of commitment to the basic principles that originally attracted many of us to the field (see Wright, 1983). Most rehabilitation professionals support the notion of facilitating independence and advocating for increased access to community resources; however, only a minority of us directly include the person with disability and his or her family in the assessment phase of rehabilitation (see Vineberg & Willems, 1971). Most assessment procedures, particularly in traditional physical rehabilitation centers, are administered routinely without investigating the consumers' and/or family members' perceptions of the need for and efficacy of the approach. Rehabilitation researchers and educators are equally prone to making the same misjudgments. Most assessment instruments have been developed without the benefit of consultation from consumers. Note, however, that the National Institute on Disability and Rehabilitation Research has recently issued a mandate that all funded research and demonstration projects use consumers from the initial development to the final write-up phase of the evaluation process. This is a welcome event, one that will have a significant impact on teams of vocational and psychosocial rehabilitation researchers and their constituencies. Considerable work will be needed, however, to have such policies adopted at the level of the U.S. Institutes of Health or Health and Welfare Canada.

Finally, it is imperative that we give greater attention to the development of utility-focused rehabilitation theories. Most rehabilitation assessment and intervention research is either atheoretical or rests on broad theoretical assumptions. If we plan to develop interventions that have a significant impact on the psychosocial and physical functioning of persons with disabilities, it is highly desirable to have a guiding conceptual framework that links target events, environments, and/or behaviors to specific treatment modalities. This goal is more likely to be achieved when we use assessments that match specific target behaviors to specific interventions. Using the FDAS as an example, we showed how theory can be used to match specific family interventions to specific family problems. The same logic can be applied to a variety of rehabilitation interventions that involve multiple problems and multiple treatment techniques. New context-specific theories need to be developed and tested, however, before we can meaningfully link specific rehabilitation problems to specific treatment modalities.

Notes

1. I thank Gary Bond, Elizabeth McDonel, and Alexandra Quittner for their useful comments and suggestions in preparing this paper.

2. Individuals with disabilities were considered at risk if they exhibited one or more of the following behaviors: (a) suicidal ideation, (b) social withdrawal, (c) aggressive behavior, (d) persistent depressive symptomatology, (e) poor school or job performance, (f) substance abuse, (g) sexual promiscuity, (h) illegal or antisocial behavior, or (i) lack of compliance with prescribed medication routines.

3. A copy of the semistructured family interview is available on request from Robert L. Glueckauf.

CHAPTER 7

Matchmaking Among Cultures: Disability Culture and the Larger Marketplace

Teena M. Wax

The effectiveness of rehabilitation assessment outcomes for people who have disabilities is likely to be a function of the degree to which these clients/consumers are included as partners in the rehabilitation service process (Healy, 1990), the use of more qualitative assessment techniques (Goldman, 1990), and the accuracy with which perspectives and expectations between rehabilitation service providers and clients are understood and shared (Ju & Thomas, 1987).

To appreciate the changing context in which rehabilitation assessment takes place, this chapter will briefly review the shifts in focus of rehabilitation services as well as describe some characteristics of the current disability constituency or "marketplace." However the context is ultimately defined, the essential ingredient of effective rehabilitation assessment outcome is likely to be determined by the degree of congruence in perspectives and expectations between rehabilitation service providers and clients with disabilities.

Among the issues affecting rehabilitation assessment outcome for clients with disabilities are the underlying values, assumptions, and biases that influence choice of assessment instruments, the type(s) of assessments conducted (e.g., qualitative or quantitative; Goldman, 1990), and results of assessment with respect to planning and implementation. This chapter will suggest a model for understanding the "ethos" of the disability marketplace as a way of improving or enhancing congruence, which in turn should lead to more effective rehabilitation assessment outcomes for this population.

Context of Rehabilitation Services

For the most part, rehabilitation service agencies and providers have been aligned with the majority or "mainstream" culture perspective about people with disabilities (Kirchner, 1984; Stubbins, 1988). Today's rehabilitation services emerged as a humanitarian response to the needs of veterans disabled by war, with a bias emphasizing the virtue of assisting those unable to provide for themselves (Eisenberg, Griggins, & Duval, 1982). Reinforcing this bias was the clinical-pathological approach of the medical model often applied during the rehabilitation process with disabled clients (Stolov & Clowers, 1981). This approach forced rehabilitation providers to diagnose and treat disabilities using assessment tools heavily oriented toward medical concepts and terminology. The "cure" for disablement was successful restoration of the individual through a combined program of medical care and job training or retraining, so the patient/client could return to remunerative employment like other "healthy" individuals.

Until the Rehabilitation Act of 1973 was passed, employers were considered the primary consumers of rehabilitation services, while people with disabilities were con sidered secondary consumers of those services (Colvin, 1983). Before that time, the major focus of rehabilitation agencies was the successful employment of war veterans and other persons with disabilities. Although clients with disabilities were the direct recipients of rehabilitation efforts (e.g., assessment, training, support services), they were seen as an (employable) "product" or "commodity" to be used by the ultimate consumer target, the employer. After the Rehabilitation Act of 1973, with its focus on independent living rather than employability, the target of rehabilitation services shifted from employers to clients themselves and their life-styles (Perlman, 1983). One example of this changing consumer market focus was increased services for clients over 65 to help them function more independently in their own homes. But, while services were now being generated for segments of the population not necessarily seeking employment or who could not be "restored" to employability, these services were also fostering a continued dependency on the rehabilitation system. Many disabled recipients of rehabilitation services also eligible to receive Supplemental Security or Supplemental Security Disability Insurance (SSI, SSDI) had sufficient disincentive to seek employment, especially at the lower levels of training or earnings—where most people with disabilities are concentrated (Asch, 1984). Within this context, rehabilitation assessment tended to proceed with the presumption that people with disabilities are beset by "limitations," and the focus of assessment tended to be on what a person *cannot* or was *unable* to do (i.e., the fundamental negative bias) (Wright & Fletcher, 1982).

Until recent years then, the rehabilitation profession has largely ignored or minimized the sociopolitical aspects of disability status (Eisenberg et al., 1982; Stubbins, 1988). Today's advances in medical technology enable people with disabilities to live longer, healthier, and more productive lives, thus broadening the nature and type of population receiving rehabilitation services. Today's laws, most recently the American with Disabilities Act (P.L. 100-336, July 26, 1990), as well as the growing disability rights movement, have shifted the dynamics of rehabilitation service provision to become more of a political negotiation process over control of resources necessary for a better quality of life. This process could be described as one of "metamorphosis" of the ideology of the relationship between the rehabilitation system and the disability constituency (DeLoach & Greer, 1981).

The Disability Marketplace Context

The 35 million people in the United States with disabilities constitute one of the most diverse and divided minority groups, cutting across ethnic, racial, religious, age, and gender lines, with a range of problems affected by environmental circumstances as well as type and severity of disability (DeLoach & Greer, 1981). Borrowing from Van Fossen's (1988) work on the structural aspects of violence in our culture, it is instructive to consider the cultural context of people with disabilities. There are often substantive differences in the norms, attitudes, and values held by people who do and don't have disabilities. In the "mainstream

TABLE 7.1

Cultural Context of Disability: Norms, Attitudes, Values, and Implications
for Consumer Behavior and Provider Assessment

Culture Criteria	Disability Culture	Mainstream Culture
Norm	Disability	Able-bodiedness
Attitude	Affirmative	Negative
	Inconvenience	Tragedy
	Entitlement	Benevolence
Value	Different	Deviant
Consumer behavior	Impression management	Stigma management
Assessment perspective	Disabled person in disability context	Disabled person in non-disability context
Assessor assumptions	Fundamental positive bias: clinical pathology	Fundamental negative bias: cultural diversity

culture," able-bodiedness is the norm (e.g., hearing and sight within normal range, unassisted ambulation and mobility), whereas, in the "disability culture," the presence of a disability characteristic is a key aspect of identification or affiliation (Table 7.1). Generally speaking, the attitude of this society's able-bodied majority toward those who are different—disabled—tends to be negative, and able-bodied people tend to view disability as a tragedy (Wright, 1983). By contrast, some people with disabilities may consider disability to be an inconvenience to be dealt with while transacting business in the mainstream world, as exemplified by research conducted by Higgins (1980) with deaf people. Because attributes of able-bodiedness (youth, slenderness, and so on) are accorded higher value than those of disability, it follows that, the greater the disability, the more devalued the person and the more negatively viewed by others. While some people who have disabilities tend to regard them as a matter of uniqueness or difference rather than as a tragedy or deviance (Funk, 1987; Griggins, 1982), it must be pointed out that often members of one disability group may share societal attitudes toward members of a disability group different than theirs (e.g., people who are deaf and those who are blind tend to avoid each other; DeLoach & Greer, 1981).

Given a cultural context in which people with disabilities experience continued disadvantages by being regarded as deviant, devalued, and tragic (Asch, 1984; Schneider & Anderson, 1980), they are often faced with the task of stigma management (Table 7.1). Stigma management is the act of mitigating the impact of disability on any interaction with the larger society. Goffman (1963), DeLoach and Greer (1981), and others illustrate how this is effected. They also suggest that the responsibility for initiating this effort at mitigation usually devolves onto the person with disability. By contrast, a person with a disability may choose to embellish its characteristics to create an affiliation with similar others, as anecdotally illustrated by DeLoach and Greer (1981). Higgins (1980) also describes, for example, characteristics of deaf persons that enhance their status in the Deaf Culture, including degree and severity of hearing loss, use of American Sign Language, experience with residential school experience, and even the hearing status of one's parents. As sort of a "flip" side of stigma management, the term *impression management* (Table 7.1) is offered to describe this process of creating or maximizing the impression created by disability characteristics to gain a possible social or economic advantage.

Perhaps the most radical shift in ideology is that being imposed by the growing disability rights constituency. By definition, *constituency* implies the distribution or allocation of societal resources like status or power to particular groups of people (Higgins, 1985; Kirchner, 1984; Stubbins, 1988). By perceiving disability as social or economic disadvantage rather than as a biological or medical failing (Asch, 1984), constituents can adopt an entitlement rather than a beneficiary stance in what Kirchner (1984) proposes to be a "minority activist" market model.

As a result, rehabilitation service providers will be faced with increasing demands for more equal and equitable services. Both rehabilitation researchers and providers are likely to show greater interest in designing and implementing assessment tools that reflect more accurately some of the contextual differences in experience and function of people with disabilities (Goldman, 1990; Healy, 1990; Levine, 1981; Ragosta, 1988).

Rehabilitation Assessment Issues and the Disability Constituency

In a number of respects, the field of rehabilitation has not kept pace with the disability movement (e.g., Johnson, 1987). For example, rehabilitation providers continue to describe people with disabilities as "the handicapped" in many circumstances at a time when such terminology is considered "politically incorrect." A major reason for this continued discrepancy may be perceived or actual incongruence between consumer and provider perspectives about rehabilitation services.

Borrowing from the taxonomy of client satisfaction developed by Winter and Keith (1988), Table 7.2 suggests possible agenda differences between consumers and service providers at different levels of rehabilitation service. Although providers and clients/consumers both appear to be interested in appropriate assessment of the client situation ("diagnosis"; see Table 7.2) and the formulation of a rehabilitation plan or contract, there nevertheless tend to be some differences in emphasis. The client/consumer is interested in diagnosis primarily to the extent that it can be translated into the most expeditious rehabilitation outcome. The provider has relatively more of an interest in creating conformity between the client situation and recognized categories of rehabilitation service plans for proper access to resources for implementation (Higgins, 1985). For example, a client may come in already knowing the specific make or model of a wheelchair he or she needs and be interested only in replacing the existing chair. But the rehabilitation counselor may required to conduct a more comprehensive assessment in conformity with agency policy.

At the program level of analysis, client and provider again share an interest in rehabilitation outcome; however, the client is probably more interested in perceived and actual impact of services on his or her employability or life-style, whereas the provider is often obligated to demonstrate effectiveness of services rendered, as in the number of cases that can be closed to meet agency production levels (Higgins, 1985). In some cases, providers might propose rehabilitation plans that have proven effective in the past, but that may not be suitable for the current client, to respond to administrative pressures. For instance, a rehabilitation counselor might encourage clients to attend a particular college with easier admission policies or more solvent support services whether or not the client finds employment relevant to the obtained degree (Higgins, 1985, p. 116).

From the client perspective, accountability is related both to the client's own efforts during the rehabilitation service process and

TABLE 7.2

Comparison of Perspectives: Rehabilitation Service Provider and Client
With Disability at Different Levels of Analysis

Consumer Perspective	Level of Analysis	Service Perspective
Diagnostic clarification	Clinical	Diagnostic classification
Plan/contract (outcome)		Plan/contract (process)
Effectiveness: improved life-style	Program	Effectiveness: caseload management
Perceived effort on client behalf	Accountability	Justify existence of program/service
Process/progress	Administration	Efficiency
Benefit (to life-style): immediate or long term	(Pure) Research	Professionalism
		Increased knowledge
		Increased application
		Increased efficacy

to expectations about desired results. From the provider's point of view, accountability is often related to justification of program or service existence through judicious dispensation and use of resources (Table 7.2). Kirchner (1984) summarized a number of studies indicating the pertinence of status characteristics of people with disabilities in determining whether or not they are accepted for rehabilitation services or benefits. In some cases, "high status" (e.g., more employable) clients were accepted more readily because relatively more of these clients need relatively fewer resources to achieve rehabilitation goal criteria for both client and agency (Higgins, 1985). In other cases, more complex clients were accepted more readily for services, and the differences in caseload assignment decisions appeared to be related to whether the agency goals were relatively more "utilitarian" (in the former instances) or "humanitarian" (in the latter instances).

The cost of services is also a shared concern of provider and consumer. Consumers are probably more interested in *benefit,* in terms of how accessible the offered resources are, the investment of client's own time and resources, and the degree to which there will be follow-up or continuity of support (Winter & Keith, 1988). Administrators, on the other hand, have relatively more concern for *efficiency* or *effectiveness* (Higgins, 1985), and the determinations of cost-benefit and of cost-effectiveness may not converge for clients/consumers and providers/administrators, respectively. For example, if a blind client and a sighted client with another disability are both considered eligible for a particular training program, but the blind client requires the services of a note taker and/or mobility guide to attend the program, the rehabilitation provider may feel more reluctant to allocate the funds for the blind client's program and may perhaps refer the client to a more accessible but less beneficial program.

Finally, although consumer and provider can agree on the necessity or value of research for enhancing knowledge about and application of rehabilitation service, the goals of research may differ for the two groups. Clients are probably more interested in applied research for its immediate and long-term benefits; in some cases, clients can be cooperative about pure research activities if convinced of some "trade-off" for themselves in enhanced or sustained quality of service or outcome. Although motivated by the welfare of clients, provider-researchers are sometimes diverted into avenues of inquiry that may end up having little or no benefit for rehabilitation due to funding availability or preestablished research agendas. The continuing negotiations between disability and rehabilitation groups (e.g., Council of Organizational Representatives—COR) and various federal research agencies (such as the National Institute on Disability and Rehabilitation Research—NIDRR—and the National Institute on Deafness and Communication Disorders) demonstrate the struggle to reconcile differing research priorities between researchers and relevant consumers (COR, 1989-1990; National Strategic Research Plan Task Force, 1989).

Because familiarity with particular disabilities varies so widely between consumers and rehabilitation providers, the aforementioned discrepancies have significant implications for the assessment process. Rehabilitation providers having little or no actual experience with daily or practical aspects of disability may carry assumptions or prognoses that minimize client credibility as sapient agents of their own interests (DeLoach & Greer, 1981; Healy, 1990; Rosenthal, 1963). Required steps in the process of assessment may be redundant or tedious for clients. If a client has received a diagnosis of multiple sclerosis (usually arrived at after months or even years of visits to doctors) or has a lifelong hearing loss, then being required to submit to yet another medical or audiological examination to satisfy the rehabilitation assessment process may be not only unnecessary but also insulting to the client's credibility (DeLoach & Greer, 1981).

A service provider's choice of assessment instruments may be inappropriate because of underlying cultural or language assumptions of the tests selected. For example, some tests administered to deaf people can yield misleading interpretations, because of the discrepant use of the English language or because of upbringing in the different culture of the residential school (Stewart, 1986; Zieziula, 1983). "Context-free" assessment instruments tend to force clients to look within themselves, usually for possible obstacles to employment (Healy, 1990). Context-based or observational assessment tools take into account specific resources in the employment environment that may contribute to the client's function (Goldman, 1990), perhaps even by revealing novel or idiosyncratic, but effective, strategies. As Wright and Fletcher (1982), Healy (1990), and Goldman (1990) have illustrated, a simple change in the language of assessment tools from a "limitation" to a "potential" perspective elicits very different responses from prospective clients, leading to very different rehabilitation strategies. For example, in a 300-item instrument used to assess the adjustment to disability, most items referred to negative consequences attributable to the dis- ability and few referred to positive consequences (Weinberg & Williams, 1978). Even the very titles of some instruments reflect this negative bias: The Acceptance of Disability Scale, the Handicaps Problems Inventory, and the Disability Factor Scales are al- ready slanted toward difficulties, obstacles, and limitations (Bolton, 1985a).

Bowe (1980) has suggested that these assessment tools may maintain people with disabilities in a dependent or depressed status and also maintain the status quo of uneven distribution of power. Other examples of biases that can affect assessment include overemphasizing the effects of disability on psychological or physical functioning, misinterpreting "normal" behavior of people with disabilities, stereotyping, and underestimating assets or potentials of people with disabilities (DeLoach & Greer, 1981). To illustrate, if a person is asked how being in a wheelchair is an obstacle to employment, that person is likely to respond with the myriad problems of gaining access to particular buildings, and the provider will probably mull over strategies for overcoming employer resistance or justifying funds for accommodations. But, if that same person were asked for examples about effective functioning in a wheelchair, one may discover more creative solutions. Such solutions could range from the client's having negotiated for a different job in a more accessible building to bartering with fellow employees for assistance in getting around a building or office. Finding out that a wheelchair user is an excellent cook and brings in goodies several times a week in exchange for assistance in getting around presents a more uplifting, interesting, and possibly more cost-effective scenario for rehabilitation!

While, in some cases, quality of services may suffer because providers have used inappropriate assessment instruments for clients with particular disabilities, making "reasonable accommodations" in the assessment process can yield more accurate results (Ragosta, 1988). Unfortunately, clients who assert their needs for these reasonable accommodations or who challenge the appropriateness of providers' assessment procedures may still run the risk of alienating those providers and diminishing their chances for appropriate services (Calkins, 1988). Yet the assessment process must accommodate input from the client/consumer rather than the reverse of having that input accommodate the assessment process.

Consistent with this viewpoint, Goldman (1990) has proposed the development of qualitative assessment methods to supplement to standardized instruments. Qualitative assessment is appropriate, according to Goldman (1990), when tests contain biases that disadvantage certain subgroups, for example, those related to client characteristics such as gender, age, ethnicity, and disability. The qualitative approach is closely related to the clinical approach to assessment, as opposed to the actuarial approach (Lanyon & Goodstein, 1982). Although the evidence favoring actuarial over clinical approaches is overwhelming (Dawes, Faust, & Meehl, 1989), it is nonetheless true that standardized tests developed for one population are not necessarily valid in a different population. To illustrate Goldman's (1990) point, the Independent Living Behavior Checklist (Walls, Zane, & Thvedt, 1979) may indeed yield reliable and valid indications of functioning for many individuals. If a person has not faced certain situations, or has used different approaches than that offered by the instrument, however, his or her score may be skewed—unless compensatory information is obtained by a discerning practitioner through qualitative assessment. In a similar vein, Lanyon and Goodstein (1982) argue that validity of rehabilitation assessment depends on practitioner knowledge of behavioral signs associated with particular disabilities. Despite the plausibility of their arguments, however, proponents of qualitative assessments have not produced any empirical studies supporting their claims.

Rehabilitation providers tend to be more concerned with concrete results in employability or independent living (Brown, Gordon, & Diller, 1983) than with what might be described as intermediary results, such as an appropriate match between technology and person with disability or one's attitude toward oneself or one's disability. It is important to ascertain not only what a client *can* do but also what she or he *does* do. For example, a person with paraplegia can get from one place to another, but how is it done? The fact that one uses crutches, a wheelchair, braces, or physical assistants may make a difference in rehabilitation planning. A hearing impaired person can "use" the telephone but may choose to do so with a TDD (telecommunications device for the deaf), an operator relay service, an amplifier on the phone, or a sign language interpreter. More pertinent, it is important to respect client preferences for one or more methods over others and to incorporate those preferences in the selection and implementation of assessment tools. In other words, it is important to achieve, as much as possible, congruence between the provider and client.

Ethos of the Disability Marketplace:
Creating Congruence

For the assessment process to become more effective, rehabilitation providers need to become more attuned to the psychosocial "stance" being assumed by the consumer/client (see Table 7.3). Clients with disabilities who identify themselves as being from a separate group and consider themselves affiliated with a disability culture (segregationist stance; Meyerson, 1955) may require a different assessment approach than clients who consider themselves to be unique individuals within the mainstream society (assimilationist stance; Meyerson, 1955). The same holds true for those clients who affiliate both with a separate disability culture and with the mainstream (bicultural stance; Meyerson, 1955) and those who are not yet affiliated (marginal stance; Glickman, 1986).

TABLE 7.3
Ethos of the Disability Marketplace

| | Consumer Adaptive Perspective | | | |
	Segregation	*Assimilation*	*Bicultural*	*Marginal*
Cultural perspective	Conflict of values	Congruence of values	Selective congruence of values	Uncertain or unclear values
Predicted consumer behavior	Refusal or rejection	Acceptance or compliance	Idiographic	Reluctance or resistance
Suggested assessment strategy	Cross-cultural	Traditional	Eclectic	Broad spectrum

Table 7.3 is proposed as a framework for identifying interrelationships among several consumer characteristics that may affect "market strategies" (approaches to assessment) possibly adopted by rehabilitation professionals.[1] Although these are by no means static categorizations, it is possible to identify four major styles of adaptation[2] adopted by people with disabilities, which in turn reflect particular cultural or value orientations. Glickman (1986) illustrates how culturally deaf (Deaf)[3] individuals may consider themselves part of an "ethnic minority" group with different norms, attitudes, and values. Some Deaf individuals are not interested in some of the audiological technology available to hearing impaired people. The availability of cochlear implants is a paradoxical benefit, in that, although the very treatment—as with other types of "restorative" surgery—has a positive outcome for some individuals, it also communicates a message that one is not acceptable the way one is. Some individuals who use well-designed wheelchairs find them technologically more liberating than the use of braces, canes, or walkers. Some individuals may prefer the cosmetic appeal of a prosthetic hand over the superior functional capacity of a metallic hook prosthetic.

In these cases, there may be a conflict of values (Table 7.3) between a rehabilitation provider and consumer with disability, because many providers routinely offer hearing aids to deaf people or seek medical/prosthetic assistance for those with physical disabilities presumably to help these individuals conform more closely to nondisabled standards. Another value conflict in rehabilitation assessment/planning may be about how clients wish to expend energy in the rehabilitation process. For instance, given a choice between auditory (e.g., hearing aid training and speech training) rehabilitation and attending a specific occupational training program accompanied by a sign language interpreter, some deaf clients may opt for the latter, possibly more expensive choice as fitting in better with their long-range rehabilitation goals.

Still another conflict between provider and client may arise about rehabilitation outcomes. Most providers still assume that clients wish to be rehabilitated or "restored" to functioning in the mainstream society, whereas some clients are interested in better functioning within the minority group. For example, some people who are blind are interested in social skills training, not so much for interacting with sighted people but for having a better social image in the community of blind people. A client in a wheelchair may be more interested in one that will facilitate participation in wheelchair basketball. From the ethical point of view, rehabilitation providers need to respect the integrity of the person who has a disability, and in some cases that will mean dispensing with the medical or prosthetic emphasis in rehabilitation assessment or planning. Wright (1988) has helped formulate guidelines for "nonhandicapping" language for possible adoption by the American Psychological Association; these guidelines shift focus from the disability to the person, for whom one characteristic is a disability. Rehabilitation service providers might find this focus more ethically sound in terms of assessment and planning practices. Unless providers are prepared to understand this context in which a number of their clients appear, they are likely to find that clients will refuse or reject the services being offered (Table 7.3).

A stronger congruence of values may be found between traditional rehabilitation services and people who consider themselves part of the mainstream of society or who wish to be. Typically, these individuals have acquired disabilities later in life or have disabilities that have been managed with minimal visibility or disruption in the world of nondisabled people. People who become deaf later in life, particularly those who have relied heavily on hearing for their occupations or activities, are likely to be more receptive to auditory technology and rehabilitation efforts and will also accept the necessary assessment procedures to access those services as well, in an attempt to regain or restore hearing sufficient for participation in mainstream activities (Kyle, 1987; Orlans, 1985). The concept of "normalization," a popular concept in rehabilitation services, has been used to describe the process for clients who are interested in establishing, reestablishing, or maintaining characteristics and behaviors as close as possible to the norms of mainstream society (Wolfensberger, 1972). Still another way in which congruence between provider and client/consumer can be achieved is in cases where agreement can be made about the nature and extent of reasonable accommodations needed to maintain a client's life-style (U.S. Commission on Civil Rights, 1983).

Rehabilitation providers meeting clients who might be considered "bicultural" need to recognize the skills of these clients that enable them to move between or among several cultures (e.g., Grosjean, 1982). These individuals will tend to be interested in selected aspects of rehabilitation services and not in others. Consequently, rehabilitation assessment and planning will tend to have a highly individualized nature with these clients (see Table 7.3). Eclectic approaches will probably be most effective with this group and be relatively more task oriented. In other instances, some of these individuals may be recognized leaders of their disability community and also be quite adept at securing rehabilitation services because of their knowledge of the system's parameters for such services. Some of these individuals can also become advocates or liaisons for other members of their community to help them secure appropriate services as well (Wax, 1990).

Finally, there is a group of clients/prospective consumers who tend to be largely invisible to the rehabilitation system because they maintain what might be described as a "marginal" status (Table 7.3), not really assimilated into the mainstream culture and not really part of any disability minority culture. Typically, individuals in this situation tend to withdraw from either world and may not be noticeable to the rehabilitation service community until brought in by a relative or other professional. One example of this kind of client is the suddenly disabled person who may need immediate medical attention and a significant amount of time to adapt to a new physical reality before considering the wider social aspects of this change in status. Because these clients tend to be unclear about how to identify themselves ("unclear values"; Table 7.3), rehabilitation providers may have to develop rather creative approaches toward assessment and planning with them. To illustrate, if a 70-year-old man becomes hearing impaired later in life—after a lifetime and life-style in the mainstream (hearing) world, such a person is faced with adjustment not only to the aging process and concomitant changes but also to committing himself to a program of auditory and perhaps social rehabilitation (Luey, 1980). Social rehabilitation efforts require some decisions about whether to reassimilate into the hearing world with appropriate assistive devices or to become involved with the deaf community, requiring learning sign language, use of interpreters, and learning the mores of the Deaf Culture. The demands involved in each kind of decision can make for a reluctant or resistant consumer of rehabilitation services if the provider does not take into consideration the amount of extra psychological support such a person may need. The assessment process itself is likely to feel overwhelming to this kind of individual and so may require more time and more sessions to accomplish successfully. Accommodations may also have to be made in the assessment instruments and procedures themselves to be accessible to some of these clients. These clients may require a more "broad spectrum" approach (Table 7.3) in that assessment and rehabilitation will be more rapport building, process oriented, and comprehensive in scope and may require more time and resources to complete, as opposed to the more situation-specific, problem-solving, task-oriented eclectic strategies proposed with bicultural clients.

Assessment Matchmaking: Creating Congruence

If the process of rehabilitation is to move closer to a partnership model of transaction between provider and consumer/client, the responsibility for making such a model effective must be shared by the involved participants.

In some significant ways, consumers with disabilities must follow the examples of the civil rights and feminism movements in wresting a more equitable share of access to rehabilitation resources. In the nature of things, power is not normally given to but is taken by those who also want or need it (Lerner, 1986). Individuals with disabilities must become informed about the types of power available to them, such as "purchase power," the power of judiciously used media, and coalitioning power (Bruck, 1978; Gartner & Joe, 1987). Presumably, individuals with disabilities are also the major source of expertise about living with those disabilities in the various contexts of their lives; they must make this information known to service providers in an assertive if not aggressive[4] manner. To illustrate, an assertive client may "educate" a provider about the impact of particular assessment techniques or questions and/or "negotiate" accommodations in the assessment process. Such a client may be able to talk a provider into accepting the most recent medical evaluation of a condition from an "outside" doctor rather than submitting to yet another examination using the provider's referral. An aggressive client might threaten to sue if a provider appears or acts insensitive to that client's rights or dignity or perhaps might manipulate the assessment process toward a desired goal by providing responses ascertained to be what the assessor expects or needs to hear.

It is worth repeating that rehabilitation providers must first understand the values underlying their work. More to the point, there is a need to change what Wright (1988) calls "fundamental affective bias" toward disabilities from the negative to the positive, for a more constructive conceptualization. Because of the pervasiveness of prejudice and discrimination against people with disabilities, rehabilitation service providers have a special obligation to become aware of the insidious ways in which this bias manifests itself and to take steps to correct them. As a rehabilitation professional herself, Wright (1983) offers examples of "corrective" beliefs and principles that can enhance the effectiveness of rehabilitation services to consumers with disabilities. Among them are the need to keep at the forefront the fundamental rights of people with disabilities to be full partners in the rehabilitation effort, to have substantive control of decisions about their assessment and planning, and to be participating citizens in the general life of their communities.

In a number of ways, the culture(s) of people with disabilities differ(s) from the mainstream culture of nondisabled people to the extent that knowledge and skill in cross-cultural assessment and counseling practices are desirable, perhaps even required, for the provider. Cross-cultural assessment takes into account similarities and differences in individual psychological functioning in various cultures and ethnic groups (Kagitcibasi & Berry, 1989). To illustrate, many deaf children were sent away to boarding schools (state schools for the deaf) and thus ended up with a "bicultural" experience in which faculty, staff, and other students at the school became a second family for the deaf children (Higgins, 1980). Many deaf people feel closer kinship with this "family" than with their families of origin, often because so much time during developmental years is spent at the school and because of differing language and communication structures. A rehabilitation provider conducting an assessment may assume that a deaf person's lack of involvement or noncommittal response when asked about family support indicates a deficit in that area and probably would not consider inquiring about the support network from school—if that provider were unfamiliar with the Deaf Culture (Glickman, 1986). A similar situation may exist for blind people who spend some years in residential schools for blind people. Without that knowledge, this assessment is already biased against the deaf or blind person and may also lead to a more negative "diagnosis" and more treatment, such as (unnecessary) mental health services.

It is incumbent upon the rehabilitation provider to become familiar with the constituency being served. Often, educational training and professional, development workshops are not enough, especially when different means of communicating or conducting activities are involved. It is suggested that rehabilitation providers commit themselves to personal participation in social or community activities where people with disabilities are involved (as opposed to being "five o'clock professionals"; DeLoach & Greer, 1981). Also helpful would be immersion-style internships or post-doctoral training experiences in settings where the primary service population consists of people with disabilities. The operative factor is exposure to people with disabilities who are not only clients or patients but also actively functioning, well-adjusted, and contributing members of the community, to establish for trainees the "fundamental positive bias" of people with disabilities (Wright, 1988) and for them to become familiar with everyday functioning with particular disabilities.

Such training experiences can contribute greatly to increased accuracy during the assessment process (Ju & Thomas, 1987). One example of rehabilitation research that led to the formulation of more accurate assessment techniques involved the question of patterns of use of assistive technology. Because of the proliferation of both educational and assistive technology resources, Scherer and McKee (1989) examined factors that affected the extent to which different people with disabilities would use, or resist using, these resources. Using intensive interview techniques with people from different disability groups, Scherer (1989) and Scherer and McKee (1989) found that characteristics of the disability, characteristics of the person, and psychosocial characteristics all contributed significantly to whether or not an individual would be a technology user or nonuser. Consequently, they developed two instruments—the Assistive Technology Device Predisposition Assessment (ATDPA; Scherer & McKee, 1989) and the Educational Technology Predisposition Assessment (ETPA; Scherer, McKee, & Young, 1990). While these instruments are undergoing evaluation through studies across the country, the focus of this research is to develop mechanisms of early identification of potential mismatches between persons with disabilities with technological resources.

In this way, the incidence of inappropriate use or nonuse of available technological resources can be minimized. Put another way, the focus of this research is to maximize the accuracy of assessment of people with disabilities with respect to technology use, relying on the information and "expertise" of the prospective consumers themselves.

This kind of research confirms the need for rehabilitation providers to accept the shift of power and resources involved in moving to more of a partnership model with consumers. As DeLoach and Greer (1981) suggest, providers need to be more open to criticism, be able to assess the validity of that criticism, and be more willing to negotiate directly with consumers. Feedback from consumers cannot be discounted, even though many do not have formal knowledge of the rehabilitation process: They are experts about the reality of their own life experiences with disability.

Concluding Remarks

Understanding and achieving congruence with the consumer perspective is an essential component of conducting an accurate and effective rehabilitation assessment process. Both rehabilitation provider and consumers with disability alike share some responsibilities toward achieving that goal. With current legislation and policies protecting the rights of people with disabilities now in place and about to be implemented in the foreseeable future, the need for equal and effective partnership between provider and consumer has never been greater or more desirable.

Notes

1. Underlying the constructs presented in Table 7.3 is a fundamental obligation to respect the integrity, dignity, and rights of consumers with disabilities. For example, the right to self-determination underscores the ethical principle of autonomy; included also are the right to privacy and the right to "folly" (the right to make decisions contrary to recommendations of providers; Beachamp & Childress, 1979).

2. Formulations of these styles of adaptation of people with disabilities are borrowed from the earlier work of Meyerson (1955), which was also later modified by Higgins (1980) and Glickman (1986).

3. Approximately 2 million people are identified as culturally deaf ("Deaf," spelled with a capital D), and many of these individuals consider the use of hearing aids as "antithetical" to the Deaf Culture, where the use of American Sign Language is the primary means of communication. People who are part of the deaf community but not culturally deaf are identified as "deaf" without the capital "D" (Padden, 1980; Vernon & Andrews, 1989).

4. Studies have been conducted comparing sex and disability role stereotypes with respect to behaviors and characteristics. For example, what may be considered "assertive" behavior in men may be considered "aggressive" in women (Broverman, Broverman, Clarkson, & Rosenkranz, 1972; Vash, 1982). In other studies, characteristics considered unpleasant or impolite may in fact be desirable or necessary in certain contexts (e.g., Sussman, 1986).

CHAPTER 8

Issues in Evaluating the Cost-Effectiveness of Neuropsychological Assessments in Rehabilitation Settings

ALFRED W. KASZNIAK
JENNIFER J. BORTZ

Within the interdisciplinary team approach to rehabilitation, a major role of the rehabilitation psychologist is in assessment of the cognitive and emotional status of rehabilitation candidates. In principle, such assessments help to establish intervention goals and provide a baseline against which a patient's future abilities may be compared (Kemp, 1985). Increasingly, neuropsychological assessment has come to play an important part in rehabilitation assessment, particularly within neurorehabilitation settings (Alfano & Finlayson, 1987). As concluded by Cope (1982), commenting on the Santa Clara Valley Medical Center Head Injury Rehabilitation Project, "The psychological distress of patients and families is significantly more limiting than the physical" (p. 8). Indeed, among rehabilitation programs geared toward patients who have suffered head injury, stroke, or other disabling neurological illness, neuropsychological assessment has come to be considered a necessary component (Alfano & Finlayson, 1987; Caplan, 1982; Christensen, 1989; Lezak, 1987; Prigatano et al., 1983). Lezak (1987, p. 43) has recommended that "the seemingly infinite variations in deficit patterns between patients, even when the underlying neuropathological condition appears to be quite similar, requires that each patient-candidate for rehabilitation be given a thoroughgoing neuropsychological evaluation if treatment planning is to be appropriate for the patient's needs, strengths, and limitations."

Clinical neuropsychology has traditionally been viewed as primarily concerned with neurological diagnosis, having been developed in neurology and neurosurgery settings, where identification of pathology is the focus (Diller, 1987; Lezak, 1983). Recently, however, a number of factors have converged to result in the field of clinical neuropsychology becoming more concerned with prognosis, rehabilitation, and patient care (Costa, 1983; Kreutzer, Leininger, & Harris, 1990; Rourke, 1982; Tupper & Cicerone, 1990a). Among these factors has been the increased awareness of the large numbers of individuals who are disabled by head trauma (Bryden, 1989; Levin, Benton, & Grossman, 1982), stroke (Foulkes, Wolf, Price, Mohr, & Hier, 1988; Gresham et al., 1975), and other neurological disorders. Medical advances in diagnostic techniques and emergency trauma care, coupled with population growth, have resulted in increasing numbers of individuals disabled by brain trauma (Klauber, Marshall, Toole, Knowlton, & Bowers, 1985). Of an estimated 500,000 head injuries per year, 100,000 die, 50,000 to 100,000 survive with severe impairments that prevent independent living, and more than 200,000 suffer continuing problems that interfere with daily living skills (Kalsbeek, McLaurin, Harris, & Miller, 1980). Similarly, although stroke mortality rate has been declining since the turn of the century (Whisnat, 1984), increased life expectancy over the past several decades has resulted in an overall increase in years of disability from stroke and other chronic diseases (McKinlay, McKinlay, & Beaglehole, 1989). These trends have been accompanied by an increased public demand for treatment of persons disabled by neurological trauma or disease and a resultant increase in the number of facilities specializing in neurorehabilitation (Diller, 1987; Trexler, 1987). Further fueling the interest of clinical neuropsychologists in rehabilitation assessment has been the advent of computerized neuroradiologic procedures that have reduced the need for neuropsychological assistance in the detection of brain damage and lesion localization (Diller, 1987; Wedding & Gudeman, 1980).

Trexler (1987) notes that neuropsychological assessment in rehabilitation serves four different purposes: (a) establishment of the existence of cognitive deficits, (b) establishment of the relative magnitude of insult, (c) estimation of the patient's ability to return to his or her previous life-style, and (d) suggestion of remediation programs. Alfano and Finlayson (1987) add the caution: "It is imperative that neuropsychological assessment identify not only the precise nature and extent of an individual patient's deficits, but that it also delineate areas of relative (residual) strength that might be capitalized on in the rehabilitation setting" (p. 107).

The questions to be addressed within this chapter are: (a) To what extent does the effectiveness of neuropsychological assessment justify its cost within the rehabilitation enterprise? and (b) What approach to, and application of, neuropsychological assessment is most effective at the least cost? In other words, is neuropsychological assessment in rehabilitation cost effective? As will be seen, a clear answer to these questions is not possible on the basis of the available data. A major goal of this chapter is therefore a delineation of issues that must be considered to address these questions adequately in the future. The following section begins with an overview of theoretical issues in cost-effectiveness and benefit-cost analyses, defining necessary terminology and examining how relevant constructs might be implemented to address the questions at hand. This introduction is followed by a review of available research that forms a partial data base of information that will be necessary to determine the cost-effectiveness of neuropsycho-logical assessment.

An Overview of Theoretical Issues in Benefit-Cost and Cost-Effectiveness Analyses

In economics, cost is the difference in monetary return "between the use of a scarce resource in one way and its use in a promising alternative" (Johnston, 1987). Costs are not the same as charges. Costs can be assessed by defining variables that characterize different resources consumed in delivery of a service and then by determining the values for those variables (Yates, 1985). There is a need to distinguish between *accounted costs* and broader *social costs*. Accounted costs include both direct and indirect costs. *Direct costs* include costs for personnel, facilities, operations, and so on that are specific to the cost objective. *Indirect costs* are those due to a variety of causes, often related to more than one cost objective (Johnston, 1987; Johnston & Keith, 1983). *Social costs* refers to the value of all of the resources (both monetary and otherwise) used in delivering a benefit (Yates, 1985). Included within social costs is the *opportunity value* or *cost*, which refers to how much resources would have been worth if they would have been put to the best alternative use (Thompson, 1980). In computing costs, it is also necessary to consider the concept of *discounting to present value*. Because a dollar in the future is generally not worth as much as a dollar now, the value of future monetary loss or gain must be reduced by a certain percentage for each future year (Johnston, 1987). This percentage is referred to as the *discount rate*.

Different interest groups typically have different perspectives on how cost variables are to be defined and on the importance of different cost variables. It is not unusual for these different perspectives to result in conflicting cost estimates (Yates, 1985), and the perspective of the individual analyzing costs must therefore be considered (Fischhoff, 1977). Yates (1985) distinguishes between operations, societal, and client perspectives. The *operations perspective* focuses upon those costs typically listed in accounting ledgers (e.g., materials, equipment, personnel, and facilities). Although the operations perspective employs readily accessible information in assessing costs, the resulting estimates may be incomplete. For example, hidden costs might include donated equipment and materials, facilities for which the program does not pay, and volunteers' time. The *societal perspective* attempts to more accurately measure the value of all resources used in delivering a service. Thus, within the societal perspective, the opportunity value of resources consumed would be considered. For example, the value of a volunteer's time might be estimated by determining what benefits might have been derived from investment of that time in some other activity. The *client perspective* includes consideration of both the money that the client pays for a service as well as the time the client is required to invest in it. From the client perspective, one would wish to estimate variables such as income lost during the time devoted to receipt of the service, and the psychological costs (to the client and his or her significant others) associated with receipt of the service.

For purposes of evaluating neuropsychological assessment in rehabilitation settings, the cost constructs just described might be implemented as follows: First, although charges are not synonymous with costs, they may provide an estimate of one resource consumed by the delivery of neuropsychological assessment, if appropriately adjusted. It is common to apply a ratio adjustment to charges (e.g., costs = .75 times charges for Medicare patients; see Johnston, 1987). Johnston (1987), however, has argued that in some circumstances, such as with hospital cost allocation schemes that are manipulated to maximize reimbursement, charges can yield a better estimate of social costs and resource consumption than accounted costs. Putnam and DeLuca (1990) have provided data on charges for neuropsychological assessment, based upon a survey of 872 members of the Division of Clinical Neuropsychology of the American Psychological Association. Of these respondents, representing all geographic regions in the United States, 34% worked in private practice only, 37% in a primary employment setting (e.g., university or nonuniversity hospital/medical center, independent rehabilitation center, or government agency/facility), and 29% in both. The majority of respondents (54% of those in primary employment and 73% of those in private practice) billed for their neuropsychological assessment services at an hourly rate. For the sake of simplicity and brevity, only the data on charges for adult patients will be reviewed. Hourly rates differed little between those in primary employment versus those in private practice, with the mean being $105 and $100, respectively. The average number of hours per neuropsychological assessment also differed little between the two groups, with a mean of 6 hours for those in primary employment and 7 hours for those in private practice. Thus total average charges for a neuropsychological assessment would fall between $630 and $700. These figures are in reasonably close agreement with the mean charge of $753 indicated by those 18% of respondents who use a fixed rate per patient for the billing of neuropsychological assessment.

If we are willing to assume, for the moment, that a ratio adjustment to the charges documented in the Putnam and DeLuca (1990) survey (i.e., charges × .75) are a reasonable estimate of the actual direct costs (i.e., for personnel, facilities, operations, and so on) and indirect costs (i.e., related to more than one cost objective) of neuropsychological assessment, and that no other hidden accountable costs exist, then we can estimate an average accounted cost of between $472 and $565 ($630 × .75 and $753 × .75, respectively). Were we to limit ourselves to an operations perspective, we might accept this as a reasonable present cost estimate for neuropsychological assessment. This would, however, neglect those additional social costs that must be estimated if we are to include societal and client perspectives. From a societal perspective, we must ask about the opportunity value of the resources expended. One obvious resource is that of the neuropsychologist's time. The 872 neuropsychologists in the Putnam and DeLuca (1990) survey spend, on average, 46% of their clinical time doing neuropsychological assessment. The remaining clinical time is divided between neuropsychological treatment (13%), neuropsychological consultation (13%), and other neuropsychological activities (29%). Kreutzer et al. (1990) point out that clinical neuropsychologists within community rehabilitation teams are likely to serve in a variety of roles, particularly when the availability of adjunct services is limited. Such roles include not only assessment but also individual, group, and family psychotherapy, cognitive remediation therapy, substance abuse evaluation and treatment, consultation with other rehabilitation professionals, serving as an expert witness in litigation, and serving as a patient advocate. Further, as documented by a recent questionnaire survey (Sweet & Moberg, 1990), of 144 psychologists with Diplomate status in clinical neuropsychology by the American Board of Professional Psychology (ABPP) and 145 randomly selected non-ABPP members of the Division of Clinical Neuropsychology of the American Psychological Association, 89% spend some amount of their professional activity in research and/or teaching. As might be expected, the percentage is somewhat greater for ABPP than for non-ABPP neuropsychologists. For nearly 25% of those in the Sweet and Moberg survey, research/teaching occupied more than 40% of their time.

Estimating the opportunity cost of the neuropsychologist's time had it been put into treatment rather than assessment services, might be possible. The Putnam and DeLuca (1990) survey reported the mean hourly rate of their sample for treatment services to be $94. Thus the opportunity cost for a neuropsychological assessment that consumes 6 hours of the psychologist's time, had this time been spent in direct treatment services, would range from $49 to $142 (accounted assessment cost of between $472 to $565 minus an accounted cost of $423—or $564 × .75—for the equivalent amount of time spent in treatment service delivery). It should be noted, however, that this opportunity cost estimate makes the assumptions that the neuropsychological assessment actually consumes a full 6 hours of the psychologist's time and that the time not spent on assessment would be devoted to treatment services. As noted above, some of most neuropsychologists' time is spent on research and/or teaching activities. Assigning a monetary value to such activities is by no means clear cut, and there would be hot debate over the question of whether research/teaching or treatment service would be a better alternative use of the neuropsychologist's time. Further complicating matters, the Putnam and DeLuca (1990) and Sweet and Moberg (1990) surveys reveal that a substantial number of clinical neuropsychologists, particularly those in primary employment settings, use technicians to conduct at least some part of the test administration. The varying use of technicians across employment settings, as well as the marked variability in their reported hourly rates of pay, is problematic for any effort to accurately estimate the opportunity cost of neuropsychological assessment.

The client perspective must not be neglected in estimating neuropsychological assessment costs. As noted above, the average length of a neuropsychological assessment is between 6 and 7 hours. Typically, this assessment would require at least two separate evaluation sessions (Lezak, 1983). Thus the client who is gainfully employed might be facing 9 to 11 hours, counting commuting time, lost from work. The data necessary to estimate the opportunity costs of neuropsychological assessment, from a client perspective, are not currently available. First, it would be necessary to know what percentage of neuropsychological assessment clients actually do miss time from work during their evaluations. For neuropsychological assessment in rehabilitation settings, it would seem likely that only a relatively small portion of clients would be actively employed at the time of the evaluation. Second, it would be necessary to have data on the cost of missed work for those who are employed. It should be noted, however, that those clients who are employed would not be the only ones for whom the client perspective would require estimating opportunity costs of neuropsychological assessment. Those involved in an inpatient or outpatient rehabilitation program potentially would be losing time from rehabilitation activities during their participation in the assessment. Again, data necessary for estimating the cost of such missed rehabilitation time are not available. Illustrative of the complexity of this problem is Keith's (1988) summary of systematic observations, over a 20-year period, at Texas and California rehabilitation facilities, documenting that patients spend a significant portion of the workday alone and not in treatment. Keith also discusses the ways in which staff considerations of convenience and constraints imposed by reimbursement systems limit the optimal use of patient time.

Finally, consideration must be given to the psychological cost to the client and his or her significant others that may be associated with participation in neuropsychological assessment. Given the challenging nature of various tasks typically employed in neuropsychological testing, and the likelihood of neurorehabilitation clients experiencing failure on a number of these tasks, the possibility of frustration and anxiety is clearly present. Complications arise, however, in the varying degree to which individuals with neurological damage or disease have a preserved awareness of their deficits and the ability to accurately appreciate task failure (see Anderson & Tranel, 1989; McGlynn & Kaszniak, 1991a, 1991b; McGlynn & Schacter, 1989; Prigatano & Schacter, 1991).

Benefit-cost analysis compares the benefits of an activity with the costs of producing the benefits (Scott & Sechrest, 1992). Benefit-cost analysis provides a method by which all monetary factors relevant to a decision can be synthesized into a single number. Benefits are typically expressed either as increases in income or as savings in expected expenditures. This definition of benefit has been referred to as the *human capital approach* (Wortman, 1983). Yates (1985) describes four major types of benefit that have been examined in benefit-cost analyses. *Actual income benefit* is the actual income experienced by an individual as a result of receiving a particular service. This could be directly measured as salary, health and other "fringe" benefits, and employer tax payments. *Inferred income benefit* can be deduced from data on nonmonetary measures of employee productivity. For example, increased lifetime income might be estimated from current measures of effectiveness of client performance (Yates, 1985). *Actual cost-savings benefit* requires measurement over long time periods of monetary outlays required for those receiving the target service compared with those who have not received the service. *Inferred cost-savings benefit* can be deduced, in short-term analyses, from data on trends in monetary outlay differentials. The results of a benefit-cost analysis can be expressed in terms of return on investment, as a benefit/cost ratio, or as net benefit (benefit minus cost) (Johnston & Keith, 1983; Thompson, 1980). Because benefit-cost analysis values all benefits and costs in the same, typically monetary, units, projects or programs of different kinds can be compared (Wortman, 1983). As emphasized by DeJong (1987), approaches to estimating cost savings are likely to become increasingly important in today's changing health care market.

A small number of benefit-cost analysis studies of medical rehabilitation exist in the literature. Johnston and Keith (1983) critically reviewed all studies available prior to 1980. Johnston (1987) reviewed those few subsequent studies and provided detailed guidance concerning methods and problems in benefit-cost analyses.

It is conceivable that benefit-cost analyses could be performed for neuropsychological assessment in rehabilitation. Data concerning actual or inferred income and cost-savings benefit data would be needed for those rehabilitation clients who did versus those who did not have an assessment performed. The selection of appropriate data for these benefit measures would depend upon the particular purpose of neuropsychological assessment for which the analysis is being performed. Returning to Trexler's (1987) list of purposes for neuropsychological assessment in rehabilitation (i.e., establishment of the existence of cognitive deficits, establishment of the relative magnitude of insult, estimation of the patient's ability to return to his or her previous life-style, suggestion of remediation programs), each different purpose would suggest the collection of somewhat different data. At the least, however, it can be argued that assessment procedures that do not have any effect on treatment have no benefit. Relatively expensive (i.e., approximately $700) assessment batteries should make some difference. In medical settings, not all tests and procedures have been proven beneficial by that criterion.

A major problem in relying exclusively upon benefit-cost analysis for making policy decisions in rehabilitation is that the theorized effects of intervention often present problems for assigning monetary values. How are we to determine the monetary value of improved quality of life, reduced suffering, or quality of care? Although techniques such as shadow pricing (i.e., assigning monetary value to goods that are not actually transacted on a market) are used in economics, they do not lend themselves well to the kinds of outcomes that are often of greatest interest to rehabilitation professionals. For this reason, cost-effectiveness analysis is typically preferable.

Cost-effectiveness analysis is distinguished from benefit-cost analysis in that costs and benefits need not be expressed in the same units (Johnston & Keith, 1983; Scott & Sechrest, 1992). Costs are typically expressed in monetary units, while effectiveness may be expressed in such variables as functional status, health status, quality of life, or quality of care, for which one may be unable or unwilling to assign a monetary value. Cost-effectiveness analyses are usually employed to decide which of two or more services is least costly in achieving the same benefit (Scott & Sechrest, 1992). One of the greatest barriers to cost-effectiveness research in the rehabilitation field is the difficulty of simplifying complex human outcomes in the operationalization of effectiveness (Johnston, 1987). As noted by Scott and Sechrest (1992), cost-effectiveness studies often achieve this conceptual simplification by ignoring many complexities of estimating benefits. Some innovative approaches to simplification of outcome have been proposed, however, such as multiattribute utility analysis (see Thompson, 1980) and the use of Delphi techniques (consensus reached by a panel of experts) to determine the relative importance of different outcome measures (e.g., DeJong, Branch, & Corcoran, 1984; DeJong & Hughes, 1982). This latter (Delphi) procedure is currently being employed by the task force to develop a uniform national data system for medical rehabilitation (Hamilton, Granger, Sherwin, Zielezny, & Tashman, 1987), jointly established by the American Congress of Rehabilitation Medicine (ACRM) and the American Academy of Physical Rehabilitation (AAPMR).

A number of published articles concerned with the effectiveness of rehabilitation programs for stroke and head injury patients have recently appeared (e.g., Dombovy, Sandok, & Basford, 1986;

Haffey & Johnston, 1989; Lehmann et al., 1975; Prigatano et al., 1983; Rappaport, Herrero-Backe, Rappaport, & Winterfield, 1989). The information necessary for cost-effectiveness analysis remains scant, however (e.g., Cope & Hall, 1982). Although no relevant studies have been published to date, it is clearly conceivable to apply cost-effectiveness analysis to neuropsychological assessment in rehabilitation settings. The approach to such analysis will be dictated, to a large extent, by the application of theory regarding the relationship of assessment to rehabilitation process and outcome.

The Role of Theory in Guiding the Operationalization of Variables Within Cost-Effectiveness Analyses

To know what outcome or effects to identify within cost-effectiveness analysis, a *theory of assessment* is needed. As discussed by Scott and Sechrest (1992), a theory can be considered to have three major functions: It describes what happens (descriptive); it explains why something happens (explanatory); and it predicts what will happen if one of the components is altered (predictive). Benefit-cost and cost-effectiveness analyses are most concerned with the predictive function of theory.

The general goal of all rehabilitation interventions is to bring the individual to a maximal (for that patient) level of functional independence. Rehabilitation efforts have historically stressed return to family life and work as indices of success. Rehabilitation success criteria of return to premorbid work and family roles may, however, be inappropriate for many rehabilitation clients (e.g., the elderly, retired stroke patient; the severe head injury patient who was premorbidly without family or steady employment). Thus attempts to operationalize functional independence, typically focusing upon physical and instrumental activities of daily living (ADL), have developed (Granger, Hamilton, Keith, Zielezny, & Sherwin, 1986), such as the Functional Independence Measure (FIM; Hamilton et al., 1987) created by the task force to develop a uniform national data system for medical rehabilitation.

Thus one theoretical linkage between psychological assessment and intervention procedures in rehabilitation must focus upon how psychological assessment measures relate to functional independence. For some areas of psychological assessment in rehabilitation, this theoretical linkage has been explicitly stated, although the validity of hypothesized relationships often has not been convincingly documented. For example, depression is frequently evaluated, with self-report or observational procedures (e.g., Kay & Silver, 1989; Lezak, 1989), under the assumptions that depression is a frequent response to the losses suffered by patients who are rehabilitation candidates and that presence and degree of depression is related to poorer adjustment to disability and lower motivation within rehabilitation programs (e.g., Hyman, 1972; Kemp, 1985).

The increased prevalence of depression in neurologically and physically disabled persons has been empirically demonstrated (e.g., Blazer, 1982; Blazer & Williams, 1980; Jacobs, 1988; Turner & McLean, 1989). Further, some research is available demonstrating the relationship of reactions following disability (e.g., due to spinal cord injury), particularly depression, to various measures of later adjustment (Kemp & Vash, 1971). The relationship of depression to motivation for rehabilitation has not been consistently documented, however. Indeed, it remains possible that apparent depression, at least that observed in the initial period of rehabilitation, might sometimes be related to rehabilitation motivation in a direction opposite to that theoretically predicted. For example, Myers, Friedman, and Weiner (1970) studied a group of 25 girls (age 9 to 16 years) with scoliosis being treated by a Milwaukee brace. Although not objectively documented in the study, it was the authors' impression that those girls who showed crying and apparent withdrawal and depression, when the brace was initially recommended, manifested a better ability to tolerate the brace than those girls who did not show this initial response. Similarly, Torkelson, Jellinek, Malec, and Harvey (1983) reported that the greatest improvement in levels of adaptive physical functioning following rehabilitation of 32 traumatic brain injury patients was related to higher levels of depression (as judged by rehabilitation professionals) at time of program admission.

In examining the theoretical linkage between neuropsychological assessment and rehabilitation, it is necessary first to ask whether neuropsychological assessment has any relationship to level of functional independence. As noted above, functional independence, within the field of rehabilitation, has typically been defined in terms of social and occupational functioning indices and measures of physical and instrumental activities of daily living. Several studies have documented the relationships between neuropsychological assessment and such measures of functional independence. For example, lower levels of intelligence test performance and other neuropsychological deficits have been shown to be related to lower levels of long-term social and economic adjustment among psychiatric patients (e.g., Gilberstadt, 1968; Glick & Sternberg, 1969; Klonoff, Fibiger, & Hutton, 1970; Pollack, Levenstein, & Klein, 1968). Heaton and Pendleton (1981) reviewed several studies examining the relationship of neuropsychological assessment to measures of independent living and self-care, vocational functioning, and academic achievement among patients with a variety of disorders. They found evidence for composite scores, derived from various measures of global neuropsychological test performance, to be predictive of the vocational, academic, and daily functional adaptation indices. For example, Newnan, Heaton, and Lehman (1978) recontacted 78 patients (with various disorders) who had received neuropsychological evaluations and questioned them about their employment during the prior 6 months. Of this group, 25 had been chronically unemployed, and the remaining 53 were asked about job stability, wages earned, and hours worked in addition to being administered the Minnesota Job Requirements Questionnaire. The patients' scores on the Halstead-Reitan Neuropsychological Battery, the WAIS, and the MMPI were highly correlated with subsequent employment status (i.e., employed versus chronically unemployed), income, and the level of skills required in the jobs they held.

Research focused on diagnostically homogeneous patient groups has also found evidence for relationships between neuropsychological assessment and measures of functional independence and social adjustment. In a short-term study of the outcome of severe closed head injury, as reported by patients' relatives, neuropsychological assessment measures were found to be significantly related to ratings of social adjustment (McKinley, Brooks, Bond, Martinage, & Marshall, 1981). For stroke patients, several studies have shown neuropsychological test results to be predictive of improvement, following rehabilitation, in self-care and ambulation as well as of whether a patient is discharged to home or institutional care (Anderson, Bourstom, Greenberg, & Hildyard, 1974; Ben-Yishay, Gerstman, Diller, & Hass, 1970; Bourstom & Howard,

1968; Lehmann et al., 1975; Lorenze & Cancro, 1962). McSweeney, Grant, Heaton, Prigatano, and Adams (1985) studied 303 patients with obstructive pulmonary disease (COPD) and associated neuropsychological impairment in comparison with 99 control subjects matched on sociodemographic variables. They found that neuropsychological measures from an expanded version of the Halstead-Reitan Battery were predictive of the quality of everyday-life functioning (assessed by both self-report and relatives' observations) for the COPD group. Those more complex, multifunctional neuropsychological tasks were found to be the best overall predictors of life functioning, while more specific neuropsychological tests served as better predictors of specific life functions (e.g., the aphasia screening test was the best predictor of communication skills).

Acker (1990) has provided a comprehensive review of these and a number of other studies of what she calls the "ecological validity" of neuropsychological tests and concludes that there is justification for cautious optimism in applying neuropsychological assessment to the prediction of a variety of everyday functioning indices. Acker also notes, however, that predictive robustness is seen not only for the better known comprehensive neuropsychological batteries but also for tests as simple as copying the Bender-Gestalt (Bender, 1938) figures. This observation raises important questions from a cost-effectiveness perspective. If simple and brief tests that can be administered by those without extensive training can provide comparable levels of prediction to that obtained when using comprehensive neuropsychological batteries, then the former obviously would be more cost effective. Unfortunately, adequate studies do not exist that *simultaneously* compare simple and brief measures with larger batteries, and different studies are sufficiently variable in the types and characteristics of patients studied as to prevent direct comparison in cost-effectiveness analysis.

Another potential application of neuropsychological assessment involves an attempt to predict differential response to rehabilitation interventions. The theoretical rationale for such a possible application is that minimal functional levels of various cognitive abilities are necessary for a patient to be able to profit from the rehabilitation effort. For example, it would be assumed that a minimal level of the ability to focus attention and maintain concentration would be necessary for a patient to benefit from any effort to retrain an old skill or teach a new one.

There does exist preliminary data to support this theoretical proposition. For example, Ben-Yishay, Piasetsky, and Rattok (1987) have reported on an evaluation of their Orientation Remedial Module (ORM) in a 6-year outpatient study of 40 chronic, severely head injured young adults. The program involved five computerized exercises, delivered in sequence, which were designed to produce a cumulative enhancement of the individual's levels of alertness, attention, and concentration. Each of the five exercises represented distinct hierarchies in a theorized continuum of attentional skills. It was found that the patient group progressed from initially impaired performance to within the average normal range on all of the tasks in the sequence. Mean scores obtained after task-specific training, in all five instances, showed significant improvement and remained relatively stable thereafter. In support of their hierarchical theory of the relationship between the five attentional skill domains, training on one task did not appear to affect performance on other tasks hypothesized to be "higher" in the hierarchy. Further, pretraining performance on the fifth and most attentionally complex task had the largest magnitude and greatest number of significant correlations with performance on a battery of neuropsychological tests designed to assess memory, psychomotor skill, perceptual integration, and abstract reasoning. Similar data, supporting the efficacy of attention training in a hierarchically organized cognitive rehabilitation program, are provided by Sohlberg and Mateer (1987, 1989).

Given such data, Ben-Yishay and colleagues (1987) argue for the value of assessing intactness of basic attention as implemented by their ORM methodology. The unanswered question, from a cost-effectiveness perspective, however, is whether some alternative, briefer, less instrument intensive, and therefore less expensive, means of assessing the same attentional constructs would be equally effective (see Sohlberg & Mateer, 1989, pp. 111-120). To address this question, a study empirically comparing the ORM method with a less costly alternative would be necessary. The challenging aspects of such a study would involve design and selection of effectiveness criteria. A within-subjects design would appear preferable, comparing the alternative attentional assessment approaches applied to the same individuals. As shown by Ben-Yishay et al. (1987), however, attentional skills can change with practice, and practice on one task could alter performance on the other, thus requiring that order effects be taken into account. In choosing effectiveness criteria, care would also need to be exercised. Using other psychometric tasks to which the attentional measures will be related is insufficient if the real goal is to determine the cost-effectiveness of the attentional measures as predictors of adaptive behavior or ability to profit from rehabilitation efforts. Issues in selecting measures of everyday adaptive functioning have been discussed by several authors of the chapters in this volume, and an excellent review of many of these issues can be found in McSweeney (1990) and other chapters in the Tupper and Cicerone (1990b) volume as well as in Johnston (1987).

One important and often overlooked problem in selecting measures of everyday adaptive functioning for use with neurologically damaged patients concerns sources of systematic bias in reporting. If self-report measures are used, it must be remembered that patients with head injury, stroke, or other neurological illness may have impaired awareness of deficits (for review, see McGlynn & Schacter, 1989). Further, as shown in recent research (e.g., Anderson & Tranel, 1989; McGlynn & Kaszniak, 1991a, 1991b), the degree of impaired awareness can vary with type of disease, disease severity, and nature of the task regarding which the person's awareness of impairment is inquired. Family members may also vary in systematic biases that affect rating of their patient's functional status. Some family members, particularly soon after the traumatic brain injury, may deny or minimize the severity of their patient's injury, while others may be devastated and exaggerate severity (Brooks, 1991). Many family caregivers of head injured, stroke, or other neurological patients experience considerable stress in their caregiver role and often manifest depressive symptoms, as documented in a growing literature (for review, see Brooks, 1991; Lezak, 1988). A depressed family caregiver might be expected to exaggerate the severity of his or her patient's cognitive or emotional deficits, because other research has shown that depressed persons tend to remember mood-congruent (i.e., negative) information more accurately than mood-incongruent (i.e., positive) information (Matt, Vazquez, & Campbell, 1992). Finally, all of the measurement considerations that have been discussed in the current volume must be applied to the selection or creation of functional status measures.

In addition to their application in predicting functional status or response to rehabilitation, neuropsychological assessments also have been proposed as a means of prescribing individually tailored approaches to rehabilitation. To what extent has the theoretical relationship between neuropsychological assessment and the specifics of rehabilitation for brain injured persons been made explicit? The answer to this question is dependent to a large extent on the particular rehabilitation facility and its orientation. Obviously, some facilities have relatively fixed rehabilitation programs into which most patients are fit. Within such programs, the role of neuropsychological assessment in guiding rehabilitation planning would be minimal, and the theoretical linkage between the two would be irrelevant. Within other settings, an individualized approach to rehabilitation is at least advocated, and it is here that we find the theoretical rationale linking assessment to rehabilitation activities must be more fully described.

Theory concerning the relationship between neuropsychological assessment and rehabilitation activities is dependent upon theory concerning the nature of functional recovery. It has been well documented that some recovery following cerebral trauma or nonprogressive disease does take place (see Finger, 1978; Finger & Stein, 1982; Scheff, 1984; Stein, Rosen, & Butters, 1974). Several different theories have been proposed to account for such recovery, however (e.g., Diller & Gordon, 1981; Luria, 1963; Meier, Strauman, & Thompson, 1987; Miller, 1984). Because different theories concerning functional recovery imply substantially different approaches to rehabilitation, it is useful to briefly review the major differences between these theories.

Miller (1984) has categorized theoretical explanations of recovery into three major groups that he designates as (a) artifact theories, (b) anatomical reorganization, and (c) functional adaptation. As described by Miller, artifact theories share in common the assumption of two components contributing to the impairment initially observed after brain damage. First, a lesion destroys particular cerebral tissue, with loss of those aspects of function dependent upon the destroyed area. This is thought of as the primary deficit and is assumed to be permanent. Second, the insult also produces largely temporary physiological disturbances in other parts of the brain that are not involved in the primary deficit. These result in secondary behavioral deficits. Therefore the task, as perceived by "artifact theorists," is to explain the mechanisms involved in production of secondary deficits and their resolution. Any detailed examination of possible mechanisms in the production and resolution of secondary deficits is beyond the scope of this chapter. Candidate mechanisms that have been suggested by various theorists include (a) edema (increase in tissue water content) in tissue adjacent to a lesion (Schoenfeld & Hamilton, 1977), which resolves spontaneously with time, and (b) diaschisis (von Monakow, 1914, as translated by Pribram, 1969, pp. 27-36), a form of "shock" or inhibition (Luria, 1963) that occurs in brain sites adjacent to or distant from the location of a lesion. For current purposes, the important point is that artifact theories posit the recovery of secondary deficits to involve a resolution of these temporary physiological disturbances.

Anatomical reorganization, or "restitution," theories assume that, when damage occurs to one brain area, recovery can take place by other brain regions taking over the functions originally subserved by the damaged locus. Possible mechanisms underlying reorganization include (a) denervation supersensitivity (Ungerstedt, 1971), in which denervated postsynaptic neurons show enhanced sensitivity to neurotransmitters, and (b) the sprouting of axon collaterals in response to damaged adjacent neurons (Moore, 1974), with accompanying formation of new synapses (reactive synaptogenesis).

Functional adaptation, or "substitution," theories posit that the person sustaining brain damage might be able to relearn the ability to achieve a goal by means other than those originally employed and now impaired by the damage. Various rehabilitation efforts have been based upon a substitution theory. These include using melodic intonation (Albert, Sparks, & Helm, 1973) with aphasic patients (presumably engaging the specialized abilities of the right cerebral hemisphere) and visual imagery (again, presumably right- hemispheric) strategies with left-hemisphere stroke patients showing verbal memory deficits (e.g., Gasparrini & Satz, 1979).

A review of the literature concerned with specific testing of these theoretical positions on recovery of function is clearly beyond the scope of this chapter. It should be noted, however, that the three theory groups described by Miller (1984) are not mutually exclusive. It is certainly possible that all three general phenomena may be operating in the recovery of function of any particular brain damaged individual. Further, each of the three theory groups does have some supporting evidence (see Finger & Stein, 1982; Miller, 1984). The theory groups do, however, suggest rather different roles for neuropsychological assessment.

The artifact theories would suggest that neuropsychological assessment be employed primarily as a means of following the patient over time to reveal when recovery of secondary deficits is complete and the unaltered primary deficits remain. No prescriptive role for neuropsychological assessment would be indicated by the artifact theories, and no specific rehabilitation approach defined. Therefore any benefits attributable to assessment would be limited to whatever advantages inhere in knowing the extent of long-term dysfunction. These might include savings from rehabilitation efforts forgone because of no expected improvement and relief to patient and family in having certain knowledge.

The anatomical reorganization theories would suggest that neuropsychological assessment focus upon a precise definition of the impaired function or functions so that rehabilitation efforts could "exercise" these functions through various task practice methods. Alternatively, the functional adaptation theories would indicate that neuropsychological assessment place greatest emphasis upon identifying intact functional systems capable of mediating behavioral goals originally subserved by damaged functional systems. Although there have been preliminary efforts at articulating the specific prescriptive relationships between neuropsychological assessment and rehabilitation efforts motivated by either the anatomical reorganization or the functional adaptation theories (e.g., Christensen, 1989; Luria, Naydin, Tsvetkova, & Vinarskaya, 1969; Reitan, 1988), greater specificity is required before useful cost-effectiveness research could be undertaken. Cost-effectiveness evaluation, it should be noted, would involve comparisons of two or more methods of assessment, probably against a criterion of speed or cost of rehabilitation. Benefit-cost evaluation would compare assessment versus no assessment against a monetized criterion.

Summary and Conclusions

Two questions motivated the review of literature contained in this chapter: (a) To what extent does the effectiveness of neuropsychological assessment justify its cost within the rehabilitation enterprise? and (b) what approach to, and application of, neuropsychological assessment is most effective at the least cost? Emphasis was placed upon the advantages of cost-effectiveness and benefit/cost perspectives for the evaluation of neuropsychological assessment in rehabilitation. Attention was drawn to the problems and complexity of these perspectives, particularly in defining the full range of both accounted costs (i.e., from an operations perspective) and social costs (i.e., from societal and client perspectives) of neuropsychological assessment and in defining indices of the effectiveness (including monetary value) of such assessment. Finally, an argument was presented for the important role of neuropsychological theory in guiding the implementation of variables with cost-effectiveness analyses of neuropsychological assessment in rehabilitation. The theoretical linkage between neuropsychological assessment and rehabilitation was examined through review of empirical studies on the relationship of neuropsychological measures to functional independence. The relation between neuropsychological assessment and theoretical explanations of functional recovery after brain damage was also explored.

Resource limitations in rehabilitation, both monetary and human, are a reality that is not likely go away any time within the foreseeable future. A major importance of benefit/cost and cost-effectiveness perspectives is that they remind us of the need for accountability. This chapter has attempted to define the kind of research that will be necessary to increase the future accountability of neuropsychological assessment within rehabilitation settings.

CHAPTER 9

Training Psychology Graduate Students in Assessment for Rehabilitation Settings

TIMOTHY R. ELLIOTT

Although assessment is traditionally considered one of the hallmarks of applied psychology, it is also a topic that can quickly raise concerns when applied to underrepresented and underserved populations. It is no surprise, then, that special considerations are warranted when conducting psychological evaluations with persons who have physical disabilities.

Exactly how these considerations are communicated to new generations of psychologists is a matter worth pondering. As of this writing, no formal recommendations have been forwarded to psychology training programs for preparing doctoral students in clinical and counseling psychology to work either with persons with physical disabilities or in the settings where rehabilitation services are delivered. Although accrediting bodies routinely recommend that training sites provide experiences with special populations, guidelines are seldom available to expedite this recommendation. Consequently, many professionals and consumers are justifiably concerned that training in psychological assessment practices with persons who have physical disabilities is receiving limited attention.

This chapter reviews several salient issues pertaining to the preparation of psychology graduate students for rehabilitation work. Historical trends will be discussed, and the educational expectations of training programs in clinical and counseling psychology accredited by the American Psychological Association (APA) will be considered. A brief review of current assessment practices will follow. Recommendations for integrating training experiences into clinical and counseling psychology doctoral programs will then be offered.

Historical Perspectives

Despite the current demand for psychologists in rehabilitation, psychologists have not always been warmly received by the rehabilitation community. In the period from 1955 to 1969, rehabilitation professionals expressed suspicions that psychologists generally knew little about the vocational concerns of persons with disabilities (Olshansky & Hart, 1967). Some viewed psychologists as having a peripheral role in rehabilitation assessment, perhaps helpful in understanding "deep-seated problems," such as unconscious processes or reality contact, or in interpreting psychiatric reports (Allen, 1958). Others believed that assessment with pencil-and-paper measures should be handled by psychometrists; psychologists could administer and interpret projective devices (Muthard & Salomone, 1969) and intelligence tests (Gill, 1972). In general, psychologists were viewed as consultants. Psychological assessment reports were not considered particularly relevant to the actual needs of the vocational rehabilitation specialist (Cull & Hardy, 1972).

Psychologists were eventually criticized for not appreciating the negative impact of the environment on persons with disability. Psychologists are often trained to assume a problem-focused view, emphasizing the negative aspects of each client and disregarding situational and environmental influences on behavior (Shontz & Wright, 1980; Wright & Fletcher, 1982). Wright and Fletcher (1982) argue that this attitude is found in psychological assessments with most clientele. Wright (1983) has been the most vocal in urging a field-theory perspective in rehabilitation generally and in assessment specifically.

Relatedly, psychological opinions about behavioral disorders among persons with disability displayed a remarkable lack of agreement. With a paucity of practicing psychologists and psychological research in the developing years of rehabilitation, many mental health specialists leaned heavily on impressionistic models of adjustment to disability. These models borrowed extensively from Freudian concepts of stagelike dynamics in reaction to acute loss. Reasoning from these models culminated in assumptions about client affective states. For example, it was presumed that all persons who acquired severe physical disabilities (e.g., spinal cord injuries) would become depressed soon after injury onset, and this depression was considered adaptive and even necessary for optimal adjustment (Nemiah, 1957; Siller, 1969a). Conversely, many other psychologists assumed that emotional disorders found in psychiatric clientele traditionally served by psychologists did not occur among medical patients (Belar, 1988). From this perspective, depression and anxiety reactions were not recognized and were subsequently left untreated as clinicians believed these were transitory states that would pass with time.

Wright (1960) criticized the flaws in the psychodynamic perspective, noting that most people expect stigmatized persons to be preoccupied with their physical conditions and to mourn their losses. Several studies have documented that rehabilitation staff, medical personnel, and people in general overestimate the degree of personal distress actually reported by persons with physical disability (Mason & Muhlenkamp, 1976; Westbrook & Nordholm, 1986). Yet these criticisms were not heeded, and many practicing clinicians uncritically embraced stage models of adjustment following disability.

Clinical assumptions about adjustment following acquired physical disability were made in the absence of systematic data collection or empirical research and without the use of standardized instruments or criteria for affective disorders (Frank, Elliott, Corcoran, & Wonderlich, 1987). Funded research from state and federal sources focused on vocational aspects of rehabilitation, so little support was available for the kind of empirical research needed to study affective reactions following acquired disability. Although some empirical investigations of depression and anxiety in rehabilitation appeared in the literature, these studies were neither systematic nor theory based.

The lack of theory-based research, conceptualizations, and interventions may have been influenced by the dearth of psychologists in rehabilitation generally. For many years, the gradual demand for psychologists in rehabilitation was met not by psychology training programs but by graduate programs with a distinct emphasis on vocational rehabilitation. Few psychology programs, up to the current time, have taken up rehabilitation as a specialty area (Leung, Sakata, & Ostby, 1990). When rehabilitation has been so defined, it has usually been in counseling psychology programs, the majority of which are housed within schools of education. With few exceptions, rehabilitation specialties (rehabilitation counseling, rehabilitation psychology, and so on) have been divorced from the scientific traditions of academic psychology.

Rehabilitation counseling has provided an invaluable service in advancing our knowledge about job placement, counseling, and vocational adjustment of persons with disability. Many of the founding and current members of Division 22 (Rehabilitation Psychology) in the American Psychological Association earned degrees in rehabilitation counseling (Jansen & Fulcher, 1982; Neff, 1971). Training programs in rehabilitation counseling emphasize the applied techniques needed to meet the rigors of vocational rehabilitation in the marketplace. These programs do not often provide training in the core areas of psychology, nor do they always provide rigorous scientific training. Consequently, few professionals from this discipline had been trained in the use of psychological theories to view clinical problems and pose empirical questions for study. In fact, vocational rehabilitation specialists openly questioned the relevance of training in core psychological areas (Olshansky & Hart, 1967).

Probably the most vocal criticism of psychological services in rehabilitation has come from consumers. It is not uncommon to read anecdotal accounts of adjustment following disability and notice salient criticisms of psychologists and other mental health workers (e.g., Caywood, 1974). A recent survey of the Paralyzed Veterans of America documents the most negative opinions about psychologists and psychological services to date (Paralyzed Veterans of American, 1988). Respondents to this survey reported psychology to be the most unhelpful service available to them. Such criticisms warrant an examination of the preparation of psychologists for work with persons with acquired physical disability.

Issues in Graduate Training

For many reasons, most doctoral programs in clinical and counseling psychology pursue APA accreditation. First, APA grants approval to programs reviewed by a representative committee. APA approval certifies that the program meets educational and training guidelines, including education in the core areas of psychology. Second, students from APA-approved academic programs have greater access to internship sites, particularly those that are APA approved. The APA-approved internship is presumed to be the most thorough and comprehensive applied experience for counseling and clinical doctoral students. Third, most state boards licensing and governing the practice of psychology favor graduates from APA-approved programs and internships. Licensure is sought by psychologists for certification, third-party reimbursements, professional privileges, and career advancement. By law, certain tests are to be administered only by licensed psychologists or under the supervision of one. Graduates of programs that are not APA approved often experience difficulties pursuing licensure.

Education in the professional and scientific aspects of psychology is germane to rehabilitation psychology (Elliott & Gramling, 1990). Supervised experiences in practica and internship rotations provided in clinical and counseling psychology doctoral programs are also valuable to those who will later work in rehabilitative settings. These programs should expose students to as many diverse populations as possible, including persons in racial minorities, in alternate sexual life-styles, and with "handicapping conditions" (APA, 1980).

Despite the APA recommendation, many APA training programs may not provide adequate preparatory experiences with persons who have these "handicapping conditions." A survey by Spear and Schoepke (1981) found that many APA training programs were not providing basic information to students about persons with disability. More recently, Leung et al. (1990) surveyed 197 APA-accredited programs in clinical and counseling psychology and found that rehabilitation-relevant course work, content, and clinical experiences were absent in half of the programs. A similar trend was observed by Parker and Chan (1990), who surveyed the educational backgrounds of psychology service directors in rehabilitation settings accredited by the Commission on Accreditation of Rehabilitation Facilities (CARF). More than 80% of the respondents had doctoral degrees either in clinical or counseling psychology, and only 4% identified rehabilitation as their specialty area at the doctoral level. Furthermore, less than half of the directors described themselves as "rehabilitation psychologists."

Collectively, these survey results raise compelling issues. It is doubtful that many psychologists in rehabilitative settings have received extensive training in rehabilitation principles and values (e.g., Wright, 1972). Many training programs and internship sites advertised under rubrics such as "behavioral medicine" or "clinical health psychology" prepare students for servicing persons with disability (Society of Behavioral Medicine, 1988). It is uncertain whether the work performed by these psychologists is compromised by their lack of training in traditional rehabilitation approaches.

Current Training and Functioning of Psychologists in Rehabilitation

For many years, leaders in rehabilitation psychology have argued that psychologists should be aware of the unique person-environment issues affecting persons with disability so as to provide proficient service to these individuals. This recommendation was formally stated by the Princeton conference on rehabilitation psychology (Wright, 1959). Through the years, however, many psychologists became interested in health and medical issues and began to provide services to persons in health care settings, including persons with acquired physical disabilities and other chronic, debilitating conditions. Generally, these psychologists were unaware of the emphasis on the field-theory perspectives stressed at the Princeton conference. Furthermore, the boundaries separating rehabilitation psychology from the currently emerging specialty areas (e.g., health psychology, behavioral medicine) were ambiguous to those involved in clinical training (Edelstein & Brasted, 1983; Klippel & DeJoy, 1984).

Shontz and Wright (1980), in an effort to define rehabilitation psychology, stated that students should be trained in the principles, values, theories, history, and social psychology of persons with disability as originally recommended at the Princeton conference

(Dembo, Diller, Gordon, Leviton, & Sherr, 1973; Wright, 1972). Specifically, the field-theory perspective—in which client behavior is seen as a function of the person-environment interaction—was proposed as the guiding theoretical basis for rehabilitation psychology. According to this view, clinicians must consider the role of the environment when assessing client behavior, and interventions for effecting environmental changes should be entertained. Leung (1984), reasoning from the field-theory perspective, recommended that students must learn to modify existing assessment practices to take into account the unique impact of the environment on persons with disability and also learn to make assessment procedures relevant to the needs of these persons.

Strict reliance upon a field-theory perspective for psychological assessment in rehabilitation has some notable shortcomings. First, Grzesiak (1981) questioned whether such an adherence was crucial for adequate functioning in rehabilitation. He argued that "psychological services to the physically disabled do not differ in any substantial way from services provided to patients or clients in other settings" (Grzesiak, 1979, p. 511). He pointed out that graduate students in psychology are adequately prepared to conduct assessments of intellectual functioning, organic status, personality, and psychopathology among rehabilitation clientele.

The emphasis on person-environment perspectives is embedded in the basic tenets of rehabilitation psychology. As Grzesiak (1981) notes, however, it has not been empirically confirmed that psychologists taking such perspectives are actually more skilled than other psychologists in working with persons with disability. Preliminary experimental evidence indicates that graduate students in APA-approved clinical and counseling psychology programs do not display stereotypical biases in their expectations for depression in a client with disability (Elliott, Frank, & Brownlee-Duffeck, 1988).

Second, correlational research indicates that predisability behavioral patterns are related to indices of adjustment following acquired physical disability. An emerging program of research suggests that preinjury patterns of substance use and use of alcohol at time of injury are significantly related to substance use among persons with spinal cord injuries (Heineman, Goranson, Ginsburg, & Schnoll, 1989; Heineman, Mamott, & Schnoll, 1990). These behaviors may in turn compromise self-care skills and health status among these individuals. Field-theory concepts may be useful in understanding person-environment interactions, but this particular theoretical perspective should not obfuscate the importance of assessing predisability behavioral patterns that have a major impact on psychological and medical adjustment following acquired disability (e.g., substance abuse, social judgment, impulsivity, social adjustment predisability). In other words, both environmental and personality factors are important.

Psychologists in rehabilitation settings devote more time to assessments than to any other clinical activity (Jansen & Fulcher, 1982). Recent surveys of clinicians in rehabilitative and other health care settings indicate that psychologists rely heavily on interview methods (Piotrowski & Lubin, 1990; Williams & Mourer, 1990). Piotrowski and Lubin (1990) surveyed practicing health psychologists to learn the specific instruments preferred with medical populations. The most frequently used instruments were the Minnesota Multiphasic Personality Inventory (MMPI), the Symptom Checklist 90/Revised (SCL-90R), and the Millon Clinical Multiaxial Inventory (MCMI). Pain was most frequently measured with the McGill Pain Questionnaire. Popular measures of neuropsychological functioning included the Wechsler Memory Scale, the Bender-Gestalt Visual Motor Test, and the Halstead-Reitan Neuropsychological Battery. Most frequently used measures of affect included the depression scale of the MMPI, the Beck Depression Inventory (BDI), and the State-Trait Anxiety Inventory. Substance abuse was often assessed by the MacAndrew Alcoholism Scale on the MMPI and the Michigan Alcoholism Screening Test (MAST).

The results of these surveys reveal that psychologists tend to use established means of assessment in working with people with disability. Certain caveats regarding these methods should be noted. Interview methods—the most preferred assessment procedure— are fraught with errors in clinical judgment and decision making. Meehl's (1954) classic statement on this method demonstrated that actuarial devices are superior to clinical methods in general. More recent applications pertinent to rehabilitation continue to show that clinicians' judgments are highly unreliable and inconsistent, regardless of level of experience and training (Faust et al., 1988; Wedding & Faust, 1989).

Another issue concerns the utility of the MMPI in rehabilitation. MMPI scores have been correlated with a variety of important variables among persons with disability, including impulsivity (Fordyce, 1964), self-care and rehabilitation performance (Malec & Neimeyer, 1983; Richards, 1981), and behavioral reactions to pain syndromes (Fordyce, 1976). The MacAndrew scale from the MMPI has also been related to substance use patterns among rehabilitation clientele (Rohe & Basford, 1989). But the MMPI can easily overestimate the level of distress among persons with acquired physical disability, because many items tap legitimate somatic concerns (Kendall, Edinger, & Eberly, 1978; Taylor, 1970). Scores on the hypochondriasis, depression, and hysteria scales are prone to be artificially elevated among persons with chronic medical conditions, because these scales contain many items that may measure somatic features of the physical condition (Pincus, Callahan, Bradley, Vaughn, & Wolfe, 1986). Similar problems have been detected in SCL-90R profiles produced by patients with chronic pain and spinal cord injuries (Buckelew, Burk, Brownlee-Duffeck, Frank, & DeGood, 1988).

The Beck Depression Inventory has a number of items that may also measure symptoms of disease or disability rather than psychological functioning (Peck, Smith, Ward, & Milano, 1989). Other evidence suggests that, although somatic items on depression scales may bias prevalence estimates of depression among patients with chronic physical conditions, correlations between depression scores and other psychological variables are not likely to be adversely inflated (Blalock, DeVellis, Brown, & Wallston, 1989).

The measurement of depression among persons with chronic physical conditions is a particularly tricky enterprise, given the interaction between psychological variables and the course and nature of physical problems (House, 1988; Kathol, 1985; Romano & Turner, 1985). Standardized interview methods adhering to strict diagnostic criteria appear to be the most promising and conservative methods for determining affective disorders in rehabilitation (Frank et al., 1987; Frank, Kashani, Wonderlich, Lising, & Visot, 1985; Gans, 1981; Kashani, Frank, Kashani, Wonderlich, & Reid, 1983; Turner & McLean, 1989).

It appears that clinical interviews and the popular psychometric instruments are the most preferred assessment procedures by psychologists in rehabilitation settings. It is unclear, however, whether psychologists are aware of the biases and shortcomings that exist in these methods. Each method can be useful. But failure to observe and work within the limitations posed by each method can result in erroneous conclusions and recommendations. For effective and reliable assessment procedures in rehabilitation, graduate training should include exposure to field-theory perspectives and clear instruction in the appropriate use of psychometric and interview methods.

Recommendations for Training Graduate Students in Psychology

The validity and reliability of assessment procedures in rehabilitation psychology understandably warrant our concern. As we have briefly surveyed the history of psychology in rehabilitation and current practices in clinics and training programs, the number of problems and shortcomings with assessment appears to obviate our ability to conduct meaningful psychological evaluations, let alone prepare students for this task. As psychologists, however, it is important that we reframe problems into challenges and be reminded that we offer skills in synthesizing basic patient information from theoretical perspectives that can benefit the rehabilitation process for client and staff. It is all too easy to fallaciously assume that persons with acquired disability are more alike than different simply by virtue of having a disability.

There are considerable and meaningful differences between (a) a 22-year-old urban youth who has acquired paraplegia in a gun battle after a "misunderstanding" with others concerning street drugs and (b) a 44-year-old Air For ːe colonel with a Ph.D. in history who, while jogging in Georgetown on a rainy day, acquired paraplegia when struck by an automobile. At first glance, many staff members may intuit some of these differences. But, as psychologists, we should be able to anticipate and assess individual characteristics directly pertinent to rehabilitation and adjustment, including preinjury level of social adjustment, social support systems, past educational and vocational histories, social problem-solving strategies, goal-directed behavior, impulsivity, and interpersonal styles. Such information can and should be communicated to staff and patient in a manner that facilitates the rehabilitation process for *each* patient.

In general, training in clinical assessment should engender critical thinking skills among graduate students, so that students can entertain several possible explanations of client behavior from different perspectives. The role of the environment in influencing client behavior should be considered, whether the client is an adult with a physical disability or a college student complaining of test anxiety. Graduate students should consider several valid—if not competing—explanations for client behavior in terms of individual difference variables, racial identity and acculturation issues (if applicable), gender role concerns, family dynamics, or other possible considerations. To borrow a concept from statistics, students should consider the "degree of variance accounted for" by each pos- sible explanation so as to offer meaningful recommendations and interventions.

Several definitive recommendations for enhancing these skills among graduate students can be implemented. The following recommendations are made primarily for implementation in clinical and counseling psychology doctoral programs.

1. Students should be provided core training in psychology. For too long, psychologists in rehabilitation have felt "isolated" from mainstream psychology (Jansen & Eisenberg, 1982). Students trained in core areas of psychology will ideally be grounded in the science and profession of psychology and then function as psychologists in rehabilitation. This core training should supply students with a firm grasp of intervention and assessment skills. Core training also provides instruction in biological, cognitive-affective, and social bases of behavior; in personality, statistics and research methodology, history and systems of psychology, scientific and professional ethics; and in minority and cross-cultural issues. Background knowledge in these areas is prerequisite for competent psychological practice in any setting and with any population.

2. Students should be trained in the use of a variety of assessment methods as well as in the unique strengths and limitations of each. This recommendation is ideally incorporated into every assessment course and practicum site in approved programs. We cannot naively assume that the current level of training in these programs is adequate across all programs for competent assessment of persons with physical disability. Students should learn the classic and contemporary means of conducting psychological evaluations with clients from as many diverse populations as possible. In addition,

students (a) should be aware of alternative ways of assessing intelligence and personality characteristics among persons with auditory, visual, and physical limitations (Eisenberg & Jansen, 1983); (b) should be aware of the limitations of clinical interview assessment and predictions based on such methods (Meehl, 1954); (c) should be well versed in the sources of bias in popular instruments like the MMPI and the BDI that may adversely alter interpretations with persons from underserved and underrepresented populations; (d) should possess skills in the efficient assessment of substance use and abuse; (e) should have the ability to conduct brief mental status examinations; (f) should have a background in family dynamics and developmental issues in the assessment of individuals; (g) should appreciate the fundamental importance of referral questions for assessment and how to appropriately address referral questions in assessment while understanding how results may be used by the referral agency; and (h) should learn the impact of person-environment interactions and situational determinants of behavior in the self-report and behavioral assessment of all clients (Wright & Fletcher, 1982).

Basic competencies and knowledge in each of these areas enrich assessment procedures in any setting and with all clientele. They are fundamental in the competent assessment of persons with physical disability.

3. Students interested in working with medical populations should receive some practicum and internship experience in psychiatric environments servicing persons with severe behavioral disorders. At first glance, this recommendation seems tangential to the roles and functions of a psychologist in a rehabilitation setting. Yet, learning basic assessment techniques with persons who have behavioral disorders and who are typically served in psychiatric settings can prove invaluable. Exposure to this type of population can advance recognition of behavioral disorders in medical settings. Students should not be trained under the myth that true behavioral disorders are not observed in medical settings (Belar, Deardoff, & Kelly, 1987). Failure to assess and intervene with aberrant behavioral problems can result in negative consequences for the patient, the health care staff, and the credibility of the psychologist.

4. Students interested in working with persons in medical settings—including rehabilitation—should receive either advanced practicum or internship experiences in the use and limitations of assessment devices. Students who wish to serve persons in medical and health care environments in general should receive advanced supervised training in the utility of assessment procedures. This can include traditional and novel methods. For example, students can learn to apply measures such as the MMPI with chronic pain and spinal cord injury patients, provided they also learn the limitations and biases that can occur in the test results. Students should also learn alternative means of collecting data pertinent to specific populations, such as behavioral methods in chronic pain rehabilitation (Fordyce, 1976), measures of outcome such as patient activities of daily living (Granger, Albrecht, & Hamilton, 1979), health status variables that have behavioral components (e.g., urinary tract infections, decubitus ulcers), certain medical tests and procedures (e.g., urine volumes; Ganguli, 1983), and issues regarding client expectations for control and rehabilitation (Dana, 1984). Training should include instruction in conducting neuropsychological screenings and in making appropriate referrals or providing more detailed assessments as appropriate. Furthermore, students need to be able to communicate comprehensible recommendations to health care staff regarding patient motivation, personality, career concerns, and behavior.

Psychologists in medical settings often erroneously assume that a physical impairment is the overriding source of distress in a patient's life (Wright, 1983). This assumption ignores individual differences that are important considerations in clinical interventions (Auerbach, 1989). Students should be alert to the stressful events experienced by clients receiving rehabilitative services. Stressors may be highly subjective and significantly related to patient adjustment (Frank & Elliott, 1987; Turner, Clancy, & Vitaliano, 1987).

Because clinical judgment is often prone to error, it is crucial that students become aware of basic research on adjustment specific to the immediate clientele. Knowledge of research in the particular content area improves clinical assessment skills, the ability to recommend meaningful strategies for group and individual interventions, and awareness of variables related to patient behavior and adjustment. For example, patients with spinal cord injuries

(SCI) who have more internal expectancies for control have been found to be less depressed, be less distressed, and have more skills relevant to daily living than patients with more external expectancies (Frank et al., 1987; Umlauf & Frank, 1983). Social problem-solving strategies (Elliott, Godshall, Herrick, Witty, & Spruell, 1991) and goal-directed behavior (Elliott, Witty, Herrick, & Hoffman, 1991) are also predictive of psychological adjustment following SCI. Psychologists should observe the interpersonal skills of the client, because these are important in psychosocial adjustment (Dunn & Herman, 1982). Social support has been positively related to adjustment after SCI (Schulz & Decker, 1985); more recent research indicates that interpersonal and coping styles can interact with certain types of support to influence both positive and negative outcomes (Elliott, Herrick, & Witty, 1992; Elliott, Herrick, et al., 1991). A significant minority of persons with SCI report problems with chronic pain (Elliott & Harkins, 1991; Mariano, 1992). Many pain assessment techniques used with other clinical populations can be adapted for use with persons who have varying types of paralysis (Wegener & Elliott, 1992). Other persons with SCI may have problems with closed head injuries or substance abuse; these problems often accompany injuries sustained in high impact accidents (Trieschmann, 1988). Different coping strategies may characterize distressed clients with SCI (Buckelew, Baumstark, Frank, & Hewett, 1990). Therefore a comprehensive psychological assessment of a person with a newly acquired SCI should evaluate the person's level of general problem-solving ability, interpersonal skills, available social support systems, expectancies for control in the rehabilitation process, and behavioral manifestations of pain and neuropsychological deficits.

Given the interdisciplinary nature of rehabilitation, the student must learn to work efficiently in professional teams. Psychologists often instruct health care staff in the proper use of psychological services and the way in which referral questions are asked of psychologists. In addition, psychologists must communicate effectively with clientele and health care staff. Field-theory perspectives are vital in this regard. Rehabilitation units are high stress, low reward environments for staff, and tense patient-staff interactions are common. Useless labels are often coined by staff to describe and anticipate patient behavior (*angry, unmotivated, depressed*). Such terminology may reveal more about the staff member than the patient. Maintaining client confidentiality while making helpful suggestions to staff and honoring staff integrity can severely tax the psychologist. Students committed to clinical positions in rehabilitation should seriously consider further intensive training during the internship and postdoctoral years in areas of interest. Other excellent suggestions relevant to assessment practices in rehabilitation can be found in Wedding and Faust (1989).

5. Students interested in working with persons in medical and health care settings should learn to integrate diagnostic and assessment data within meaningful models. Currently, it has been acknowledged that psychological adjustment among persons with chronic, debilitating physical conditions is influenced by myriad factors. Several models incorporating biological, social, environmental, and personal factors have been articulated for spinal cord injury (Frank, Umlauf, et al., 1987), rheumatoid arthritis (Anderson, Bradley, Young, McDaniel, & Wise, 1985), multiple sclerosis (Devins & Seland, 1987), and chronic pain (Flor, Birbaumer, & Turk, 1990). Of these models, the most succinct and comprehensive has been proposed by Dennis Turk and his colleagues. From this perspective, assessment of persons with physical disabilities should be conducted along three axes: biomedical, psychosocial, and behavioral (Turk & Rudy, 1987). The first axis includes any data regarding the person's physical condition, including information from physical examinations, laboratory tests, and assessments of functional mobility, strength, daily activities, and other dimensions as relevant. The second axis—psychosocial—involves the actual psychological assessment of affect, personality, cognitive styles, coping mechanisms, and other relevant personal characteristics such as mental functioning and intelligence. The last dimension—the behavioral axis—pertains to the observable behavior of the person, including overt behaviors in the rehabilitation unit, behaviors observed by others in the person's environment, the behavioral responses of significant persons in the client's life, client activity levels, and recreational and prescription drug usage. In this latter dimension, psychologists take into account interactions between the person and environment. The resulting conclusions and recommendations based on systematic data collection across these realms ideally would prove more reliable and valid than reliance on any one particular dimension.

Concluding Remarks

The above recommendations can be incorporated into current clinical and counseling training programs without unfairly taxing students or faculty or without compromising the quality of psychological service to persons with physical disabilities. It remains to be seen whether training programs will improve preparatory experiences for students to work competently with persons who have physical disabilities. Failure to address this need may result in further frustration for psychologists and consumers of rehabilitative services.

PART IV

Improving the Quality and Integrity of Rehabilitation Assessment Practices

CHAPTER 10

Psychosocial Rehabilitation Assessment: A Broader Perspective

DAVID S. CORDRAY
GEORGINE M. PION

Assessment is conducted for a variety of reasons and in numerous ways. In the context of rehabilitation services, it is most frequently undertaken as a means of determining a level (or levels) of functioning within individuals. When such assessments are followed by a prescription involving subsequent courses of action (e.g., therapy and training), additional assessments may be undertaken to establish whether a desired change in functioning occurred. If an acceptable level of functioning has been achieved over the course

AUTHORS' NOTE: Some of the concepts described in this chapter have evolved in part from our participation in a national evaluation sponsored by the National Institute on Alcoholism and Alcohol Abuse (NIAAA). One key component of this endeavor includes the support of 14 research demonstration projects on alcohol and other drug abuse interventions for homeless persons (NIAAA, 1991), along with an evaluation of the collective effort. Members of the National Evaluation Team who have contributed to the overall evaluation plan and its execution include Robert Orwin, Joseph Sonnefeld, and Laurie Teraspulsky (R.O.W. Sciences, Inc.); Friedner Wittman (CLEW Associates); Howard Goldman and Susan Ridgely (University of Maryland); Robert Huebner, Harold Perl, and Jack Scott (NIAAA). In accordance with contractual obligations, no site-specific data have been used in this chapter, and all methodological and programmatic examples are hypothetical and should not be attributed to any individual site and its experiences.

of treatment, clients may be released or they may enter into subsequent treatment phases. As emphasized in other chapters in this volume, given the importance of these channeling and transition decisions, it is necessary that assessment procedures be of appropriate technical quality, following acceptable psychometric practices.

Much of the emphasis in rehabilitation is on ways to improve the quality of individual-level assessment. Although this emphasis is appropriate, it is somewhat narrow in several ways. For example, when assessment is used to make decisions about channeling clients into specific service regimens (i.e., "matching" client needs with specific intervention strategies), there is often a large knowledge gap (depending upon the area) about what works best for specific types of clients. Under these circumstances, assessment concepts ought to be broadened to incorporate questions about treatment effectiveness. Stated somewhat more crudely, assessment of individual-level functioning is of limited value *unless* we know whether subsequent interventions are effective. This notion is not new, of course. Asking questions about treatment effectiveness, however, does raise a series of additional assessment issues. This chapter, in an effort to broaden the concepts of assessment within psychosocial rehabilitation, highlights assessment of intervention parameters. In making the case, we begin by providing an overview of some age-old (but nevertheless important) methodological and programmatic assessment issues.

Treatment Effectiveness Assessment

Syntheses of prior research, more often than not, conclude that the evidence on treatment effectiveness is mixed; that is, some proportion of the available studies report positive findings, a fraction suggest no differences, and there may even be a minority insinuating that an intervention is actually harmful to its recipients (relative to usual or customary care). As previously shown by Bond and Boyer (1988) and others, such heterogeneity of results also characterizes the field of psychosocial rehabilitation.[1]

At first glance, the presence of heterogeneous results would seem to pose no problem. After all, the scientific process is intended not only to "weed out" those interventions possessing little merit but also to retain strategies that seem beneficial. Under optimal circumstances, where control over the interventions, assignment process, and methods of assessment is high, results generated by traditional experimental methods can be generally trusted. In examining interventions that incorporate psychosocial rehabilitation approaches, however, experimental control often is difficult to achieve. Thus the process of discovering "what works for whom and under what conditions" is far more challenging and vulnerable to several sources of uncertainty. More to the point, determining what course of treatment ought to be provided once a diagnosis is made is far from clear, regardless of the technical quality of the client-level assessment process.

To increase the level of confidence that can be placed in the veracity of results generated by impact assessments of psychosocial rehabilitation strategies, whether they are positive, negative, or no difference, much can be learned by adopting a perspective that simultaneously incorporates consideration of research design, assessment, *and* programmatic (or intervention) issues. Planning studies that optimize the integrity of these domains should increase the chances of obtaining trustworthy and useful evidence on intervention efforts. In terms of implementation, this entails choosing a comprehensive set of research tactics that map onto the complexities of actual assessment conditions, interventions, and service delivery systems in which they are nested. Most of these research tactics to be discussed involve a network of assessment concerning individual characteristics that goes beyond establishing levels of functioning and features of the intervention.

A Partial Accounting of Variability

Although reviews of between-study differences routinely denote numerous potential reasons for "explaining" the heterogeneity in results, the literature to date has been relatively fragmented. The usual practice has been to identify selected features of the intervention/assessment process but stop short of furnishing an overall framework for how those pieces fit together. Some exceptions do exist in terms of explicit attention paid to the interrelationships among factors (e.g., Boruch & Gomez, 1977; Lipsey, 1990; Sechrest et al., 1979). The implementation details, however, remain in need of further articulation.

Judgments as to the success of an intervention traditionally have been based on reviews concerning the quality of the research design and methodology underlying results, that is, the strength of the basis for causal attribution (Cordray, 1990). Studies that rely on randomized experiments or high quality quasi experiments are viewed as producing trustworthy findings. It is not uncommon, however, to find heterogeneity in results even when there is homogeneity in research quality. Does this mean that results are equally trustworthy? Are the results specific to the context or method and therefore not generalizable? From a strict research perspective, answers to these questions seem straightforward, but these are not the appropriate questions. What we need to know is why heterogeneity exists in results across studies that claim—at least on the surface—to be testing the same general intervention, on clients with the same levels of functioning, and so on.

Distinguishing results solely on the strength of the basis for causal attribution (e.g., weak versus strong) represents only part of the picture. Part of the heterogeneity problem can be better understood by scrutinizing more closely the features of interventions. In particular, two separable notions have begun to chip away at our "black-box" conception of treatments. Namely, it has become more apparent that interventions are processes that vary in *strength* and *integrity*. Although these features generally assume a continuous form, each feature has been simply dichotomized as weak or strong for the purposes of clarity. Figure 10.1 shows eight possible design/treatment scenarios. As we shall demonstrate, attending to all of these sources of variability can work toward unraveling the mystery surrounding observations of study differences in effect sizes and even the direction of effects.

As should be obvious from Figure 10.1, there are often very good and compelling reasons for between-study differences in results. Thus a comprehensive understanding of treatment effects requires the conjoint consideration of programmatic and research design features. In this section, we first review some of the major methodological and programmatic-based sources of uncertainty that contribute to heterogeneity.

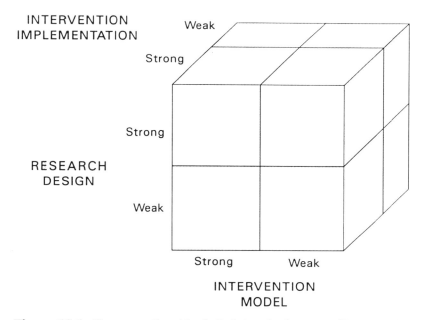

Figure 10.1.   Factors to Consider in Judging the Success of Interventions

Methodological Features and Sources of Fallibility

Regarding the basis for causal attribution, the fallibility of research methods (e.g., diagnostic assessment, assignment procedures, and statistical analyses) is readily apparent to any seasoned services researcher. Experience has told us that fallibility comes in several forms and is predictable under certain circumstances. For example, a chief culprit for no-difference findings is lower than expected sample sizes within conditions. This has become such an obvious problem that we now have the "Sechrest Rule,"[2] which can be liberally translated: "As soon as the ceremonial ribbons inaugurating a new treatment program are cut, 50% of the target population disappears." This "vanishing act" can be attributed to a myriad of implementation factors (e.g., insufficient recruitment of clients into the study, preassignment refusal by clients to accept the intervention or alternative conditions). Other possible suspects for weak causal attribution include insensitive measures, within-group heterogeneity of clients (e.g., differential severity of disorders), attrition from measurement, and "dropping out" of the intervention, to name a few. When considered individually, these transgressions may appear trivial, only involving a small fraction of the sample at each point of the assessment process. As we move from recruitment to final assessment, however, these various processes accumulate, posing the potential threat that statistical power will be insufficient to detect an effect—even if it is there.

Statistical power aside, inadequate control over plausible rival explanations within a given study (i.e., poor research design configurations), on a case-by-case review, often leave us with the impression that little faith can be placed in the results—positive, neutral, or negative. The use of true experimental designs, of course, facilitates appropriate inferences, but these are fragile entities that can easily devolve into quasi-experimental assessments due to the pressures of field conditions. To the extent that proper statistical models cannot be confidently applied, the causal inference is muddied at best. In the worst case, it becomes impossible to distinguish intervention failures from those implied by these methodological transgressions. This is only part of the picture, however. If program implementation is not carefully assessed (i.e., monitored) as part of the overall evaluation plan, the results of the study, regardless of whether the research design is strong or weak, are potentially confounded and still subject to heterogeneity.

Programmatic Features: Strength and Integrity

Interventions themselves are subject to a variety of external pressures that dampen their strength and integrity (Yeaton & Sechrest, 1981). By *strength,* we mean the intensity of the intervention relative to the magnitude of the problem that it is intended to correct. Relative strength of an intervention can also be defined in comparison with customary or usual care conditions. For example, if case management services provided to homeless substance abusers typically (under usual care circumstances) involve a ratio of 1 case manager for every 75 homeless clients, an intervention that reduces this ratio to 1:10 is a relatively strong service delivery alternative.

The integrity of an intervention should be distinguished from its strength; namely, the former refers to the *faithfulness* with which the intervention reflects its original conceptual model (i.e, the rationale for change or the theory that "explains" why the intervention ought to work), irrespective of the strength implied by the conceptual model. It should be obvious that, if the integrity of an intervention is incomplete, its strength is diluted in practice. When this happens, null results fail to distinguish between "theory", or model, failure and implementation failure (Lipsey, 1991). We return to these concepts in subsequent sections.

Although factors jeopardizing treatment integrity surface in many different types of social programs, the likelihood of their occurrence (at least at some level) may be exacerbated for psychosocial interventions that are targeted at individuals with multiple problems, that are committed to delivering multiple services (e.g., social skills training, enhancement of job skills, and mental health services) to address the range of problems, and/or that require participation by several different providers. Simply stated, under these conditions, there are additional opportunities for the original plan to be "watered down" in some way.

A Few Caveats

It is difficult to characterize prototypical methodological (design and assessment) and programmatic issues in psychosocial rehabilitation as a field partly because its substantive boundaries are far from clear.[3] As such, describing modal practices is next to impossible. The modal case may not necessarily generalize to other areas, or it easily may be dismissed as irrelevant. One approach to methodological issues in psychosocial rehabilitation then is to recognize these differences and tailor the discussion to the subclusters implied by these three dimensions—clients, interventions, and organizations. Another tactic—the one we have chosen here—is to capitalize on the "comprehensive case" or those forms of rehabilitation research that are most complex. By specifying the comprehensive case, it is possible to articulate how all the pieces *might* fit together. The importance of any particular segment within the comprehensive case can be considered (or ignored) on a situation-by-situation basis.

What, When, and How of Assessment

Simply exhorting investigators to devote closer attention to both methodological and programmatic issues can be interpreted at worst as "bordering on the obvious" and at best as another reiteration of previous counsel regarding what constitutes good practice. In the remainder of this chapter, however, our intent is to advance one step further by more explicitly demonstrating how best to work toward such integration. In general, this implementation occurs via three broad research activities: (a) in planning and designing both the intervention and the evaluation, that is, before the intervention is implemented; (b) in monitoring program implementation and the degree to which the research design has remained intact; and (c) in reporting the results of the impact assessment. To aid our discussion of these three strategies, Figure 10.2 provides a graphic representation of both the critical programmatic and the methodological features embodied in assessing the effectiveness of psychosocial rehabilitation interventions.

This integrated model is not new. Rather, it draws upon and integrates at least two well-established literatures. First, it draws upon the idea that careful articulation of the intervention model enhances our a priori understanding of how the intervention should work at both the operational and the conceptual levels. Here, we borrow concepts on and experiences with intervention articulation from Chen and Rossi (1983), Rutman (1980), Wang and Walberg (1983), Weick (1980), and Wholey (1977). Although such strategies are well known, prior discussions have generally overlooked how the research process fits into the overall scheme. Second, design issues are well understood; we draw upon the methodological literature for this part of the model. Those who have contributed greatly to our understanding of the research process have done so, however, by focusing on methodological features—the intervention being represented as merely an "X" in the classic Campbell and Stanley design configurations. Our model rectifies this by incorporating both sets of considerations into the same pictorial rendering.

What to Assess: Elements of the Model

As illustrated by Figure 10.2, the assessment process is far more elaborate than implied by conventional consideration of

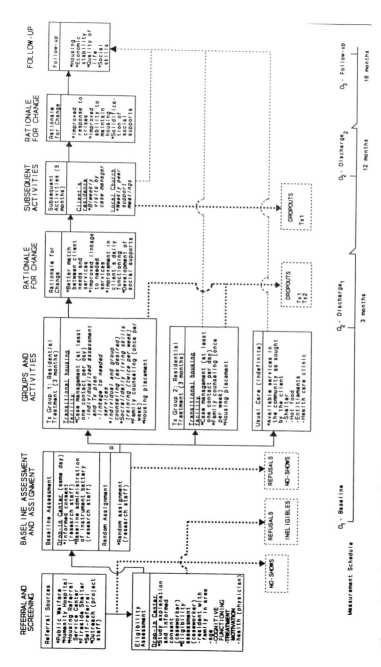

Figure 10.2. Integrated Methodological and Problematical Model: A Hypothetical Example

individual levels of functioning. The overall assessment and research design must map onto the structure and operations of the program throughout all its stages—from the moment an individual is identified as a potential client (which may be an informal or loose form of assessment) to his or her last recorded contact (i.e., the last scheduled assessment of participant outcomes). This comprehensive view of the assessment process can be roughly categorized into seven major components:

1. *Referral sources.* These include all possible "feeders" into the project such as community organizations, the individuals themselves (i.e., self-referrals), and more proactive outreach efforts undertaken by project staff (e.g., actively "beating the bushes" for potential participants).

2. *Screening assessment.* Not all persons identified as potentially eligible for participation in a study may be members of the true target population for a particular intervention. For example, the nature of some individual's problems may be too severe for consideration (e.g., a history of violent behavior that may endanger others) or not sufficiently serious to justify the use of limited project resources (e.g., an individual who is literally living "on the streets" and has no place to go may be more in need of services than a person who chooses to temporarily live in a shelter until he and his roommate "patch up" an argument). Thus there is a screening process, however cursory, to determine the eligibility of individuals for services. This process can be altered over time, as shown in the figure, by relaxing or tightening criteria (e.g., changing the minimal threshold for cognitive functioning and adding a screener for level of treatment motivation).

3. *Baseline assessment and assignment.* The crux of any evaluation design is the nature of the assignment process. Furthermore, the baseline assessment is essential for establishment of client needs, suitability, and preintervention standing on important variables. As stipulated in the figure, it is important to know the sequencing of assessment and assignment, who is responsible for each, and the context in which they occur. As one example, the potential opportunities for sabotaging the assignment process must be acknowledged through proper specification of staff, location, timing, and actual procedures.

4. *Groups and activities.* Fundamental to the evaluation design is an explication of the key ingredients that distinguish intervention(s) from comparison groups *and* their common elements. Ideally, these descriptions should denote the setting in which an activity occurs, who is designated to deliver the service, its required frequency and/or duration, and what it entails (e.g., individual or group counseling). These latter elements become the basis for establishing the strength of the intervention relative to its bases for comparison. For example, a treatment activity (relative to a comparison) may differ in terms of its frequency (number of times delivered per week), intensity (e.g., a face-to-face meeting with a case manager versus a brief telephone contact), or nature of activities (e.g., a goal-setting session with a client verus housing placement).

5. *Rationale for change.* Although not always well articulated, interventions do not "spring out of the blue"; rather, they are grounded in some notion about why the services to be delivered should remedy the targeted problem(s). To determine whether the mechanisms underlying the stated rationale are initiated by the intervention, assessment is needed.

6. *Subsequent activities.* Some interventions involve multiple phases through which all clients must progress, and each phase differs along the dimensions previously identified. Others provide more flexible opportunities (e.g., upon discharge, a participant can choose to attend or not attend program alumnae support group meetings and events).

7. *Final outcomes and follow-up.* The raison d'être of any impact assessment is collecting sound information on the outcomes of interest. The critical components include issues surrounding the optimal timing of each measurement wave (e.g., How long after discharge should the first follow-up occur?) and when change should be expected to occur on which variables.

When and How: Planning and Monitoring

Planning should not be approached in the abstract. Rather, it should be grounded in at least two ways. First, as reflected in Figure 10.2, the form of the treatment intervention needs to be articulated in sufficient detail to be capable of specifying what is *unique* about the intervention (i.e., its active ingredients) and what it has in common with the control condition; a *rationale for change* should also be posited (i.e., how the intervention is expected to work). These assessments, in turn, provide a foundation for the development of a measurement scheme that allows for tracking of the implementation of the intervention conditions.

This form of articulation and subsequent measurement is rare, and for very good reasons. Lipsey, Crosse, Dunkle, Pollard, and Stobart (1985) show that theorizing, itself, is relatively rare in juvenile justice intervention efforts. Mowbray and Herman (1991) concur in terms of mental health treatment strategies. Our experience suggests that much of what passes as the basis for an intervention is highly atheoretical, but this does not mean that the intervention developers do not also lack a rationale for why they believe the intervention will be successful. Clearly, it may be too much to ask that all studies have a full-blown theoretical rationale underlying them. Simply being clear on what is being tested by descriptively assessing treatment conditions, however, may constitute a major step toward increasing our understanding of how interventions work (or fail to work).

The second critical aspect of the planning process should incorporate a realistic characterization of the context within which the intervention is to be implemented. As can be seen in Figure 10.2, not only is client flow dependent upon knowing a great deal about the service system that surrounds the intervention, but knowledge concerning the types of services already in place (and therefore potentially overlapping) is also critical in specifying the potential "relative" strength of the proposed intervention. Furthermore, the rationale for the intervention, in part, delimits the scope and content of the baseline and follow-up assessment process. All of these issues influence, in turn, the estimation of effect size and the sample size needed to detect meaningful estimates of treatment effectiveness.

The planning process is filled with uncertainty. As most of us recognize, systematic planning in community-based research is based on incomplete information. After all, if we knew enough to perfectly plan all aspects of a study, it probably would be the case that the study does not need to be conducted. Professional experience, prior research, and the use of good sense within the planning process can increase the odds of success, but only to a degree.

And, although uncertainty can be lessened by merely being more clear about the nature of the intervention and its context, our characterization of the process appears to *increase* uncertainty by pointing out, explicitly, the numerous pieces of the puzzle that cannot be or are not known in advance.

Studies are rarely, if ever, planned and launched (or set adrift) while the researcher sits back and waits for the results to come in. Rather, the integrity of the intervention and the research design needs to be routinely assessed and adjusted as necessary. Furthermore, novel psychosocial interventions are even more dynamic than fixed treatment protocols, reacting to the ebbs and flows of internal and external forces, making assessment that much more important. Just as forecasters have trouble predicting the short-range future, systematic planning has its limits. As such, the monitoring function within this type of research is critical. It is through the specification of a plan and the monitoring of its fit with the services system and its integrity that the chances of interpretable evidence resulting are likely to be bolstered. In essence, monitoring is the fallback strategy for planning failures.

It is obvious that many aspects of the program/methods model need to be taken into account as part of planning and monitoring, and some are presumably more critical than others. Where, then, are the "softest spots" in the system, and what can be done to improve the odds that the program/research will be successful (or at least interpretable)? In our experience, the so-called soft spots in intervention research involve client flow, treatment specification, and power estimation. The following sections examine each in more detail.

Client Flow

As noted early, the "Sechrest Rule" implies that half the clients "vanish" as soon as treatment doors are opened. Where do they go? What, if anything, can be done to reduce this leakage? As a starting point for answering these types of questions, the modeling process depicted in the lower portion of Figure 10.2 delineates critical points in the client-flow process. For many intervention areas (e.g., job training), determining the number of eligible participants who might be served is relatively easy (e.g., checks are processed for recipients or permanent agency records of individuals served exist). Deriving estimates of the size of subgroups of at-risk populations (e.g., the homeless) is more difficult for several reasons. First, definitions of target populations are often vague. For example, it is extremely difficult to know the number of homeless individuals in a particular catchment area, given that definitions of the condition vary, ranging from literally homeless to precariously housed (e.g., "doubled up" with friends); methods of ascertainment are crude (e.g., service use records and self-report); and multiple services are used by this transient population (see Cordray & Pion, 1991; Wright, 1991). Given that a substantial amount of effort is required to unduplicate lists maintained by service agencies, obtaining even an order of magnitude estimate is often not a simple task, and resorting to professional "guesstimates" is quite common. Consequently, a partial explanation for the Sechrest Rule is that some potential participants never existed at the onset but were rather a result of wishful thinking, duplicated counts, or both.

Interventions are generally targeted at subgroups with particular types, levels, or constellations of dysfunction (e.g., homeless alcohol abusers *with* persistent and severe mental health disorders). The level of diagnostic care needed to accurately find individuals with specific disorders is exceptionally high, requiring considerable training, professional skill, and resources. To the extent that initial estimates of the size of the population do not take these attributes into account, the actual eligible pool will be reduced. Continuing with the homeless example, diagnosing their level of mental health disorders is still a relatively uncharted area and subject to great variability in estimates of prevalence. Lehman and Cordray (1991), in a reanalysis of prior estimates of the prevalence of mental health problems, substance abuse, and dual diagnoses (mental health *and* substance abuse problems) among the homeless, reveal that the size of the prevalence estimates depends heavily on the sensitivity and specificity of the diagnostic assessment methodology. Although approximately 50% of homeless persons have some form of diagnosed mental health problem, only about 20% have severe and persistent mental health problems. Without knowing the composition of the population, interventions targeted at the latter group could seriously overestimate the demand for their services, exceeding the Sechrest Rule's leakage of 50% by a great deal.

The Sechrest Rule suggests that clients disappear from the initial pool of eligibles. Figure 10.2 identifies numerous other points in the client-flow process that are vulnerable to client loss as well as the need for additional assessment (e.g., to model the influence of postassignment attrition). Some of these may be more directly under the control of the researcher (e.g., assignment and entry into the intervention) whereas others are not (e.g., decisions by a client to continue or not continue in the program for its intended duration). The magnitude of the influence of "leakage" from one point in the process to the next on the overall sample is not well documented. As stated above, one thing is certain—the influence is cumulative across stages of the client-flow process.

As a simple exercise, Figure 10.3 shows the cumulative effect of two levels of seemingly trivial "leakage" (from one stage to the next) and some preliminary data from our monitoring of the NIAAA homeless projects. In the first case (line A, Figure 10.3), we assume that the proportion of clients flowing from one stage to the next is .90. In the second case (line B), this proportion is set at .80. Five "points of leakage" are designated in our program/methods model. Applying the .90 and .80 transition probabilities across these nodes of the client-flow process (as depicted in Figure 10.2) suggests that the cumulative effect of leakage is quite dramatic; namely, even if leakage is seemingly minimal (.1) at each stage, over the study's time line, the cumulative effect is quite high—roughly a 40% loss. Reducing the transition probabilities to .8 (also seemingly high) reduces the number of clients who complete all phases of the intervention by nearly 70%.

Our monitoring of the early stages of a sample of the NIAAA homeless projects suggests that transition probabilities are not uniform across stages of the client-flow process. As shown in Figure 10.3 (line C), the greatest loss in clients is due to their ineligibility, unwillingness to be assessed (baselined), and limited retention in the interventions. That is, about half of the clients who were contacted by project staff were deemed eligible; about 60% of those deemed eligible consented to be assessed and assigned to interventions; and about half remained in the intervention for its intended duration. For those phases of the client-flow process that are most directly under the control of the researchers, transition probabilities are .93 and 1.0 (between assignment and

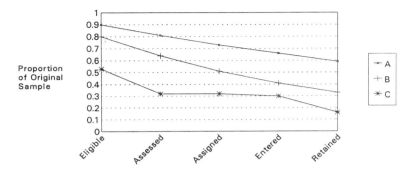

Progressive Stages in the Client Flow Process

Figure 10.3. Influence of Client Loss Over Successive Stages of the Client-Flow Process

NOTE: A assumes that the proportion of clients moving from one stage to the next is .9. B assumes that this proportion is .8. C is based on the preliminary aggregate data from eight sites participating in the NIAAA project.

entering the intervention and between baseline assessment to assignment, respectively). As can be seen, the cumulative effect of leakage (some of which was planned for as part of the original site-level proposals) reduces the number of clients who receive a full dose of the intervention to about one sixth of the original size of the population pool. Programmatic efforts to enhance retention and willingness to participate in the intervention (after eligibility has been determined) are currently under way as a result of these early warning signals.

Treatment Specification

Many forms of psychosocial rehabilitation involve diagnosis of an individual's level of functioning, the planning and delivery of tailored treatment regimens, and coordination among several service activities. In contrast to drug trials or other interventions that entail standardized treatment protocols following diagnosis, the form, duration, and intensity of the "treatment" that is to be delivered in psychosocial interventions can vary on a case-by-case basis. This form of tailoring does not mean that interventions are idiosyncratic. Rather, they usually involve an overarching model (in the broadest sense) or treatment philosophy that dictates (or at least directs) the clinical course. As such, two forms of treatment specification are required: (a) elaboration of the conceptual or philosophical model and (b) designatation of the specific menu of services that are available to clients (as needed). Using the terminology in Figure 10.2, the "rationale for change" involves this description of the model or philosophical orientation of the intervention strategy, and "groups and activities" denotes the catalog of possible services that are implied.

The treatment descriptions in Figure 10.2, however, are only part of the story. As previously argued, the strength and integrity of a psychosocial rehabilitation intervention must also be established. To accomplish this, we must move beyond mere description. Determining the strength and integrity of an intervention requires making comparative judgments according to evaluative criteria and principles. That is, we must assess whether an intervention ever was of sufficient potency to be capable of effecting the desired outcomes and whether the treatment as implemented adhered to its original model. With regard to the latter, the literature on program implementation provides much useful guidance in terms of identifying appropriate practice (e.g., Brekke, 1987; Kettner, Moroney, & Martin, 1990; Roberts-Gray & Scheirer, 1988). At the same time, how best to judge treatment strength remains relatively uncharted territory. The relationships depicted in Figure 10.4 may be useful in offering some preliminary thoughts for how to arrive at these judgments concerning treatment strength.

As shown, the etiology of the problem that an intervention is intended to address, of course, constitutes a major factor in judging the appropriateness (i.e., the plausibility that it might work) of any ameliorative efforts (path *a* in Figure 10.4). In addition, understanding the causal origins of a problem (e.g., homelessness) furnishes a way to ground judgments concerning the strength of an intervention model (path *c*), gas implemented. Developing interventions based on evidence about the nature of the problem is a formidable challenge that investigators must confront. Let us sidestep this for a moment to provide some commentary on areas that are challenging but less imposing.

As a point of departure, assessing treatment integrity involves a relative comparison between the model as planned and the treatment services as delivered (path *b* in Figure 10.4). As such, two

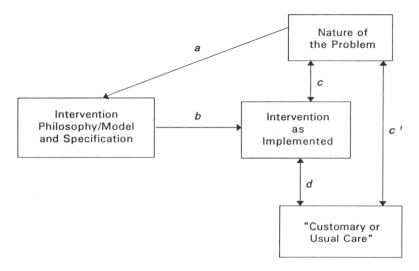

Figure 10.4. Treatment Integrity and Strength

types of assessment are needed. In its simplest form, this assessment entails a comparison of the description of the model and services that were *planned* versus the same set of descriptions concerning *what actually transpired*. For example, if a model for case management prescribes that an individualized treatment plan (ITP) be developed by the case manager for each client within 1 week of treatment entry, then such a document should be contained in each client's case file. With regard to more "demanding" intervention models, the integrity judgment becomes increasingly complex. That is, if the model specified that each client was to receive an ITP *and* this plan of needed services should be delivered in the "least restrictive environment," both the presence of a plan and the appropriateness of the service setting(s) must be assessed. An intervention then may receive a perfect score on the first "test" but be judged as below standards on the second criteria. This suggests that the development of assessment models for judging integrity must consider ways of differentially weighting the importance of program components.

As suggested above, judging the strength of an intervention is formidable for two reasons: (a) The origins of a problem are not always sufficiently understood to assure that a limited set of proper courses of action exist; and (b) it is exceedingly difficult to transform a multivariate set of intervention activities into a dosage level.[4] Similar to judgments of integrity, however, the strength of an intervention can be cast as a relative judgment. We can circumvent the epistemological quagmire of rendering a judgment for path *c* by recognizing that most intervention studies involve comparison groups composed of individuals who receive "usual care" or customary services rather than no treatment or services. Because usual care or circumstances represent actions intended to address the same problems, they too can be characterized as possessing some degree of strength (path *c'*). By closely examining the unique and common features that distinguish each condition—akin to the "method of difference" logic of experimental control (Boring, 1954)—it is possible to derive an index of "relative strength" within any intervention study (path *d*). Our hypothetical example displayed in Figure 10.2 illustrates how relative strength between alternative treatments can be characterized, using comprehensive descriptions of unique services (those elements in italics) and common services available to each group. When sufficient descriptive evidence on routine service provision (i.e., usual care) is available through existing agency records or pilot data, an a priori judgment of relative strength is possible. Obviously, when this is lacking, post hoc assessments become the only recourse. With a little effort (e.g., pilot testing), this dependence can be reduced.

The Dynamics of Intervention Research: Monitoring and Controlling Treatment Drift

Similar to other social programs, the successful implementation of psychosocial rehabilitation interventions that adhere closely to their intended models is dependent on a whole host of factors, including the availability of qualified staff, acquisition of appropriate physical facilities, cooperation of other service providers in the community, and political views. Furthermore, even when fully implemented, rehabilitation interventions do not operate in a vacuum but are part of a services delivery system that is volatile (e.g., Rossi & Freeman, 1989). Obviously, such "environmental" fluctuations can affect the program's continued ability to achieve full-scale implementation (e.g., linkages with other providers can be eroded due to staff and administrative turnover). Moreover, contextual shifts also can affect changes in what constitutes "usual or customary care"; for example, available services can be eliminated by state and local funding cuts, and new treatment options can become available to those assigned to the "usual care" condition by funding opportunities. As such, one's ability not only to determine the impact of an intervention but also to judge the "relative strength" of an intervention by comparing it with "usual or customary care" (path *d*) can be hampered. We refer to these alterations as "treatment drift," that is, the extent to which groups converge (or diverge) over the course of the study. This "volatility" of the treatment and its intended bases for comparison can result from four different scenarios.[5]

"Watering down" of the intervention of interest. A problem commonly discussed in the literature (e.g., Rossi, 1978) involves the situation where the delivery of the intervention is "incomplete" or "diluted." The precipitating factors are several and can be attributed to difficulties encountered in services delivery, client receipt of the services, or both. For example, some intervention models involve the use of staff with certain expertise (e.g., individuals who have specific clinical training and who are willing to be "live-in" counselors), and difficulty may be encountered in hiring qualified individuals due to budget constraints (e.g., low salaries) or applicants' unwillingness to reside in a facility. Consequently, if rapid crisis intervention and the establishment of strong counselor-client relationships are key ingredients of the intervention, access to a counselor for only 8 rather than 24 hours a day introduces problems in implementation. Because the client receives a lower-than-intended "dose," the "distance" between the treatment and "usual care" conditions shrinks. As is obvious, assessments as to both the integrity and the strength of the treatment are adversely affected.

Enhancement of "customary or usual" care. Commitment to remedying a target population's problems (e.g., those experienced by homeless individuals with serious mental problems) typically is not unique to the group involved in the intervention being studied. As such, the simple fact that a new program exists (i.e., the intervention) may serve as a catalyst to existing agencies, spurring them to revise their existing services to resemble those of the innovation (e.g., the assignment of a specific case manager to each client rather than having a "whoever is available" procedure) or to develop new components that are potentially as effective as those incorporated by the program of interest. In addition, both public and private sponsors of "usual care" introduce changes through revisions in program regulations (e.g., expanding services to be reimbursed by Medicaid) or funding new initiatives to be carried out by "usual care" providers.

Contamination or leakage. The basis for comparison also can be diminished by client and/or provider behaviors that work toward eliminating distinctions between the services provided in each condition. For example, consider a study with a target population (e.g., homeless) in which individuals from two city shelters are assigned either to the experimental group (those who receive a specially structured curriculum for daily living skills) or to a group that receives no special care. Here, the danger looms that participants of each group have the opportunity to intermingle during certain activities (e.g., meals) and what was learned by the experimental group can be communicated to their "usual care" counterparts. Contamination also can occur by permitting the same set of intervention staff (e.g., specially trained case managers) to provide services not only to the experimental group but also to the usual care clients (even on an occasional basis to help evenly distribute caseload across all agency case managers).

Strength of "common ingredients" relative to "unique" components. In some cases, it may be plausible that the "unique" elements of the intervention pale relative to their commonly shared components with the usual care condition in terms of expected potency. The consequence is that the probability of detecting differences in outcomes is reduced. For example, consider a substance abuse treatment program designed for homeless women and children that permits the families to remain "intact" during the mother's treatment. The program receives external funding to test the addition of a new component—the provision of supported work. If allowing women to be with their children is the critical element for engagement and completion of treatment, the likelihood of finding no added value of supported work is increased.

Social experimentation involves testing whether potentially innovative treatments actually outperform customary or usual care configurations. As such, implementation failures, treatment drift, and all other operational difficulties that might surface should be part of the assessment of treatment efficacy. It might be said that a good idea that cannot withstand the pressures of the real world is probably not a good idea after all. On the other hand, some forms of drift are due to premature imitation (e.g., upgrading the usual care). In this case, before the "verdict is in" regarding the intervention's efficacy, bits and pieces are being unsystematically adopted by other settings. This may or may not be good practice, and several alternatives seem sensible. At the very least, careful accounting of changes in service packages, across groups, is necessary. At the other extreme, close monitoring and thoughtful technical assistance might provide sufficient resources to maintain or optimize the original plan. Although conventional wisdom suggests that holding interventions constant is unrealistic and may be akin to wrestling with a bear, some confrontations are worthwhile. Perhaps the more important issue is this: Where should our energies be placed?

Client Flow, Drift, and Power

One main contention of this chapter is that the joint consideration of programmatic (e.g., treatment drift) and methodological issues (e.g., sample size resulting from the client-flow process) is essential for increasing the overall quality of impact assessments. Failure to plan for client loss across critical stages of research process can have substantial consequences for the overall design, seriously undermining the chances of detecting an effect of the intervention. As an illustration, returning to our hypothetical intervention depicted in Figure 10.2, suppose the expected effects size of the comparison between the first intervention and the "usual care" is four tenths (.40) of a pooled standard deviation. For a two-tailed test (alpha = .05 and statistical power of .80), a sample size of 100 per group would be required. A loss of 25 clients (per group) reduces statistical power to .68 (a 15% reduction) and statistical power dips to .50 (a 38% loss) when the processes associated with client flow decrease the sample by half (in both groups).

The recognition that the attained sample size will be the product of a chain of transition probabilities provides a useful starting point for the planning process. Here, "backward mapping" of the client-flow process, taking into account the expected loss at each stage, can provide realistic initial (as part of recruiting) sample sizes. Doubling the recruitment effort (if feasible) at the "front end" increases the chances that the attained sample size will be sufficient (of course, internal and external validity can be threatened by various forms of client loss, and these cannot be compensated for by simply increasing sample sizes). Although acknowledging these sources of loss during the planning process is important, actual monitoring of the client-flow process over the course of the project is essential. We have found it useful to establish a management plan that entails monthly recruiting goals, along with methodological (enhanced outreach) and programmatic (e.g., removing barriers) modifications to correct and account for shortfalls. Lipsey (1991) provides sage advice on how to increase design sensitivity through a variety of means.

Client retention in the intervention has a compounding effect on statistical power. It also complicates the causal inference process by potentially introducing pre- and postassignment selection biases. Assuming that this latter problem can be handled as part of the statistical analysis (i.e., modeling) phase of the study (see Cordray, 1986), it is possible to get a sense of the separate influence of partial receipt of treatment on statistical power. Altering the example from above, suppose retention was .75 (that is, 75% of the clients received the full dose, and the average effect size is .40). Assume that the clients who did not receive the full dose dropped out of the intervention immediately after being assigned. If we also assume that this subgroup received no benefit from the intervention (the effect size for them would be .00) and that the pooled standard deviation is unaffected by partial receipt of the intervention, the new effect size would be .30 (or .75 × .40 = .30). With the same sample sizes as above, effective statistical power would be no more than .56, or a 30% reduction, as compared with the initial plan (because of an increase in variance due to partial exposure, the power would be lower than stated here; see Lipsey, 1991). If retention were 50% in the intervention group, the effect size would be .20, and the achieved statistical power would be no more than .30 (a 63% reduction).

Given this line of reasoning, it is relatively easy to consider the impact of the treatment drift described in an earlier section. Returning to Figure 10.4, recall that path *d* was designated as the relative strength of the intervention versus a comparison or control condition. If the treatment and control conditions become similar (either qualitatively or quantitatively) over the course of the study, statistical power is greatly reduced. As with retention, the influence of treatment drift is multiplicative (also see Boruch & Gomez, 1977).

Because of the interdependencies among methodological and programmatic elements of services research, it is difficult to provide precise estimates of their separable influence on the sensitivity of the overall design. Coupling the results of the simple examples above with the algebra underlying the Boruch and Gomez (1977) augmented formulation for statistical power in true experiments, however, it is fairly clear that treatment strength and integrity play a much greater role in dampening results than classically viewed methodological features of the design. Efforts to maintain treatment integrity and full receipt should be given high priority.

Summary

We began this discussion with the idea that assessment in psychosocial rehabilitation should be broadened to include treatment parameters. Further, we noted that evidence on treatment effectiveness is generally mixed. Implicit in this focus is a concern about the trustworthiness of these patterns of results. Is the evidence on positive effects correct? Do no-difference findings really mean that the intervention has no merit? As shown, there are numerous methodological and programmatic sources of uncertainty that promote such heterogeneity and uncertainty. To date, an almost lavish amount of attention has been directed at the technocratic features of services research; more attention is now needed with regard to the programmatics of interventions. An interpretive perspective that integrates features of the research and the intervention is offered as a way of sorting prior results and for improving future conduct.

In our view, broadening the assessment process involves integrated planning and monitoring of client flow, explicit treatment specification within and across groups or conditions, and treatment drift. Currently, application of this perspective is handicapped by the lack of information on simple issues such as expected client flow, retention rates, and other transition probabilities. Furthermore, based on our reading of reports recounting prior studies, such reports are woefully inadequate in their descriptions of what happened inside and outside the "black box" labeled as treatment. More complete reporting is needed (see Cordray & Sonnefeld, 1985). In particular, additional attention must be directed at describing (a) how many "participants" were encountered at each stage of the client-flow process; (b) what services were and were not delivered in each condition (e.g., see Figure 10.2); (c) the amount of treatment that participants in each group received; and (d) how the interventions and their bases for comparison changed over time. To the extent that this information is assiduously collected and reported, planning and execution of future studies will be enhanced.

Notes

1. Our use of the term *psychosocial rehabilitation* in this chapter coincides with that provided by the International Association for Psychosocial Rehabilitation Services (1985), which characterizes this approach as "the process of facilitating an individual's restoration to an optimal level of independent functioning in the community . . . [that] seeks a comprehensive approach to the provision of vocational, residential, social/recreational, educational, and personal adjustment services" (p. 111). As Cnaan, Blankertz, Messinger, and Gardner (1988) point out, this generic definition has encompassed a variety of approaches and target populations.

2. The origins of this rule are actually somewhat unclear. We have also heard it referred to as the Boruch Axiom. It is probably the case that they both thought of it independently.

3. As Cnaan et al. (1988) have noted, psychosocial rehabilitation has been referred to by various labels (e.g., psychiatric rehabilitation and psychoeducation), applied to a range of target populations (e.g., people with head injuries, individuals with psychiatric problems, and prisoners), and involved various mixtures of services. Moreover, even when interventions are aimed at the same population and seek to deliver the same set of services, they may be structurally implemented in different fashions.

4. To be concrete, consider a very simple analogy. Aspirin is labeled as having a specified strength of its active ingredient (e.g., 500 mg). Whether this is a strong or weak dosage depends upon the severity of one's headache. For those normal types of headaches that result from trying to write a chapter, 500 mg of aspirin is a strong intervention. If the chapter is not finished on time and causes migraine headaches, the same 500 mg dosage is judged to be weak.

5. Our discussion of "treatment drift" is based on a collaborative analysis with Rob Orwin (R.O.W. Sciences, Inc.). It should be noted that additional threats to maintaining the distinctiveness of study groups exist but are not a result of *treatment drift* per se. First, some impact studies examine two treatment alternatives rather than a comparison of an intervention with a "customary care" or "no treatment" condition. In this case, the ability to detect differences (path *d*) is impeded by the possibility that both treatments may perform equally well. Without a counterfactual group, no-difference findings are highly plausible and may lead to the erroneous inference that the interventions do not work. Second, in contrast to changes in the services provided by a group, shifts may occur in terms of unanticipated disparities between the intended and enrolled participants of a target population. These typically result from problems associated with identifying the appropriate target population (e.g., some homeless persons may be too cognitively or physically disabled to benefit from interventions that focus on job training or housing placement) or selecting participants (e.g., screening for those who are committed to treatment and who might improve "on their own" or as a result of almost any type of service). Lipsey (1991) refers to this as a client × treatment interaction.

CHAPTER 11

Evaluating the Measurement Properties of Rehabilitation Assessment Instruments

JEFFREY B. BROOKINGS
BRIAN BOLTON

In evaluating the construct validity of rehabilitation assessment instruments, an important issue is *factorial validity,* the extent to which the items and relationships among them are consistent with the underlying theoretical construct or constructs they are hypothesized to measure. A second important issue, *factorial invariance,* concerns the equivalence of the scale's factor structure across two or more populations and is of special interest to rehabilitation psychologists, given the frequency with which measures normed on other populations (e.g., the Minnesota Satisfactoriness Scales) have been used for assessment of rehabilitation clients' employment functioning.

Until recently, studies of the factorial validity and factorial invariance of psychological measures were conducted using exploratory factor analysis (EFA). EFA is quite useful in situations where the researcher has no a priori factorial hypothesis but seeks instead to identify (i.e., "explore") the previously unknown factors underlying associations among measured variables, such as questionnaire items (for detailed discussions of EFA methods, see Gorsuch, 1983, 1988).

In studies of published measures, however, there is always at least one a priori factorial hypothesis: the factor structure reflected in the recommended scale or subscale scoring procedure. Also, subsequent studies may produce findings that suggest additional factor models for consideration. In these situations, tests of alternative factor models—using recently developed confirmatory factor analysis (CFA) methods—are preferable to EFA, where there are limitations on the types of factor models that can be specified and ambiguity in the evaluation of competing solutions (see Hertzog, 1989).

In a broader context, CFA can be viewed as one element of the latent variable analysis procedures that constitute structural equation modeling (SEM). Briefly, SEM involves (a) a measurement model, which specifies relationships between measured and latent variables (i.e., factor loadings) and is assessed using CFA, and (b) a structural model, which posits causal relations among the latent variables. The role of CFA, then, is to identify latent variables, which are examined subsequently in relation to other latent variables to provide evidence on a variety of scale properties, including convergent and discriminant validity, predictive validity, and so on (see Bentler, 1988; Loehlin, 1987). The principal strength of SEM methods over other multivariate procedures, such as multiple regression and path analysis, is the assessment of latent variables represented by multiple indicators, which removes measurement error from the regression coefficients estimated in the structural model.

In this chapter, we will focus on CFA, using three examples, to illustrate the utility of the procedure for investigating the factorial validity and factorial invariance of multiscale inventories used in rehabilitation assessment. The analyses described here were conducted using the most popular of the CFA computer programs: LISREL (Jöreskog & Sörbom, 1984). Other software packages for performing CFA, including EQS (Bentler, 1985) and LISCOMP (Muthén, 1987), however, are available as well.

Model Specification

CFA of a multiscale inventory using LISREL entails specifying three matrices that are analogous to the factor pattern matrix,

TABLE 11.1
Pattern of Fixed and Estimated Parameters for the GATB Subscales

GATB Subscale	Cognitive	Perceptual	Psychomotor	Error/ Uniqueness
Factor loadings:				
Verbal (V)	X	0	0	X
Numerical (N)	X	0	0	X
Spatial (S)	0	X	0	X
Form (P)	0	X	0	X
Clerical (Q)	0	X	0	X
Motor (K)	0	0	X	X
Finger (F)	0	0	X	X
Dexterity (M)	0	0	X	X
Factor correlations:				
Cognitive	1			
Perceptual	X	1		
Psychomotor	X	X	1	

NOTE: Zeroes and 1s represent parameters fixed by hypothesis, and Xs represent parameters estimated by LISREL.

factor correlation matrix, and communalities from an EFA. Table 11.1 shows these three matrices for a CFA of the General Aptitude Test Battery (GATB; U.S. Department of Labor, 1982a). The data for this example are from a sample of 1,025 vocational rehabilitation clients.

The three columns in the center of the upper portion of Table 11.1 reflect the hypothesized subscale structure of the GATB. The columns of the matrix represent latent variables (i.e., factors) and the rows represent measured variables, which may be items, item "parcels," or, as in this example, subscales. Zeroes indicate parameters fixed at zero and Xs represent parameters that are free and estimated by LISREL. The model specified in Table 11.1, which was derived from previous research on the GATB by Hunter (1980), is a three-factor "simple structure" model; that is, each subscale is hypothesized to load on only one factor.

Directly below the subscale target matrix is the factor variance/ covariance matrix, which contains estimates of relationships among the latent variables. The matrix in Table 11.1 reflects an oblique factor model; all of the factor covariances are free and estimated. Also, the elements on the principal diagonal, the factor variances,

TABLE 11.2

Correlation Matrix and Descriptive Statistics for the GATB Subscales

GATB Subscale	V	N	S	P	Q	K	F	M
Verbal (V)	—							
Numerical (N)	620	—						
Spatial (S)	442	413	—					
Form (P)	471	517	549	—				
Clerical (Q)	573	626	387	689	—			
Motor (K)	330	366	191	449	530	—		
Finger (F)	250	313	281	475	403	477	—	
Dexterity (M)	231	292	232	454	423	617	662	—
Mean	85.8	79.4	91.7	92.1	96.9	82.9	73.9	81.0
SD	15.7	33.7	30.7	33.3	16.2	21.8	26.4	30.1

NOTE: Decimals are omitted from the correlation coefficients. $N = 1,025$. All correlations are statistically significant ($p < .05$, two tailed).

are fixed at 1. This was done because, in CFA, it is necessary to fix one parameter for each latent variable, either a factor loading or the factor variance, at some nonzero value, to establish the scale of the factor and identify the model (Long, 1983). Also, fixing the factor variance at 1, as we did in this example, produces a "standardized" solution, which transforms the factor covariances to correlations to facilitate interpretation.

Finally, the far right-hand column of Table 11.1 is a vector of error/uniquenesses for each measured variable. These values are a combined estimate of unreliable variance (error) and reliable variance not shared with the other measured variables (uniqueness) and are equivalent to 1 minus the communality.

Descriptive statistics and the correlation matrix for the eight subscales are presented in Table 11.2. It is generally recommended that CFAs be performed on variance/covariance matrices (Cudeck, 1989), particularly if the researcher is interested in assessing the invariance of the parameter estimates (e.g., factor loadings) across populations. In this example, however, the analyses were based on the correlation matrix to simplify interpretation of the results.

Estimated factor loadings, error/uniquenesses, and factor correlations for the three-factor model are shown in Table 11.3. All of the parameters are within acceptable ranges (e.g., error/uniquenesses > 0), and all are significantly different than zero ($p < .05$).

TABLE 11.3
Parameter Estimates for the GATB Three-Factor Model

GATB Subscale	Cognitive	Perceptual	Psychomotor	Error/ Uniqueness
Factor loadings:				
Verbal (V)	.760	0	0	.423
Numerical (N)	.816	0	0	.334
Spatial (S)	0	.558	0	.689
Form (P)	0	.815	0	.336
Clerical (Q)	0	.843	0	.289
Motor (K)	0	0	.715	.489
Finger (F)	0	0	.750	.437
Dexterity (M)	0	0	.853	.273
Factor correlations:				
Cognitive	1			
Perceptual	.855	1		
Psychomotor	.464	.669	1	

NOTE: Fit indexes: χ^2/df = 13.95; RMSR = .05; TLI = .88. Zeroes and 1s represent parameters fixed by hypothesis. All estimated parameters are statistically significant (p <.05).

The factor correlations, which represent correlations among the latent constructs (assuming error-free measurement), are highly similar in pattern and magnitude to those reported by Hunter (1980) for 23,428 workers from the general adult working population.

Assessment of Overall Model Fit

The χ^2 test statistic is a global indicator of a model's ability to reproduce the sample correlation matrix. A *nonsignificant* χ^2 indicates a good fitting model, but the statistic is extremely sensitive to sample size. Almost any model will be statistically rejected if the sample size is large. For example, the χ^2 for our three-factor model is 237.13 (df = 17), which is significant at the .001 level.

Conversely, a poor fitting model may produce a nonsignificant χ^2 if the sample size is small enough. Therefore assessments of model fit and comparisons of alternative models require the use of substantive and practical criteria, in conjunction with indexes of model fit (see Marsh, Balla, & McDonald, 1988, for a comprehensive evaluation of CFA fit indexes). Three of the most frequently reported fit indexes, shown at the bottom of Table 11.3 for the three-factor GATB model, are as follows:

1. The χ^2/df ratio provides information on the relative fit of alternative models to the data. Various authors have suggested values ranging anywhere from 2.0 to 5.0 as representing adequate fit. Because the ratio is based in part on the χ^2 statistic, however, it too is highly sensitive to sample size, hence the large χ^2/df value (13.95) for the three-factor GATB model.

2. The root mean square residual (RMSR; Jöreskog & Sörbom, 1984) is a measure of average residual correlation, that is, the average difference between the values in the sample correlation matrix and the correlations implied by the model. Based on Cole's (1987) suggestion that values ≤ .10 indicate an acceptable fit, the RMSR of .05 is supportive of the three-factor representation of the GATB.

3. The Tucker-Lewis Index (TLI; Tucker & Lewis, 1973) scales the χ^2 from 0 to 1 and reflects the proportion of covariance explained by a model. Zero represents the fit of a null model (Bentler & Bonett, 1980), which assumes that the measured variables are uncorrelated, and 1 represents a perfectly fitting model. Larger values therefore indicate better fit, and the .88 computed for this example compares favorably with the values (.85 to .90) recommended by researchers. Of the fit indexes evaluated by Marsh et al. (1988), the TLI was most independent of sample size.

The fit indexes reported in Table 11.3 for our three-factor model illustrate several important issues for researchers to consider when using CFA. First of all, different indexes may lead to different conclusions about a model. The χ^2/df value (as well as the χ^2 test statistic reported earlier) would lead to rejection of the three-factor model, while the RMSR and TLI suggest that the model should be accepted.

A second issue is that, until recently, there was little guidance in the literature regarding the "best" index or indexes to use. Fortunately, Marsh et al. (1988) identified the factors, including model fit, that influence the various fit indexes, so that researchers can select *combinations* of indexes that compensate for the shortcomings of the individual indexes. Finally, because the various fit indexes are interpreted using "rules of thumb," rather than specific statistical criteria, the evaluation of model adequacy must always involve the researcher's substantive knowledge of a scale and the construct it is intended to measure.

Applications of CFA in Rehabilitation Assessment

Until recently, few CFA studies of assessment instruments have been reported in the rehabilitation literature. In this section, we summarize briefly the results of two published studies to illustrate the application of CFA for the purpose of assessing the psychometric adequacy of rehabilitation assessment instruments. (Interested readers should consult the primary sources for more detailed descriptions of the studies.) We conclude with a look at some recent developments in CFA and covariance structure modeling techniques and the implications of these developments for investigations of rehabilitation assessment instruments and prediction of vocational rehabilitation outcome.

The U.S. Employment Service Interest Inventory

Our first example is a CFA of the U.S. Employment Service Interest Inventory (USES-II; U.S. Department of Labor, 1982b) for 732 adult clients (502 males, 230 females) at a comprehensive medical and vocational rehabilitation institution (the USES-II is described in Bolton & Brookings, this volume; details of these analyses are reported in Brookings & Bolton, 1989). The primary purpose of the analysis was to determine whether the 12-scale structure of the USES-II, which evolved from analyses of samples drawn from the general adult population, would obtain also for vocational rehabilitation clients. This is an important issue because the 12 interest categories serve as the primary organizing basis for the occupational information presented in the U.S. Department of Labor's (1979) *Guide for Occupational Exploration* (GOE); therefore confirmation of the 12-scale structure for vocational rehabilitation clients is an important first step in validating the Department of Labor's vocational counseling system for this population.

A secondary objective was to use hierarchical confirmatory factor analysis (HCFA) to determine whether there is a meaningful second-order organization of the 12 scales. The purpose of HCFA is to assess the extent to which a hypothesized higher order factor (or factors) accounts for correlations among the first-order factors. As used here, the technique involves factor analyzing the matrix of correlations among the 12 first-order factors. The second-order models were derived from Prediger's (1976) "world-of-work map," Roe's (1956, 1985) circumplex arrangement of work fields, and Holland's (1984) hexagonal model. Of particular interest was the GOE assertion that scores on the USES-II scales can be related directly to the six interest areas contained in Holland's model.

The CFAs provided strong support for the 12-factor model for both males (χ^2/df = 1.85, RMSR = .05, TLI = .92) and females (χ^2/df = 1.45, RMSR = .06, TLI = .92). All of the estimated factor loadings (i.e., those not fixed at 0) were statistically significant (p <.05) and large (mean target loadings were .76 and .75 for males and females, respectively). Also, the interfactor correlations were generally low to moderate, indicating that all 12 factors were clearly defined. Finally, results of the HCFAs indicated that none of the hypothesized second-order models provided an adequate fit to the data.

On the basis of these results, it was concluded that (a) the 12-factor model provided the most accurate and parsimonious representation of the USES-II for vocational rehabilitation clients; (b) the results supported the use of the Department of Labor's Counselee Assessment/Occupational Exploration System with rehabilitation clients; and (c) vocational counseling strategies based on the assumption that USES-II scores can be translated directly into Holland categories are not warranted.

The Minnesota Satisfactoriness Scales

Our second example is a CFA of the Minnesota Satisfactoriness Scale (MSS; Gibson, Weiss, Hendel, Dawis, & Lofquist, 1970) items for 174 workers with severe handicaps to employment (for a description of the MSS, see Bolton & Brookings, this volume; for details on the analyses reported here, see Brookings & Bolton, 1991).

There is considerable evidence that the MSS is a reliable and valid measure of the satisfactoriness construct. Even though the MSS has been used in several studies of workers with disabilities, there have been no factor analyses of MSS ratings for this population.

The analyses, then, addressed two primary issues: (a) the factorial validity of the MSS four-subscale/General Satisfactoriness scale structure for workers with severe handicaps to employment, using CFA and HCFA, and (b) the factorial invariance of the MSS, assessed by conducting parallel HCFAs of data for the MSS developmental sample (i.e., a sample of 2,373 workers without handicaps used in the *development* of the MSS) and by comparing overall model fit and parameter estimates for the two populations.

In addition to the null model, the following factor models were evaluated: (a) a one-factor General Satisfactoriness model, based on the relatively large interitem correlations reported in the MSS manual (ranging from .10 to .86, mean $r = .35$); (b) a four-factor oblique model with latent variables corresponding to the MSS subscales; and (c) a hierarchical model with a second-order factor hypothesized to account for covariances among the four first-order factors. The hierarchical model corresponds directly to the four subscale/General Satisfactoriness scale scoring scheme recommended by Gibson et al. (1970) and therefore represents the "target" model. As with the USES-II example, however, we focused initially on the MSS first-order factor structure prior to evaluating the second-order target model.

Fit indexes for the analyses of the client and developmental data indicated that, for both samples, the four-factor and second-order models were superior to the one-factor model, even after the greater parsimony of the one-factor model was taken into account. These results provided strong support for the factorial validity of the MSS for workers with severe handicaps to employment and for the invariance of this structure across populations. Also, because both the four-factor and second-order models fit the data better than did the one-factor model, it was concluded that scoring the MSS as a unidimensional scale only would result in the loss of potentially useful information contained in the four subscales. Therefore rehabilitation researchers and counselors using the MSS should follow the recommended procedure of scoring the four subscales *and* the General Satisfactoriness scale.

Recent Developments in CFA Methodology

CFA and the software packages used to implement it are constantly evolving; consequently, new developments in the technique are appearing almost daily. One example of this rapid evolution is an issue addressed in this chapter: factorial invariance. In the LISREL manual, Jöreskog and Sörbom (1984) described a series of four tests used to determine the correspondence of factors across populations. More recently, Drasgow and Kanfer (1985) pointed out several problems that may arise in invariance tests as a result of violations of distributional assumptions and recommended adaptations in the procedure to overcome these problems. Finally, Byrne and her colleagues (Byrne, Shavelson, & Muthén, 1989) have provided researchers with detailed procedures to follow in assessing the invariance of measuring instruments, and Byrne's (1989) nonmathematical introduction to LISREL includes the data matrices and LISREL program input needed to duplicate all of the analyses reported in her book.

HCFA is another procedure receiving increased attention in the measurement literature. Marsh and his colleagues (e.g., Marsh, 1987; Marsh & Hocevar, 1985) have published a number of HCFA studies using LISREL; Hertzog (1989) has provided an excellent primer on evaluating hierarchical models; and Rock, Bennett, and Jirele (1988) described several procedures that are useful for assessing the invariance of higher order factors.

A third area that has produced rapid developments in CFA methodology is the assessment of convergent and discriminant validity via multitrait-multimethod (MTMM) designs. Cole (1987) described the advantages of CFA over EFA for separating trait and method variance in MTMM studies, and Widaman (1985) outlined a CFA-based procedure for evaluating convergent and discriminant validity of psychological measures (see also Byrne, 1989). Subsequently, Marsh and Hocevar (1988) noted weaknesses in the analysis of MTMM data using the "traditional" CFA approach (e.g., the inability to separate measurement error from uniqueness) and proposed HCFA as a means of overcoming these weaknesses.

Finally, as noted earlier, the latent variables identified via CFA can then be examined in relation to other latent variables (i.e., in a structural model) to provide evidence on various scale or subscale properties. Lewis and Bolton (1986), for example, used CFA to identify three latent independent variables (educational attainment, work values, and opportunity structure) and one latent dependent variable (occupational attainment) for a sample of 380 vocational rehabilitation clients. Next, they assessed structural models representing causal effects of the latent independent variables on the latent dependent variable. Of the three latent independent variables, educational achievement had the largest effect on occupational attainment.

Comments on CFA

CFA represents a powerful and potentially useful methodology for assessing the psychometric adequacy of rehabilitation assessment instruments. It has numerous advantages over EFA for analyzing published instruments, as the examples described in this chapter demonstrate, and is embedded in a broader methodology for assessing causal models of vocational rehabilitation outcomes. A cautionary note is in order, however. The legitimacy of some procedures (e.g., the "sensitivity analyses" advocated by Byrne et al., 1989), which involve successive iterations and reestimations of a particular model, is debatable (see Cliff, 1983). In any event, it is clear that, as the number of post hoc modifications of a model increases, the study moves rapidly along the continuum from confirmatory to exploratory. In this regard, Gorsuch (1988) has noted that confirmatory factor analysis is a poor exploratory technique. Finally, the most important ingredient in the psychometric evaluation of rehabilitation assessment instruments is still sound research design. No statistical procedure will yield meaningful results from a poorly designed study.

Summary

Procedures for using CFA to evaluate the factorial validity and factorial invariance of rehabilitation assessment measures were described via a numerical example. Then, recently published studies of rehabilitation assessment instruments were presented to illustrate the application of CFA to vocational assessment and counseling with rehabilitation clients. Specifically, it was shown how the results of CFAs led to concrete recommendations for scoring the MSS and interpretation of USES-II scale scores for vocational counseling. Other topics covered included recent developments in CFA methodology, the role of CFA in addressing broader issues involving latent variable analysis, and some limitations of the procedure.

CHAPTER 12

Measurement in Rehabilitation: From the Beginning to What End?

LEE B. SECHREST

I have to begin this chapter with a disclaimer of any particular expertise in rehabilitation psychology. I did not even know there was such a field until a few years ago when Robert Glueckauf brought me into contact with it. On the other hand, after some of the reading I have done recently, I have begun to feel a little like Molière's famous doctor who was surprised to learn that he had been speaking prose all his life without knowing it. I still disclaim any expertise, but I have been interested in problems having to do with chronic mental illness, training of severely mentally retarded persons, reform of crim nal offenders, and treatment of drug addiction. I simply did not know that all of that is part of rehabilitation psychology. My reading has helped me to understand the very broad range of problems included under the rubric of rehabilitation psychology and something of the common threads that link all those problems. Nor was I fully aware that the populations to be served span virtually all age groups, all social classes, all racial, ethnic, and linguistic groups—and most all of most other dimensions along which people differ.

I make a point of all this because it throws into such sharp relief the enormity of the measurement problems that face those who work as rehabilitation psychologists. The problems and their solutions cannot be boiled down to a few simple ideas or principles that can be offered as expert—I am tempted to say glib—advice to those in the field by those outside it, whatever their expertise in measurement.

In the pages that follow, I will discuss a variety of measurement problems in general terms and try to extrapolate to rehabilitation as an area of application. In some cases, I will point to issues that seem to me potentially particularly troublesome to the rehabilitation psychologist, although, again, I will be venturing beyond the limits of my knowledge and competence.

The Measurement Tasks
in Rehabilitation Psychology

The variety of measurement tasks facing the rehabilitation psychologist is formidable, probably more formidable than is usually recognized. My reading of the field is certainly that full recognition of the range of measurement tasks is lacking. Following are some of the tasks I have identified:

1. *Assessing individual clients*. This task is so obvious that I will not dwell on it save to note that the range and variety of individuals potentially in need of assessment are extraordinary.

2. *Assessing rehabilitators*. If it is to be fully effective, part of the task of rehabilitation psychology must be to assess rehabilitators—that is, service providers—themselves. Examples are afforded by Sather (1985), in relation to planning for improvement in counselor performance; MacGuffie, Misener, and Reichart (1989), in defining roles and functions of medical rehabilitation counselors; and Cullen, Clark, Cullen, and Mathers (1985), in assessing attitudes of prison guards and others toward rehabilitation. These and many other examples that could be adduced indicate the potential desirability of, or even need for, assessing rehabilitation personnel for competence, for training needs, for motivational intervention (e.g., Ursprung, 1986), and other characteristics important for adequacy of functioning in the field. Bolton (1978) warned quite some time ago, however, that assessment of counselor performance should

be done cautiously and with due regard for the complex influences on that behavior.

3. *Assessing training.* Efforts need to be directed toward assessing the effects of and otherwise evaluating training programs, such as in Ewan and Whaite (1983) and Barnes, Brook, Hesketh, and Johnson (1985). Such evaluations may require assessment of characteristics of the programs themselves as well as of specific skills and abilities toward which they are directed. In some instances, attitudes may be as important as skills (Ursprung, 1986).

4. *Assessing services.* Quality has become a major issue in the field of health services, and extensive work has been done on methods of assessing quality of those services (Brook & McGlynn, 1991). I do not get an indication of anywhere near the same level of concern for assessing quality of services in other human problem areas, including rehabilitation, but the issue certainly needs to be raised. Services of low quality may not be services at all.

5. *Assessing outcomes.* The range of outcomes relevant to rehabilitation is as wide as the range of rehabilitation problems and efforts. Vocational rehabilitation may be assessed simply in terms of job tenure, but, for some purposes, productivity at work may need to be measured (e.g., Ugland, 1982). Work productivity may need to be assessed too in relation to a wide range of performance deficits (e.g., Butler et al., 1989).

6. *Assessing environments.* Rehabilitation always occurs in environmental contexts, which may differ from rehabilitation to later circumstances of living and implementation. Mulvey, Linney, and Rosenberg (1987), for example, found that "institutionality" could be defined in terms of two dimensions representing organizational characteristics important to the quality of residential services. Moos and his associates have been especially influential in their work on assessing environments (e.g., Lemke & Moos, 1990; Timko & Moos, 1991).

7. *Assessing unusual populations and capacities.* More than those in most other fields, rehabilitation specialists may be called upon to assess unusual populations and, in relation to those populations, unusual specific capacities or skills. For example, assessment

of infants and small children is notably difficult under any circumstances, but early motor development (Piper, Darrah, & Byrne, 1989) and other prespeech behaviors are obviously challenging tasks. Often rehabilitation specialists may be called upon to make assessments of unique capacities such as gait (Sampaio, Bril, & Breniere, 1989) or interventions such as the "effect of an inhibitive weight-bearing mitt on tone reduction and functional performance in a child with cerebral palsy" (Smelt, 1989). In such circumstances, rehabilitation assessments must rely on fundamental knowledge of the principles of measurement because appropriate instruments are nonexistent and opportunities for instrument development are limited.

8. *Demonstration of applicability of standard (adapted) measures*. Assessment in rehabilitation as often as not is likely to require the use of standard instruments but also the positive demonstration of their applicability. For example, Cattell's *16PF* was adapted for use in a rehabilitation setting with a visually limited population, and it was shown that the adaptation could be made without effect on the relevance of available norms (Jones, 1983). Only infrequently will it be possible in rehabilitation applications to avoid the requirement of demonstrating the suitability of standard measures, thus adding to the burden.

9. *Assessment of patient preferences*. Although I did not encounter any instances in the literature of assessment of patient preferences, I believe that task to be an important one. If rehabilitators are not dealing with preferences now, my expectation is that they will be doing so before long, whether by choice or by demand. In medicine, it is increasingly recognized that patients may differ widely in their utilities for different outcomes, and those utilities should be honored by clinicians. For example, one of my colleagues has told me that Native American males may prefer to forgo hip replacement surgery because, after that operation, they can no longer sit cross-legged or ride a horse. Unfortunately, assessment of patient preferences is extraordinarily difficult because patients must make choices between states they may never have experienced (Sechrest & Figueredo, in press). Preferences will be no more easily assessed in rehabilitation.

None of the assessment tasks mentioned is a simple task by itself, and collectively they represent stupendous demands on the field.

Generic Problems in Assessment

I turn now to some generic problems in assessment that almost certainly apply to rehabilitation psychology. These problems have not been resolved in other fields, and they will not be easier for rehabilitation specialists.

Regrettably, the first problem is that, or so it seems to me, training in quantitative methods is receiving declining emphasis in psychology programs. Whether it is declining or not, the results of a survey of Ph.D.-granting departments (Aiken, West, Sechrest, & Reno, 1990) indicates that the level of quantitative training in most programs is minimal and, in my estimation, deficient. That is particularly true with respect to training in measurement, now almost absent from most training programs. Apparently, many programs now substitute courses in testing for what was meant in the establishment of original training standards to be reasonably rigorous training in the field of tests and measurements, that is, psychometrics. That deficiency is, in my estimation, tantamount to psychology's giving up its birthright.

For reasons of space, but also because they should not have to be repeated here, I will pass only lightly over some standard psychometric problems. For the most part, they are recognized as problems, even if the recognition is often more of a nod of acquaintance than a firm embrace.

Reliability. That measures should be "reliable" is usually mentioned in any more than a cursory discussion of measurement, but the topic is also very often treated casually. An apparently common inclination is to accept any evidence of any kind of reliability as license for any use whatsoever of the measure in question. A reliability coefficient is a quantitative estimate of the degree to which it is legitimate to generalize an observed score *across a particular characteristic of the instrument or condition of measurement.* For example, an internal consistency coefficient is an estimate of the generalizability of a score across a universe of items from which the items actually used are assumed to have been drawn at random for a population from which the sample actually studied is assumed to have been drawn at random. Thus an internal consistency coefficient, such as Cronbach's alpha, is not a warrant for assuming stability over time (test-retest) or for stability within a new population, such as a disabled population.

Moreover, a reliability coefficient is a continuous (but nonlinear) quantitative estimate of the dependability of a measure. No threshold exists at which reliability, whatever the kind of coefficient, is to be regarded as "satisfactory." Low reliability represents a strict limit on the usefulness of a measure, particularly for individual assessment. Errors of measurement (i.e., random errors) cancel each other out over a set of observations, and one can be reasonably certain that two groups that differ substantially on some measure also differ on correlates of that measure. That is not so true, however, of individual measures. The *standard error of measurement* of scores

$$SE = \sigma \sqrt{1 - r^2}$$

Thus, for example, if the standard deviation of a performance measure is 10 points, and the measure has a reliability of .8, then a person with an observed score of 50 (near the mean) can be assumed to have a (true) score that with .95 confidence lies between 38 and 62! For clinical purposes, that is a very large range of possible scores.

In research, low reliability of measures of either independent or dependent variables can have marked effects on outcomes (Sutcliffe, 1980). Even if an experimental intervention had a completely consistent effect on some dependent variable—that is, the intervention correlated perfectly with the outcome—if the outcome measure had a reliability of only .7, the proportion of variance accounted for by the intervention would have decreased from 100% to only 50%. If rehabilitative interventions are to be evaluated on the basis of objective measures of any kind—and how else would we want them evaluated?—then it is critical to pay attention to reliability of measurement of *all* measures involved. That is an important dictum because the possibility of unreliability in outcome measures is often ignored.

As should be clear, measures of reliability are not intersubstitutable. Measures of agreement between judges are not interpretable in the same way as measures of agreement over time (test-retest) or measures of agreement over different sets of items (internal consistency). Both clinicians and researchers need to specify the universe(s) across which they intend to generalize scores and then make certain that the reliability coefficient they cite pertains to that universe.

Validity. No essential distinction exists between reliability and validity. Both have to do with the legitimate generalization of observed performances (scores) to unobserved instances. Generalizability theory (Shavelson & Webb, 1991; Shavelson, Webb, & Rowley, 1989) is an approach to measurement that deserves attention in all fields. Concepts of validity usually relate to generalizations outside the specific measurement context in which performances are observed. A measure of speed on a data entry task would be valid for whatever other performances it was predictive, but it would be especially useful if it proved to be generalizable to an actual work situation.

Distinctions are often made between predictive and construct validity, but those distinctions may not be of great importance. Construct validity, however, deserves mention in the context of assuring ourselves that we know and understand what we are actually measuring. Any measure that is consistent in any way at all can be considered to be measuring *something*; the question is whether we know what that something is. An important part of the task of any researcher is to discover what it is that each of his or her measures is measuring. A given measure might turn out to have construct validity for measurement of social desirability, which might not be the preference of the investigators, but knowing that fact would be critically important if the investigator had rather hoped otherwise.

Need for theory. If we are to improve existing measures, develop satisfactory new ones, and use them all wisely, we need better theory on which to base them. The plea for better theory is so common that it gets to be regarded as tiresome, but that commonness should enhance rather than diminish the influence of the plea. Theoretical development is needed in relation to both the constructs we employ in our research and the characteristics of our measures of them. If we do not understand very well just what we mean by *rehabilitative potential* or some such term, we cannot expect to develop very satisfactory measures of it. That is, we will not be able to specify very well just how that potential should manifest itself and hence be measurable in a way that would be generalizable, say, to progress in a rehabilitation program.

Similarly, we need better theory about the ways in which constructs may manifest themselves and the implications of those ways for specific characteristics of measures. Commonly, for example, we simply tote up the number of items responded to in particular ways and assign the resulting score to a person, or we count the number of responses we observe in a period of time and assign the resulting number. That is fairly crude, or may be, given that we know so little about the functional relationships between responses and the latent traits that they represent. Note that gravitational force is proportional to the *square* of distance. A commonly used index of "ponderosity" (body mass) is weight in kilograms divided by height (in meters) raised to the power of 2 for males and 1.5 for females (Ware et al., 1980). We do not have even that level of sophistication in most of our social and behavioral measures.

Rules for deriving scores. Measurement models underlying most instruments and procedures in the social and behavioral sciences are rarely explicit. Nonetheless, an implicit model is a necessity, and it is important for those using measures to understand the assumed models. One part of any model is the rule by which scores are derived to represent performances. Fiske (1978) has described a number of different rules or models by which scoring may be accomplished. The rules by which performances are translated into numbers are rarely even mentioned, and often they appear scarcely to have been thought of, but they are important. Not all the models proposed by Fiske need to be described here, but examples may help to show the nature and potential importance of understanding how our measures are put together.

The simplest rule is *cumulative frequency*, which means that relevant behaviors or responses are counted, and the total is the score. For example, suppose a clinician notes that "on eleven occasions during the interview, Mr. F had to stop and begin his sentence again because he could not find the word he apparently wanted." The clinician is implying that all 11 of the critical instances are equally important and that the number is interpretable without respect to the number of possible occasions on which a critical response might have occurred. Reporting that a patient threatened staff members 4 times during a day is a similar example, in that the statement does not take into account the total number of interactions the patient had with staff.

A second rule is *cumulative relative frequency,* which counts the number of critical responses and assumes that they are all equally important but also uses a standard number of stimuli or occasions. Cumulative relative frequency is the most common method of scoring tests and inventories. Thus one exposes each subject to, say, 30 items and counts the number of "correct" responses. The difference between cumulative frequency and cumulative relative frequency is that, by the latter rule, the number of items or occasions is constant across subjects. If one had a standardized speech sample and scored for speech disfluencies per minute or per 100 words, one would have a cumulative relative frequency measure. The two rules are similar in that all critical responses are counted in the same way. A "true" response to "I am often nervous" is counted in the same way as a true response to "I worry a lot." Or, stumbling over one word is counted the same as stumbling over another.

A *homogeneity* model weights responses according to their value on some underlying scale, what we would call a latent variable. One possibility is an *average weighted response* rule, which requires that each response be given a value on the relevant scale and then that the score be the average value of all responses recorded. Loevinger (1966) has used that scoring rule for her measure of ego strength. Essentially, any score that is derived by calculating the average of the values of a number of responses fits the average weighted response rule. The average judged quality of the products of a sheltered work program would fit the rule; that is, all the products are assumed to be equally relevant, and the average of their values is a sufficient summary of performance.

Another possible homogeneity rule, however, would be to score performance by the *maximum response value.* The seriousness of a person's criminal record, for example, is determined by the value of the most serious crime. An accused armed robber, for

example, cannot mitigate the seriousness of that crime by pointing out that he also frequently engaged in shoplifting, bringing
the average seriousness of his crimes down to a fairly low level.
Kohlberg's conception of level of moral development focused on
the highest level displayed by a person being interviewed, not on
the average level. The level of disability for a person might be better
reflected in the most serious problem rather than in the average
of all problems. That is, however, a matter to be decided by clinicians
or researchers developing or using assessment tools.

To reiterate, a variety of assumptions must, inevitably, be made
when one attempts to derive a score to represent a performance.
The assumptions may be explicit or implicit. They are not made
less troublesome or binding by being ignored.

Meaningful metrics. The scores used to represent performances
may or may not be expressed in a metric that has any directly
interpretable meaning. The number of days a worker is absent is
meaningful; so would be the average pay earned by persons 6
months after completing a rehabilitation program. By contrast, an
improvement of 4 points on a self-esteem scale is not interpretable
in any direct way. In what ways might a person be better off by
having 4 additional points of self-esteem?

What is at issue are the behavioral implications of scores on
measures. We have a fair, but still limited, understanding of the behavioral implications of, say, IQ points. We have almost no understanding of the behavioral implications of many of our measures
such as self-esteem, anxiety, and extraversion. One study of patients in dental offices (Robertson, Gatchel, & Fowler, 1991)
found about a 10-point decrease in anxiety scores from the time
at which patients were waiting to be worked on and the time after
all work was completed. A series of such studies could help greatly
in understanding anxiety measures. Another approach has been
taken by McEwan and Devins (1983), who wanted to know whether
self-reported anxiety is noticeable by others and found that high
anxious subjects who were somatically reactive were not thought
by their peers to be as anxious as they, themselves, were. The idea
of relating scores on common inventory dimensions to peer
ratings on the same dimensions with the aim of determining "just
noticeable differences" in personality variables would be well
worth exploring. Without work of that sort, along with work on

behavioral implications, we will continue to be in the dark with respect to the useful meaning of many of our favorite clinical and research measures.

Effect size estimates. The practice of reporting outcomes of studies solely in terms of p values should long since have been abandoned. Probability values indicate almost nothing of value about a research finding (Cohen, 1990). Effect size estimates that estimate the percentage of variance of one variable accounted for by another variable at least show something about the strength of the relationship. Even better would be effect size measures reflecting behavioral implications as described previously; for example, that extent of participation in a vocational training program accounts not only for, say, 30% of the variance in posttraining income but that, for every additional week of participation, an average of 10 cents per hour of earnings could be expected. Or for every week of participation, one could expect 2 more days of work per month.

More attention should be paid to specification of the shape of functional relationships between variables because relationships may not always be linear. Some relationships may be characterized by irregularities in the form of plateaus as certain critical values of variables are reached. For example, it is quite possible that, once a person can read at the fourth grade level, no advantage in performance on other variables, such as earnings, would be realized by incremental improvements in reading. It might be that reading would have to be improved to, say, the sixth or seventh grade level before any advantage would accrue. Unfortunately, functional relationships are rarely examined and portrayed.

Premorbid measures. If one is to assess the effects of rehabilitative interventions, it is necessary to have knowledge of premorbid performance measures. The old joke about the man with the injury being delighted to hear his physician say that of course he would be able to play the violin after surgery because he had not been able to play one before is apropos. If a person had bad work habits and could not hold a job before an injury, it might be expecting too much of a rehabilitative unit to think that it should produce a dependable, model employee. Unfortunately, for most purposes, good estimates of premorbid performance are often lacking for critical variables of interest.

Dikmen, McLean, Temkin, and Wyler (1986), for example, were interested in the cognitive sequelae of closed head trauma but realized that victims of such injuries might have shown a variety of deficits before their injuries. For example, they might have suffered previous head injuries. Dikmen and her associates hit upon the ingenious notion of having each head injured person name a good friend most like him and then testing that friend's cognitive performance as a control for premorbid condition. The results produced strong evidence that recovery is more complete than had been thought, a major proportion of postinjury deficits not being actually residual but reflective of premorbid condition. Dikmen's work should be taken as a virtual prescription for the necessity of, in some manner, getting good estimates of premorbid functioning as a step in estimating effects of rehabilitation. Even a randomized experiment might be misleading because it might suggest limited effects when, in fact, whatever was achieved might have been the maximum attainable.

Reactive measures. Many problems are posed by reliance on reactive measures, by which is meant measures that, when applied, themselves change the phenomenon being measured (Webb, Campbell, Schwartz, & Grove, 1981). If people are being surveyed about their voting habits, they may exaggerate their tendencies to seek out information about candidates and issues out of a concern to appear sensible and responsible. As a mental experiment, consider what a person might report to a pollster as opposed to what that same person might report to a friend during a casual conversation.

Blood pressure, as an example, is likely to be higher when measured in a medical office setting than when measured at home ("In-Home Measurements," 1988), and drug use is likely to be underreported in most settings. Compliance with medical regimens, such as faithfulness in taking pills, has been difficult to measure because of reporting biases. Recipients of heart transplants, and probably other organs too, report positive well-being that seems out of line with their actual states, often claiming to be better off than persons never sick (Sechrest & Pitz, 1987).

Various investigators have devised methods to reduce reactivity biases. The most common ways are to assure persons of confidentiality or even anonymity in research settings. Blood pressures may be measured several times in the expectation that patients will calm down during a session. Drug use may be checked by means of urine samples, and assessment of compliance with medication regimens has been improved by microprocessors placed within devices—pill containers and so on (Byrne, Averbuch, Rubio, & Weintraub, 1990). One tactic devised by psychologists is the "bogus pipeline" that causes people to think that the person doing an assessment has a direct measure of some fundamental physiological response and therefore that they should report faithfully, such as on cigarette smoking (Murray, O'Conell, Schmid, & Perry, 1987) or alcohol use (Lowe et al., 1986).

More research is badly needed on ways of estimating reactivity biases and on ways of getting around them. Reactivity is as important in clinical as in research settings but seems to have been of less systematic concern, perhaps because clinicians believe themselves able to detect the bias when it occurs. Whether they can or not would be a useful topic for research efforts.

Clinicians as instruments. In many circumstances, clinicians themselves may be employed as instruments of assessment. For example, when clinicians are asked to make a diagnosis for research purposes, then the clinicians are being used as instruments. Clinicians may be asked to make prognostic predictions, to estimate functional deficits, and so on. When used in that way, then any and all of the concerns that might be held about any instrument—that is, psychometric properties—are applicable to clinicians. One may legitimately inquire whether clinicians are reliable in their judgments over time, whether they agree with each other, whether their judgments are in accord with other information, and so on. Whether judgments of clinicians have sufficient sensitivity and specificity is as important as for other assessment instruments.

If clinicians are to be employed in assessment, they should be trained specifically for the tasks they are to perform. They may, in fact, also need to be selected (tested) for the tasks because not all potential clinicians may have the kind of personal sensitivity and other attributes that are required to be expert. They should also be exposed to prediction tasks and subsequent feedback carefully structured to ensure the exact abilities required for later use. Dawes (in press), for example, points out that clinicians may believe that they know what characterizes people who abuse children based on extensive experience with people who have been child abusers, but, unless they have had comparable opportunities to study people who have not abused their children, their knowledge is hopelessly biased. Even if child abusers nearly always have a particular pattern on the Rorschach, that does not mean that most people with that pattern would be child abusers. Most sex abuse cases involve males, for example, but most males do not abuse children sexually. If clinicians are to be used as instruments, then they need to be individually validated as instruments. One fact that has to be remembered is that one half of all clinicians are below the median in clinical ability!

Clinical judgment. Clinicians also may be used to process information so as to synthesize it and produce overall judgments. Thus clinicians may be asked to "interpret" MMPI profiles. But they probably should not be asked to perform such tasks. Clinicians are not, in fact, very good at synthesizing information, a proposition that has been known for a long time but for just as long a time substantially ignored (Dawes, Faust, & Meehl, 1989). Goldberg (1991) has shown recently that the research literature does not support the idea that clinicians can perform the functions of the multiple regression analysis, which is what data synthesis requires. Regrettably, statistical methods for data synthesis and prediction, so-called actuarial methods, have never been much developed despite Meehl's (1954) early and persuasive arguments for them.

A story is relevant here: Once upon a time in a far-off land, an annual contest took place each year to see which member of the tribe had reared the largest pig. The custom was to assemble all the pigs in an enclosure, whereupon the judges, the elders of the tribe, would wander gravely among the pigs, conferring with each other repeatedly. Ultimately, the chief judge would announce, "Well, this looks like the biggest pig!" and the owner of that pig would then be given the prize. A bright young farmer was, however, disturbed by this procedure, although he could not articulate exactly why. Finally, he figured out an alternative method. He gathered a bunch of river stones of reasonably uniform size and procured both a log and a long plank. After balancing the plank on the log, each pig in turn would be place on the opposite end, and a pile of stones would then be placed opposite until the plank again balanced. At that point, the pile of stones for that pig would then be neatly stacked beside the pig's owner, and the next pig would then be similarly balanced. When all that was done, the judges then walked through the pile of stones until, finally, the chief judge would announce, "Well, that looks like the largest pile of stones!" And the owner standing beside that pile would be given the prize.

Too Many Instruments

Emperor Franz Josef II of Austria, responding on one occasion to a performance of Mozart's music, remonstrated, "Too many notes, my dear Mozart! Too many notes." Similarly, without any pretense of the imperial, I remonstrate, "Too many instruments!" We have hundreds of instruments (measures), probably thousands if we consider all the instruments created for research purposes. Pressures exist to give all these instruments different names, compounding the numerosity. Contrast this situation with the biomedical enterprise. The sphygmomanometer is used to measure blood pressure with a view to understanding hemostatic tension and arterial dynamics. There are no other instruments for that purpose. Body temperature is measured with a thermometer, although it may be measured in any one of several orifices. The situation in the biomedical sciences is not all that different than psychology in terms of the problems posed. No measure of blood pressure exists other than what is provided by blood pressure measuring devices. Why did psychology end up with so many measures of intelligence or authoritarianism or anxiety? One reason, I think, is that, save perhaps for a few commercially competitive tests (IQ, achievement, personality), the developmental costs of psychological instruments are low, and, because constructs are so vaguely defined, it is easy to come up with a new name for a new instrument, whatever its nature.

Do we really have as many variables as are implied by the plethora of our instruments? That is unlikely. In some ways, the Buros Mental Measurements Yearbook and similar catalogs are an embarrassment, or should be. How many different variables can there be? There are very few completely orthogonal variables, keeping in mind that a correlation of .01 would be statistically significant with $N = 40,000$ or so. Obviously, the number of correlated variables can be enormous, but then we need to account for all the correlations between variables. The currently accepted idea of the "Big Five" variables in personality suggests something of the limits in the field.

Brendan Maher once suggested to me that the best proof available that the universe is constantly expanding is the fact that we have been able to account for 100% of the variance in just about everything several times over, and we keep finding ourselves coming up short in new attempts. The fact is that very little attention is ever paid to either discriminant or incremental validity of measures. Craik (1986) has suggested that every study including any relatively new measures should also include one or more related "old" variables against which the new ones would be calibrated. That approach would also make it possible to assess incremental validity of new measures, that is, by showing that in multiple regressions they have significant beta weights after variance explained by old variables is removed. We could probably pare down our list of instruments by a good bit if we just tried.

Latent Variables and Measurement Models

Under most circumstances, in psychology, and related fields like rehabilitation, our observed, or measured, variables are not the ones in which we are interested in a literal sense. We are, instead, interested in underlying or latent variables of which the observed variables are either signs or for which they are surrogates. Thus we would not really be interested specifically in the responses of subjects to 10 particular anxiety items we might use in a study. We would be interested instead in an underlying latent variable of anxiety that we would suppose to have accounted for responses to the 10 items and that would account for many other responses of the persons studied.

Thinking in terms of latent variables requires specification of measurement models, that is, the ways in which observed variables are related to underlying variables and therefore the ways in which they are related to each other. Thus two or more observed variables may be related because they reflect the same underlying trait but also because they share a common source of extraneous variance such as might arise from common methods of measurement. The specification of measurement models requires specification also of the degree of error in measurement, which makes it possible to correct estimates of the relationships between variables for attenuation attributable to unreliable (error) measurement. Multiple regression assumes that independent (predictor) variables are measured without error; that is, regression coefficients do not reflect the effects of any measurement error and therefore are *underestimates* of the true effects. We badly need to know how to capitalize on the power of new approaches that can produce better estimates of the effects in which we are interested.

Some variables frequently employed in studies appear to be measured essentially without error, but often those variables are surrogates for some other, latent variable that is not at all to be considered as measured without error. Age, sex, income, and education are typical surrogate variables. Very seldom when age is included as a variable in a study is the investigator actually interested in the number of years that have elapsed since the person's birth. Rather, the investigator is interested in age as it reflects things that have happened to the person since birth, such as biological changes if health is at issue, certain kinds of experiences if social outcomes are of interest. Age is not perfectly correlated with either biological change or with social experience. Not all "baby boomers" had baby boomer type experiences. Some elderly persons are in very good physical condition and some are not. Income predicts whether people will buy a major appliance during the coming year; education predicts whether they are likely to buy beer or to buy wine. If income or education is used as a surrogate variable for social class, then the attenuated relationship that either has to social class will result, quite inevitably, in an underestimate of the effect of social class on the dependent variable of interest. The same consequence, underestimate of effect, will obtain for any latent variable represented in a study by an (often pale) surrogate. One useful stratagem, although it is not a solution, is to build a measurement model into analyses by using plausibly high and low values of reliability coefficients to bracket the measurement error. At least one can then get an indication of the sensitivity of the overall analytic model to measurement problems.

Variables such as sociodemographic indicators should be used in studies only with great care. That care starts with full realization of why they are used. If they are used as surrogates for other variables, the researcher needs to specify those variables and then consider the possibility of more direct measurement of them. If sex is used as a surrogate for a particular way of looking at problems as a result of a residue of life experiences that differ between the sexes, one might think of trying to develop a measure of that outlook rather than casually and inexplicitly substituting a binary indicator of quite another variable, biological sex.

Improving Measures

The measures we use in the social and behavioral sciences, including those in the field of rehabilitation, must be improved. Meehl (1986) has noted that a fundamental difference between the hard sciences and the soft ones is that, when the former are faced with a measurement problem involving an inadequate instrument, they immediately set about improving the instrument or the underlying measurement process. In the soft sciences, and that includes most of psychology, measurement problems are more likely to be met with resignation or abandonment of the problem.

The fact is that we, as a field, know what has to be done to improve our measures. What we seem to lack is the will to do so. The way is hard, not easy. It requires long, tedious, persistent effort. That sort of work is not so much fun, and the payoff is uncertain. The common complaint is that work on measurement problems does not lead to tenure. That may be true, in which case, as a manifestation of noblesse oblige, development of better measures should be a focus of interest for already tenured faculty, for the full professors.

The tools required for development and improvement of measures are available. The multitrait-multimethod matrix (MTMM), described originally by Campbell and Fiske (1959), has been available for more than 30 years, but the published instances of its use would probably not number 100. Recent advances in statistical analysis for the MTMM (Ferketich, Figueredo, & Knapp, 1991; Figueredo, Ferketich, & Knapp, 1991) should facilitate its use, but the important barriers have always been the conceptualization of problems in the first place and the effort required to collect the necessary data.

Statistical measurement models. In recent years, software required for implementing sophisticated measurement models, especially the use of structural equations, has become readily available. One critical element in the armamentarium is confirmatory factor analysis, described elsewhere in this volume by Brookings and Bolton. An example of the application of sophisticated statistical analyses to a measurement problem in rehabilitation is the work of Ludlow et al. (1983). They wanted a measure of attitudes toward the blind that would be sensitive to changes and used procedures involving analyses of residuals to identify peculiar items and calibration of both items and persons at different time periods. Their results were both useful to them and indicative of the general value of the approach.

An effective attack on measurement problems in psychology will require a more integrative, truly *psychological* approach than has been characteristic of our efforts. Improvement in measurement will benefit from applications of knowledge in such basic areas as memory, judgment, and cognition.

Litigation. Applied areas such as rehabilitation may not need to decide to devote attention to measurement. Litigation may force the case. Pullin and Zirkel (1988) have reviewed the legal issues involved in testing the handicapped and concluded that its widespread use to make critical individual decisions coupled with "growing vigilance" by the handicapped community make increased legal scrutiny highly likely. Both federal and state statutes aimed at ensuring free and equal access of handicapped persons to education, jobs, and public services provide grounds for legal action against alleged inappropriate use of tests and other measures. Such suits, except for those involving racial issues in special education testing, had not been common at the time of the Pullin and Zirkel review, but their expectation was that more suits were in the offing.

Interventions, Costs, and Benefits

Measurement problems in rehabilitation are aggravated by the diversity of intervention approaches, methods, techniques, and so on that are required. Measurements are for some purpose, and, if we are to facilitate response to treatment interventions, we must have a fine grasp on just what those interventions are and what characteristics of persons and situations might contribute to a favorable response to them. In some instances, problems may arise because, in fact, rehabilitative techniques are not well understood or may be lacking altogether. The advantage in accurate assessment that does not or cannot change any treatment decision is certainly small.

Kaszniak (in this volume) has provided a useful discussion of benefits and costs of assessments, and I do not wish to reprise his comments. I can only say, though, that I believe that benefit/cost considerations raise serious questions about the end to which measures, even if they are good ones, may be put, especially in clinical settings. Smith and I (Smith & Sechrest, 1991) have shown that aptitude × treatment interactions, those predicting differential response to treatment for persons having different characteristics, are almost certain to be small, except for obvious cases such as that deaf persons require interventions different than those for the blind. Moreover, reliable interactions require studies of very large scale, usually far larger than is customary in a field like rehabilitation.

For clinical use, most of our assessments and other measurement procedures lack the precision that one would hope for in making individual treatment decisions. Correlations in the range of .5, which is about as high as can be found in the literature, do not produce impressive increases in accuracy of prediction except at the extremes of distributions. I do not think that we ought to sink into terminal pessimism about the prospects for really useful clinical instruments, but we need to be realistic at least.

Improvement of measures for research purposes is important and feasible. Errors do not cancel each other out in clinical use; for example, one cannot claim to be, on average, correct, because an error in excluding one person from a treatment program was compensated for by an error in including another person. For research purposes, however, measures of modest validity can, if properly applied, produce groups with substantially different mean values on characteristics of interest. Other sciences have recognized the importance of measurement even when immediate, practical value is not at issue. Rehabilitation, along with other areas of applied psychology, would do well to devote a significant portion of its efforts toward improving its capacity to measure the things in which it is interested.

A final comment, which gets back to about where I began, is that rehabilitation, again along with other areas, needs to put more emphasis on training its scientists *and* practitioners in measurement. Training now is demonstrably inadequate. Improvement will require upgrading of requirements in quantitative methods and in theory of measurement. I believe that improvement will also require greater emphasis on philosophy of science so that we all understand, at a more fundamental level, what we are doing in the first place.

References

Acker, M. B. (1990). A review of the ecological validity of neuropsychological tests. In D. E. Tupper & K. D. Cicerone (Eds.), *The neuropsychology of everyday life: Assessment and basic competencies* (pp. 19-55). Boston: Kluwer Academic.

Ahlmen, M., Sullivan, M., & Bjelle, A. (1988). Team versus non-team outpatient care in rheumatoid arthritis. *Arthritis and Rheumatism, 31,* 471-479.

Aiken, L., West, S. G., Sechrest, L., & Reno, R. (1990). Graduate training in statistics, methodology, and measurement in psychology: A survey of Ph.D. programs in North America. *American Psychologist, 45,* 721-734.

Albert, M. L., Sparks, R. W., & Helm, N. A. (1973). Melodic intonation therapy for aphasia. *Archives of Neurology, 29,* 130-131.

Alfano, D. P., & Finlayson, M. A. J. (1987). Clinical neuropsychology in rehabilitation. *The Clinical Neuropsychologist, 1,* 105-123.

Alker, H. A. (1972). Is personality situationally consistent or intrapsychically consistent? *Journal of Personality, 40,* 1-16.

Allen, W. S. (1958). *Rehabilitation: A community challenge.* New York: John Wiley.

Allison, J. (1983). *Behavioral economics.* New York: Praeger.

Allison, J., & Timberlake, W. (1974). Instrumental and contingent saccharin-licking in rats: Response deprivation and reinforcement. *Learning and Motivation, 5,* 231-247.

American Educational Research Association, American Psychological Association, National Council on Measurement in Education. (1985). *Standards for educational and psychological testing.* Washington, DC: American Psychological Association.

American Hospital Association. (1989). *Survey of medical rehabilitation hospitals and programs: 1988.* Chicago: American Hospital Association.

American Psychological Association. (1980). *Accreditation handbook.* Washington, DC: Author.

American Psychological Association, Task Force on Standards for Educational and Psychological Tests. (1985). *Standards for educational and psychological testing.* Washington, DC: Author.

American Psychological Association, Task Force on Standards for Educational and Psychological Tests. (1986). *Guidelines for computer-based tests and interpretation.* Washington, DC: Author.

Anderson, K. O., Bradley, L., Young, L., McDaniel, L., & Wise, C. (1985). Rheumatoid arthritis: Review of psychological factors related to etiology, effects, and treatment. *Psychological Bulletin, 98,* 358-387.

Anderson, S. W., & Tranel, D. (1989). Awareness of disease states following cerebral infarction, dementia, and head trauma: Standardized assessment. *The Clinical Neuropsychologist, 3,* 327-339.

Anderson, T. P., Bourstom, N., Greenberg, F. R., & Hildyard, V. G. (1974). Predictive factors in stroke rehabilitation. *Archives of Physical Medicine and Rehabilitation, 55,* 545-553.

Andrews, J., Brocklehurst, J. C., Richards, B., & Laycock, P. J. (1981). The rate of recovery from stroke—and its measurement. *International Rehabilitation Medicine, 3,* 155-161.

Anthony, W. A. (1979). *Principles of psychiatric rehabilitation.* Baltimore: University Park Press.

Anthony, W. A., Cohen, M., & Farkas, M. D. (1990). *Psychiatric rehabilitation.* Boston: Boston University, Center for Psychiatric Rehabilitation.

Anthony, W. A., & Jansen, M. A. (1984). Predicting the vocational capacity of the chronically mentally ill: Research and implications. *American Psychologist, 39,* 537-544.

Antonak, R. F., & Livneh, H. (1988). *The measurement of attitudes toward people with disabilities: Methods, psychometrics and scales.* Springfield, IL: Charles C Thomas.

Arkes, H. R., & Faust, D. (1987, August). *Cue utilization in neuropsychology.* In D. Faust (Chair), Clinical Judgment in Neuropsychology: How Good Are We? Symposium conducted at the annual convention of the American Psychological Association, New York.

Asch, A. (1984). Experience of disability. *American Psychologist, 39,* 529-536.

Auerbach, S. M. (1989). Stress management and coping research in the health care setting: An overview and methodological commentary. *Journal of Consulting and Clinical Psychology, 57,* 388-395.

Baker, F., & Intagliata, J. (1982). Quality of life in the evaluation of community support systems. *Evaluation and Program Planning, 5,* 69-79.

Barnes, J., Brook, J. A., Hesketh, B., & Johnson, M. (1985). The professional psychologist as evaluator in a community agency setting. *Professional Psychology: Research and Practice, 16,* 681-688.

Batavia, A. I., & DeJong, G. (1990). Developing a comprehensive health services research capacity in physical disability and rehabilitation. *Journal of Disability Policy Studies, 1,* 37-61.

Beachamp, T., & Childress, T. (1979). *Principles of biomedical ethics.* New York: Oxford University Press.

Bear-Lehman, J., & Abreu, B. C. (1989). Evaluating the hand: Issues in reliability and validity. *Physical Therapy, 12,* 1025-1033.

Bechtoldt, H. P. (1959). Construct validity: A critique. *American Psychologist, 14,* 619-629.

Becker, R. L. (1989). *Becker Work Adjustment Profile: Evaluator's manual.* Columbus, OH: Elbern.

Belar, C. (1988). Education in behavioral medicine: Perspectives from psychology. *Archives of Behavioral Medicine, 10,* 11-14.

Belar, C., Deardoff, W., & Kelly, K. (1987). *The practice of clinical health psychology.* New York: Pergamon.

Bellack, A. S. (1979). A critical appraisal of strategies for assessing social skill. *Behavioral Assessment, 1,* 157-176.

Belmore, K., & Brown, L. (1978). A job skill inventory strategy designed for severely handicapped potential workers. In N. G. Haring & D. D. Bricker (Eds.), *Teaching the severely handicapped* (pp. 223-262). Columbus, OH: Special Press.

Bender, L. (1938). *A visual motor gestalt test and its clinical use.* New York: American Orthopsychiatric Association.

Bentler, P. M. (1985). *Theory and implementation of EQS: A structural equations program.* Los Angeles: BMDP Statistical Software.

Bentler, P. M. (1988). Causal modeling via structural equation systems. In J. R. Nesselroade & R. B. Cattell (Eds.), *Handbook of multivariate experimental psychology* (2nd ed., pp. 317-335). New York: Plenum.

Bentler, P. M., & Bonett, D. G. (1980). Significance tests and goodness of fit in the analysis of covariance structures. *Psychological Bulletin, 88,* 588-606.

Benton, A. (1974). *Revised visual retention test* (4th ed.). New York: Psychological Corporation.

Ben-Yishay, Y., Gerstman, L., Diller, L., & Hass, A. (1970). Prediction of rehabilitation outcomes from psychometric parameters in left hemiplegics. *Journal of Consulting and Clinical Psychology, 34,* 436-441.

Ben-Yishay, Y., Piasetsky, E. B., & Rattok, J. (1987). A systematic method for ameliorating disorders in basic attention. In M. J. Meier, A. L. Benton, & L. Diller (Eds.), *Neuropsychological rehabilitation* (pp. 165-181). New York: Guilford.

Bergner, M. (1985). Measurement of health status. *Medical Care, 23,* 696-704.

Berven, N. L. (1980). Psychometric assessment in rehabilitation. In B. Bolton & D. W. Cook (Eds.), *Rehabilitation client assessment* (pp. 46-64). Baltimore: University Park Press.

Berven, N. L. (1984). Assessment practices in rehabilitation counseling. *Journal of Applied Rehabilitation Counseling, 15,* 9-14, 47.

Berven, N. L., & Maki, D. R. (1979). Performance on Philadelphia JEVS samples and subsequent employment status. *Journal of Applied Rehabilitation Counseling, 10*(4), 214-218.

Bickman, L. (1987). The functions of program theory. In L. Bickman (Ed.), *Using program theory in evaluation* (New Directions for Program Evaluation, No. 33, pp. 5-18). San Francisco: Jossey-Bass.

Bickman, L. (Ed.). (1990). *Advances in program theory* (New Directions for Program Evaluation, No. 47). San Francisco: Jossey-Bass.

Bitter, J. A., & Bolanovich, D. J. (1970). WARF: A scale for measuring job-readiness behaviors. *American Journal of Mental Deficiency, 74,* 616-621.

Blalock, S. J., DeVellis, R., Brown, & Wallston, K. A. (1989). Validity of the Center for Epidemiological Studies Depression Scale in arthritis populations. *Arthritis and Rheumatism, 32,* 991-997.

Blazer, D. (1982). *Depression in late life.* St. Louis, MO: C. V. Mosby.

Blazer, D. G., & Williams, C. D. (1980). Epidemiology of dysphoria and depression in an elderly population. *American Journal of Psychiatry, 137,* 439-444.

Block, J. (1968). Some reasons for the apparent inconsistency of personality. *Psychological Bulletin, 70,* 210-212.

Bolton, B. (1978). Methodological issues in the assessment of rehabilitation counselor performance. *Rehabilitation Counseling Bulletin, 21,* 190-193.

Bolton, B. (1983). Psychosocial factors affecting the employment of former vocational rehabilitation clients. *Rehabilitation Psychology, 28,* 35-44.

Bolton, B. (1985a). Measurement in rehabilitation. In E. L. Pan, T. E. Backer, & C. L. Vash (Eds.), *Annual Review of Rehabilitation, 4,* 115-144 (New York: Springer).

Bolton, B. (1985b). United States Employment Service Interest Inventory. In D. J. Keyser & R. C. Sweetland (Eds.), *Test critiques* (Vol. 3, pp. 673-681). Kansas City, MO: Test Corporation of America.

Bolton, B. (1986). Minnesota Satisfactoriness Scales. In D. J. Keyser & R. C. Sweetland (Eds.), *Test critiques* (Vol. 4, pp. 434-439). Kansas City, MO: Test Corporation of America.

Bolton, B. (Ed.). (1987a). *Handbook of measurement and evaluation in rehabilitation* (2nd ed.). Baltimore: Paul H. Brookes.

Bolton, B. (1987b). *Manual for the Vocational Personality Report.* Fayetteville: Arkansas Research and Training Center in Vocational Rehabilitation.

Bolton, B. (1988a). *Special education and rehabilitation testing: Current practices and test reviews.* Austin, TX: Pro-Ed.

Bolton, B. (1988b). Vocational assessment of persons with psychiatric disorders. In J. A. Ciardiello & M. D. Bell (Eds.), *Vocational rehabilitation of persons with prolonged mental illness* (pp. 165-180). Baltimore: Johns Hopkins Press.

Bolton, B. (1990). Functional Assessment Inventory. In D. J. Keyser & R. C. Sweetland (Eds.), *Test critiques* (Vol. 8, pp. 209-215). Kansas City, MO: Test Corporation of America.

Bolton, B. (1991a). Preliminary Diagnostic Questionnaire. In D. J. Keyser & R. C. Sweetland (Eds.), *Test critiques* (Vol. 9, pp. 405-410). Kansas City, MO: Test Corporation of America.

Bolton, B. (1991b). Becker Work Adjustment Profile. In J. C. Conoley & J. J. Kramer (Eds.), *The eleventh mental measurements yearbook.* Lincoln: University of Nebraska Press.

Bolton, B. (1991c). Disability Factor Scales. In D. J. Keyser & R. C. Sweetland (Eds.), *Test critiques* (Vol. 9, pp. 184-192). Kansas City MO: Test Corporation of America.

Bolton, B. (1992). Rehabilitation indicators. In D. J. Keyser & R. C. Sweetland (Eds.), *Test critiques* (Vol 10). Kansas City, MO: Test Corporation of America.

Bolton, B. (in press). Retest reliability of 16 PF-E. *Multivariate Experimental Clinical Research.*

Bolton, B., & Cook, D. (Eds.). (1980). *Rehabilitation client assessment.* Baltimore: University Park Press.

Bolton, B., & Dana, R. H. (1988). Multivariate relationships between normal personality functioning and objectively measured psychopathology. *Journal of Social and Clinical Psychology, 6,* 11-19.

Bolton, B., & Roessler, R. (1986). *Manual for the Work Personality Profile.* Fayetteville: Arkansas Research and Training Center in Vocational Rehabilitation.

Bond, G. R., & Boyer, S. L. (1988). Rehabilitation programs and outcomes. In J. A. Ciardiello & M. D. Bell (Eds.), *Vocational rehabilitation of persons with prolonged mental illness* (pp. 231-263). Baltimore: Johns Hopkins Press.

Bond, G. R., & Dietzen, L. L. (1992). *SSA supported employment project for SSI/SSDI beneficiaries with serious mental illness* (Final report to the Social Security Administration, Grant No. 12-D-70299-5). Washington, DC: Social Security Administration.

Bond, G. R., & Dincin, J. (1986). Accelerating entry into transitional employment in a psychosocial rehabilitation agency. *Rehabilitation Psychology, 31,* 143-155.

Bond, G. R., & Friedmeyer, M. H. (1987). Predictive validity of situational assessment at a psychiatric rehabilitation center. *Rehabilitation Psychology, 32,* 99-112.

Bond, S., Bordieri, J., & Musgrave, J. (1989). Tested versus self-estimated aptitudes and interests of vocational evaluation clients. *Vocational Evaluation and Work Adjustment Bulletin, 22*(3), 105-108.

Bordieri, J. E., & Thomas, D. (1986). Facility based services purchased by state vocational rehabilitation agencies. *Vocational Evaluation and Work Adjustment Bulletin, 19*(3), 135-138.

Boring, E. G. (1954). The nature and history of experimental control. *American Journal of Psychology, 67,* 573-589.

Borman, W. C. (1975). Effects of instructions to avoid halo error on reliability and validity of performance evaluation ratings. *Journal of Applied Psychology, 60,* 556-560.

Boruch, R. F., & Gomez, H. (1977). Sensitivity, bias, and theory in impact evaluations. *Professional Psychology, 8,* 411-434.

Botterbusch, K. (1987). *Vocational assessment and evaluation systems: A comparison.* Menomonie: University of Wisconsin—Stout, Materials Development Center.

Bourstom, N. C., & Howard, M. T. (1968). Behavioral correlates of recovery of self-care in hemiplegic patients. *Archives of Physical Medicine and Rehabilitation, 49,* 449-454.

Bowe, F. (1980). *Rehabilitating America.* New York: Harper & Row.

Brekke, J. S. (1987). The model-guided method for monitoring program implementation. *Evaluation Review, 11,* 281-299.

Brolin, D. E. (1976). *Vocational preparation of retarded citizens.* Columbus, OH: Charles E. Merrill.

Brook, R. H., & Lohr, K. N. (1985). Efficacy, effectiveness, variations, and quality: Boundary-crossing research. *Medical Care, 23,* 710-722.

Brook, R. H., & McGlynn, E. A. (1991). Maintenance of quality of care. In E. Ginzberg (Ed.), *Health services research: Key to health policy* (pp. 284-314). Cambridge, MA: Harvard University Press.

Brookings, J. B., & Bolton, B. (1988, August). *Dimensionality of the 16-PF-E with rehabilitation clients.* Paper presented at the American Psychological Association Meeting, Atlanta, GA.

Brookings, J. B., & Bolton, B. (1989). Factorial validity of the United States Employment Service Interest Inventory. *Journal of Vocational Behavior, 34*, 179-191.

Brookings, J. B., & Bolton, B. (1991). Dimensions of satisfactoriness for workers with severe handicaps to employment. *Rehabilitation Psychology, 36*, 21-30.

Brooks, D. N. (1991). The head-injured family. *Journal of Clinical and Experimental Neuropsychology, 13*, 155-188.

Broverman, I., Broverman, D., Clarkson, F., & Rosenkranz, P. (1972). Sex role stereotypes: A current appraisal. *Journal of Social Issues, 28*, 59-78.

Brown, A., Gordon, W., & Diller, L. (1983). Functional assessment and outcome measurement: An integrative review. *Annual Review of Rehabilitation, 3*, 93-120.

Brown, M., Diller, L., Fordyce, W., Jacobs, D., & Gordon, W. (1980). Rehabilitation indicators: Their nature and uses for assessment. In B. Bolton & D. Cook (Eds.), *Rehabilitation client assessment* (pp. 102-117). Baltimore: University Park Press.

Brown, M., Diller, L., & Gordon, W. A. (1983). Functional assessment and outcome measurement: An integrative review. *Annual Review of Rehabilitation, 3*, 93-120.

Bruck, L. (1978). Disabled consumer bill of rights. In R. Goldenson, J. Dunham, & C. Dunham (Eds.), *Disability and rehabilitation handbook*. New York: McGraw-Hill.

Bryden, J. (1989). How many head-injured? The epidemiology of post head injury disability. In R. L. Wood & P. Eames (Eds.), *Models of brain injury rehabilitation* (pp. 17-27). Baltimore: Johns Hopkins University Press.

Buckelew, S. P., Baumstark, K., Frank, R. G., & Hewett, J. (1990). Adjustment following spinal cord injury. *Rehabilitation Psychology, 35*, 101-109.

Buckelew, S. P., Burk, J., Brownlee-Duffeck, M., Frank, R. G., & DeGood, D. (1988). Cognitive and somatic aspects of depression among a rehabilitation sample: Reliability and validity of SCL-90-R research subscales. *Rehabilitation Psychology, 33*, 67-75.

Butler, R. W., Anderson, L., Furst, C. J., Namerow, N. S., et al. (1989). Behavioural assessment in neuropsychological rehabilitation: A method for measuring vocational-related skills. *Clinical Neuropsychologist, 3*, 235-243.

Byrne, B. M. (1989). *A primer of LISREL: Basic applications and programming for confirmatory factor analysis*. New York: Springer-Verlag.

Byrne, B. M., Shavelson, R. J., & Muthén, B. (1989). Testing for the equivalence of factor covariance and mean structures: The issue of partial measurement invariance. *Psychological Bulletin, 105,* 456-466.

Byrne, L., Averbuch, M., Rubio, A., & Weintraub, M. (1990). Compliance (CMPL) measures via medication event monitoring system (MEMS) as an adjunct in interpreting pharmacokinetic data. *Clinical and Pharmacological Therapeutics, 47,*152.

Calkins, P. (1988, May). *Voting and disability: An emerging constituency.* Unpublished manuscript.

Campbell, D. T., & Fiske, D. W. (1959). Convergent and discriminant validation by the multitrait-multimethod matrix. *Psychological Bulletin, 56,* 81-105.

Campbell, S. K. (1987). On the importance of being earnest about measurement, OR, How can we be sure that what we know is true? *Physical Therapy, 67,* 1831-1833.

Caplan, B. (1982). Neuropsychology in rehabilitation: Its role in evaluation and intervention. *Archives of Physical Medicine and Rehabilitation, 63,* 362-366.

Caston, H. L., & Watson, A. L. (1990). Vocational assessment and rehabilitation outcomes. *Rehabilitation Counseling Bulletin, 34,* 61-66.

Caywood, T. (1974). A quadriplegic young man looks at treatment. *Journal of Rehabilitation, 49*(6), 22-25.

Chapman, L. J., & Chapman, J. P. (1967). Genesis of popular but erroneous psychodiagnostic observations. *Journal of Abnormal Psychology, 72,* 193-204.

Chapman, L. J., & Chapman, J. P. (1969). Illusory correlation as an obstacle to the use of valid psychodiagnostic signs. *Journal of Abnormal Psychology, 74,* 271-280.

Chen, H. (1990). Issues in constructing program theory. In L. Bickman (Ed.), *Advances in program theory* (New Directions for Program Evaluation, No. 47, pp. 7-17). San Francisco: Jossey-Bass.

Chen, H., & Rossi, P. H. (1980). The multi-goal, theory-driven approach to evaluation: A model linking basic and applied social science. *Social Forces, 59,* 106-122.

Chen, H., & Rossi, P. H. (1981). The multi-goal, theory-driven approach to evaluation: A model linking basic and applied social science. In H. E. Freeman & M. A. Solomon (Eds.), *Evaluation studies review annual* (Vol. 6, pp. 38-54). Beverly Hills, CA: Sage.

Chen, H., & Rossi, P. H. (1983). Evaluating with sense: The theory-driven approach. *Evaluation Review, 7,* 283-302.

Chen, H., & Rossi, P. H. (1987). The theory-driven approach to validity. *Evaluation and Program Planning, 10,* 95-103.

Christensen, A. L. (1989). The neuropsychological investigation as a therapeutic and rehabilitative technique. In D. W. Ellis & A. Christensen (Eds.), *Neuropsychological treatment after brain injury* (pp. 127-153). Boston: Kluwer Academic.

Cliff, N. (1983). Some cautions concerning the application of causal modeling methods. *Multivariate Behavioral Research, 18,* 115-126.

Cnaan, R. A., Blankertz, L., Messinger, K. W., & Gardner, J. R. (1988). Psychosocial rehabilitation: Toward a definition. *Psychosocial Rehabilitation Journal, 11,* 61-77.

Cohen, J. (1990). Things I have learned (so far). *American Psychologist, 45,* 1304-1312.

Cole, D. A. (1987). Utility of confirmatory factor analysis in test validation research. *Journal of Consulting and Clinical Psychology, 55,* 584-594.

Colvin, C. (1983). Rehabilitation in the public mind. In L. Perlman (Ed.), *Rehabilitation in the public mind* (pp. 48-56). Alexandria, VA: National Rehabilitation Association.

Cook, D. W. (1983). The accuracy of work evaluator and client predictions of client vocational competency and rehabilitation outcome. *Journal of Rehabilitation, 49*(2), 46-49.

Cook, D. W., & Brookings, J. B. (1980). The relationship of rehabilitation client vocational appraisal to training outcome and employment. *Journal of Applied Rehabilitation Counseling, 11*(1), 32-35.

Cook, J. A., Bond, G. R., Hoffschmidt, S. J., Jonas, E. A., Razzano, L., & Weakland, R. (1991). *Assessing vocational performance among persons with severe mental illness.* Chicago: Thresholds National Research and Training Center.

Cope, D. N. (1982). Conclusions. In *Head Injury Rehabilitation Project final report.* A report to the National Institute for Handicapped Research from the Institute for Medical Research, Santa Clara Valley Medical Center, San Jose, CA.

Cope, D. N., & Hall, K. (1982). Head injury rehabilitation: Benefit of early intervention. *Archives of Physical Medicine and Rehabilitation, 63,* 433-437.

Cordray, D. S. (1986). Quasi-experimental analysis: A mixture of methods and judgment. *New Directions in Program Evaluation, 31,* 9-27.

Cordray, D. S. (1990). Strengthening causal interpretations of nonexperimental data: The role of meta-analysis. In L. Sechrest, E. Perrin, & J. Bunker (Eds.), *Research methodology: Strengthening causal interpretations of nonexperimental data* (pp. 151-172). Rockville, MD: Agency for Health Care Policy and Research.

Cordray, D. S., & Pion, G. M. (1991). What's behind the numbers? Definitional issues in counting the homeless. *Housing Policy Debate, 2,* 587-616.

Cordray, D. S., & Sonnefeld, L. J. (1985). Quantitative synthesis: An actuarial base for planning research. *New Directions in Program Evaluation, 27,* 29-48.

Costa, L. (1983). Clinical neuropsychology: A discipline in evolution. *Journal of Clinical Neuropsychology, 5,* 1-11.

Cottone, R. R., Grelle, M., & Wilson, W. C. (1988). The accuracy of systemic versus psychological evidence in judging vocational evaluator recommendations: A preliminary test of systemic theory of vocational rehabilitation. *Journal of Rehabilitation, 54*(1), 45-51.

Council of Organizational Representatives (COR). (1989-1990). [Minutes]. Washington, DC: Author.

Craik, K. H. (1986). Personality research methods: An historical perspective. *Journal of Personality, 54,* 18-51.

Crewe, N. M., & Athelstan, G. T. (1984). *Functional Assessment Inventory manual.* Menomonie: University of Wisconsin–Stout, Materials Development Center.

Cronbach, L. J., & Meehl, P. E. (1955). Construct validity in psychological tests. *Psychological Bulletin, 52,* 281-302.

Cudeck, R. C. (1989). Analysis of correlation matrices using covariance structure models. *Psychological Bulletin, 105,* 317-327.

Cull, J. G., & Hardy, R. E. (1972). *Vocational rehabilitation: Profession and process.* Springfield, IL: Charles C Thomas.

Cullen, F. T., Clark, G. A., Cullen, J. B., & Mathers, R. A. (1985). Attribution, salience, and attitudes toward criminal sanctioning. *Criminal Justice and Behavior, 12,* 305-331.

Dana, R. H. (1984). Assessment for health psychology. *Clinical Psychology Review, 4,* 459-476.

Davidoff, G. N., Ring, H., & Solzi, P. (1991). Acute stroke patients: Long-term effects of rehabilitation and maintenance of gains. *Archives of Physical Medicine and Rehabilitation, 72,* 869-873.

Dawes, R. M. (1979). The robust beauty of improper linear models in decision making. *American Psychologist, 34,* 571-582.

Dawes, R. M. (1989). Experience and validity of clinical judgment: The illusory correlation. *Behavioral Sciences & the Law, 7,* 457-467.

Dawes, R. M. (in press). *Psychology and psychotherapy: The myth of professional expertise.*

Dawes, R. M., Faust, D., & Meehl, P. E. (1989). Clinical versus actuarial judgment. *Science, 243,* 1668-1674.

Dawis, R. V. (1976). The Minnesota Theory of Work Adjustment. In B. Bolton (Ed.), *Handbook of measurement and evaluation* (pp. 227-248). Baltimore: University Park Press.

Dawis, R. V. (1987). The Minnesota Theory of Work Adjustment. In B. Bolton (Ed.), *Handbook of measurement and evaluation in rehabilitation* (2nd ed., pp. 203-217). Baltimore: Paul H. Brookes.

DeJong, G. (1987). Medical rehabilitation outcome measurement in a changing health care market. In M. J. Fuhrer (Ed.), *Rehabilitation outcomes: Analysis and measurements* (pp. 261-271). Baltimore: Paul H. Brookes.

DeJong, G., Branch, L. G., & Corcoran, P. J. (1984). Independent living outcomes in spinal cord injury: Multivariate analyses. *Archives of Physical Medicine and Rehabilitation, 65,* 66-73.

DeJong, G., & Hughes, J. (1982). Independent living: Methodology for measuring long-term outcomes. *Archives of Physical Medicine and Rehabilitation, 63,* 68-73.

DeLoach, C., & Greer, B. (1981). *Adjustment to severe physical disability.* New York: McGraw-Hill.

Dembo, T., Diller, L., Gordon, W., Leviton, G., & Sherr, R. (1973). A view of rehabilitation psychology. *American Psychologist, 28,* 719-722.

Derogatis, L. R., & Cleary, P. (1977). Confirmation of the dimensional structure of the SCL-90 R study in construct validation. *Journal of Clinical Psychology, 33,* 981-989.

Devins, G. M., & Seland, T. (1987). Emotional impact of multiple sclerosis: Recent findings and suggestions for future research. *Psychological Bulletin, 101,* 363-375.

Dial, J. G., McCarron, L. T., Freemon, L., & Swearingen, S. (1979). Predictive validation of the abbreviated McCarron-Dial Evaluation System. *Vocational Evaluation and Work Adjustment Bulletin, 12*(1), 11-18.

Dikmen, S., McLean, A., Jr., Temkin, N. R., & Wyler, A. R. (1986). Neuropsychologic outcome at one-month postinjury. *Archives of Physical Medicine and Rehabilitation, 67,* 507-513.

Diller, L. (1987). Neuropsychological rehabilitation. In M. J. Meier, A. L. Benton, & L. Diller (Eds.), *Neuropsychological rehabilitation* (pp. 3-17). New York: Guilford.

Diller, L., & Gordon, W. A. (1981). Rehabilitation and clinical neuropsychology. In S. B. Filskov & T. J. Boll (Eds.), *Handbook of clinical neuropsychology* (pp. 702-733). New York: John Wiley.

Dombovy, M. L., Sandok, B. A., & Basford, J. R. (1986). Rehabilitation for stroke: A review. *Stroke, 17,* 363-369.

Donaldson, S. W., Wagner, C. C., & Gresham, G. E. (1973). A unified ADL evaluation form. *Archives of Physical Medicine and Rehabilitation, 54,* 175-180.

Drasgow, F., & Kanfer, R. (1985). Equivalence of psychological measurement in heterogeneous populations. *Journal of Applied Psychology, 70,* 662-680.

Dunlap, W. R., & Iceman, D. J. (1985). The development and validation of a set of instruments to assess the independent living skills of the handicapped. *Educational and Psychological Measurement, 45,* 925-929.

Dunn, E. J., Searight, H. R., Grisso, T., Margolis, R. B., & Gibbons, J. L. (1990). The relation of the Halstead-Reitan Neuropsychological Battery to functional daily living skills in geriatric patients. *Archives of Clinical Neuropsychology, 5,* 103-117.

Dunn, M., & Herman, S. (1982). Social skills and physical disability. In D. M. Doleys & R. Meredith (Eds.), *Behavioral medicine: Assessment and treatment strategies* (pp. 117-144). New York: Plenum.

Edelstein, B. A., & Brasted, W. S. (1983). Clinical training. In M. Hersen, A. Kazdin, & A. Bellack (Eds.), *The clinical psychology handbook* (pp. 35-56). New York: Pergamon.

Eder, R. W., & Ferris, G. R. (1989). *The employment interview: Theory, research, and practice.* Newbury Park, CA: Sage.

Efron, D. E., & Glueckauf, R. L. (1989). Pragmatics of the Tiger-Shark integrative model of family therapy. *Journal of Strategic and Systemic Therapies, 8*(1), 1-17.

Eisenberg, M. G., & Glueckauf, R. L. (1991). Introduction. In M. G. Eisenberg & R. L. Glueckauf (Eds.), *Empirical approaches to psychosocial aspects of disability* (pp. xi-xiii). New York: Springer.

Eisenberg, M., Griggins, C., & Duval, R. (1982). *Disabled people as second class citizens.* New York: Springer.

Eisenberg, M., & Jansen, M. (1983). Rehabilitation psychology: State of the art. In E. L. Pan, T. E. Backer, & C. L. Vash (Eds.), *Annual review of rehabilitation* (Vol. 3, pp. 1-31). New York: Springer.

Eisenberger, R., Karpman, M., & Trattner, J. (1967). What is the necessary and sufficient condition for reinforcement in the contingency situation? *Journal of Experimental Psychology, 74,* 342-350.

Elliott, T., Frank, R. G., & Brownlee-Duffeck, M. (1988). Clinical inferences about depression and physical disability. *Professional Psychology: Research and Practice, 19,* 206-210.

Elliott, T., Godshall, F., Herrick, S., Witty, T., & Spruell, M. (1991). Problem-solving appraisal and psychological adjustment following spinal cord injury. *Cognitive Therapy and Research, 15,* 387-398.

Elliott, T., & Gramling, S. (1990). Psychologists and rehabilitation: New roles and old training models. *American Psychologist, 45,* 762-765.

Elliott, T., & Harkins, S. (1991). Psychosocial concomitants of persistent pain among persons with spinal cord injury. *NeuroRehabilitation: An Interdisciplinary Journal, 1*(4), 9-18.

Elliott, T., Herrick, S., Patti, A., Witty, T., Godshall, F., & Spruell, M. (1991). Assertiveness, social support, and psychological adjustment of persons with spinal cord injury. *Behaviour Research and Therapy, 29,* 485-493.

Elliott, T., Herrick, S., & Witty, T. (1992). Problem solving appraisal and the effects of social support among college students and persons with physical disabilities. *Journal of Counseling Psychology, 39,* 219-226.

Elliott, T., Witty, T., Herrick, S., & Hoffman, J. (1991). Negotiating reality after physical loss: Hope, depression, and disability. *Journal of Personality and Social Psychology, 61,* 608-613.

England, B., Glass, R. M., & Patterson, C. H. (1989). *Quality rehabilitation: Results-oriented patient care.* Chicago: American Hospital Publishing.

Epstein, S. (1978). The stability of behavior: I. On predicting most of the people much of the time. *Journal of Personality and Social Psychology, 37,* 1097-1126.

Ewan, C. E., & Whaite, A. (1983). Evaluation of training programs for health professionals in substance misuse: A review. *Journal of Studies on Alcohol, 44,* 885-899.

Faust, D. (1984). *The limits of scientific reasoning.* Minneapolis: University of Minnesota Press.

Faust, D. (1989). Data integration in legal evaluations: Can clinicians deliver on their premises? *Behavioral Sciences & the Law, 7,* 469-483.

Faust, D. (1991). What if we had really listened? Present reflections on altered pasts. In D. Cicchetti & W. M. Grove (Eds.), *Thinking clearly about psychology: Vol. 1. Matters of public interest.* Minneapolis: University of Minnesota Press.

Faust, D., Guilmette, T. J., Hart, K., Arkes, H. R., Fishburne, F. J., & Davey, L. (1988). Neuropsychologists' training, experience, and judgment accuracy. *Archives of Clinical Neuropsychology, 3,* 145-163.

Faust, D., & Ziskin, J. (1988). The expert witness in psychology and psychiatry. *Science, 241,* 31-35.

Faust, D., Ziskin, J., & Hiers, J. B., Jr. (1991). *Brain damage claims: Coping with neuropsychological evidence* (Vols. 1 & 2). Los Angeles: Law and Psychology Press.

Fee, F. A., Elkins, G. R., & Boyd, L. (1982). Testing and counseling psychologists: Current practices and implications for training. *Journal of Personality Assessment, 46,* 116-118.

Feldman, D. J., Lee, P. R., Unterecker, J. U., Lloyd, K., Rusk, H. A., & Toole, A. (1962). A comparison of functional oriented medical care and formal rehabilitation in the management of patients with hemiplegia due to cerebrovascular disease. *Journal of Chronic Diseases, 15,* 297-310.

Ferketich, S. L., Figueredo, A. J., & Knapp, T. R. (1991). The multitrait-multimethod approach to construct validity. *Research in Nursing and Health, 14,* 315-320.

Feynman, R. P. (1985). *Surely you're joking, Mr. Feynman!* New York: Norton.

Figueredo, A. J., Ferketich, S. L., & Knapp, T. R. (1991). More on MTMM: The role of confirmatory factor analysis. *Research in Nursing and Health, 14,* 387-391.

Finger, S. (Ed.). (1978). *Recovery from brain damage: Research and theory.* New York: Plenum.

Finger, S., LeVere, T. E., Almli, C. R., & Stein, D. G. (1988). *Brain injury and recovery.* New York: Plenum.

Finger, S., & Stein, D. G. (1982). *Brain damage and recovery: Research and clinical perspectives.* New York: Academic Press.

Fischhoff, B. (1977). Cost benefit analysis and the art of motorcycle maintenance. *Policy Science, 8,* 177-202.

Fischhoff, B. (1980). For those condemned to study the past: Reflections on historical judgment. In R. A. Schweder & D. W. Fiske (Eds.), *New directions for methodology of behavioral science: Fallible judgment in behavioral research* (pp. 79-93). San Francisco: Jossey-Bass.

Fischhoff, B. (1982). Debiasing. In D. Kahneman, P. Slovic, & A. Tversky (Eds.), *Judgment under uncertainty: Heuristics and biases* (pp. 422-444). Cambridge, UK: Cambridge University Press.

Fisher-Beckfield, D., & McFall, R. M. (1982). The development of a competence inventory for college men and evaluation of relationships between competence and depression. *Journal of Consulting and Clinical Psychology, 50,* 697-705.

Fiske, D. W. (1978). *Measuring the concepts of personality.* Chicago: Aldine.

Flor, H., Birbaumer, N., & Turk, D. C. (1990). The psychobiology of chronic pain. *Advances in Behavior Research and Therapy, 12,* 47-84.

Fordyce, W. E. (1964). Personality characteristics in men with spinal cord injury as related to manner of onset of disability. *Archives of Physical Medicine and Rehabilitation, 45,* 321-325.

Fordyce, W. (1971). Behavioral methods in rehabilitation. In W. S. Neff (Ed.), *Rehabilitation psychology* (pp. 74-108). New York: American Psychological Association.

Fordyce, W. E. (1976). *Behavioral methods for chronic pain and illness.* St. Louis: C. V. Mosby.

Fortune, J., & Eldredge, G. (1982). Predictive validation of the McCarron-Dial Evaluation System for psychiatrically disabled sheltered workshop workers. *Vocational Evaluation and Work Adjustment Bulletin, 15*(4), 136-141.

Foulkes, M. A., Wolf, P. A., Price, T. R., Mohr, J. P., & Hier, D. B. (1988). The stroke data bank: Design, methods, and baseline characteristics. *Stroke, 19,* 547-554.

Frank, R. G., Beck, N., Parker, J., Kashani, J., Elliott, T., Haut, A., Smith, E., Atwood, C., Brownlee-Duffeck, M., & Kay, D. (1988). Depression in rheumatoid arthritis. *Journal of Rheumatology, 15,* 920-925.

Frank, R. G., & Elliott, T. (1987). Life stress and psychologic adjustment following spinal cord injury. *Archives of Physical Medicine and Rehabilitation, 68,* 344-347.

Frank, R. G., Elliott, T., Corcoran, J., & Wonderlich, S. (1987). Depression following spinal cord injury: Is it necessary? *Clinical Psychology Review, 7,* 611-630.

Frank, R. G., Kashani, J., Wonderlich, S., Lising, A., & Visot, L. (1985). Depression and adrenal function in spinal cord injury. *American Journal of Psychiatry, 142,* 252-253.

Frank, R. G., Umlauf, R., Wonderlich, S., Askanazi, G., Buckelew, S., & Elliott, T. (1987). Differences in coping styles among persons with spinal cord injury: A cluster-analytic approach. *Journal of Consulting and Clinical Psychology, 55,* 727-731.

Freedman, B. J., Rosenthal, L., Donahoe, C. P., Jr., Schlundt, D. G., & McFall, R. M. (1978). A social-behavioral analysis of skill deficits in delinquent and nondelinquent adolescent boys. *Journal of Consulting and Clinical Psychology, 46,* 1448-1462.

Frey, W. D. (1984). Functional assessment in the '80s: A conceptual enigma, a technical challenge. In A. S. Halpern & M. J. Fuhrer (Eds.), *Functional assessment in rehabilitation* (pp. 11-43). Baltimore: Paul H. Brookes.

Fry, R. (1986). *Work evaluation and adjustment: An annotated bibliography.* (Available from the Materials Development Center, School of Education and Human Services, University of Wisconsin—Stout, Menomonie, WI 54751)

Fuhrer, M. J. (1987a). Overview of outcome analysis in rehabilitation. In M. J. Fuhrer (Ed.), *Rehabilitation outcomes* (pp. 1-15). Baltimore: Paul H. Brookes.

Fuhrer, M. J. (Ed.). (1987b). *Rehabilitation outcomes: Analysis and measurement.* Baltimore: Paul H. Brookes.

Funk, R. (1987). Disability rights: From caste to class in the context of civil rights. In A. Gartner & T. Joe (Eds.), *Images of the disabled, disabling images.* New York: Praeger.

Gaffney, L. R., & McFall, R. M. (1981). A comparison of social skills in delinquent and nondelinquent adolescent girls using a behavioral role-playing inventory. *Journal of Consulting and Clinical Psychology, 49,* 959-967.

Gangu. ` R. (1983). Medical assessment. In M. Hersen, A. Kazdin, & A. Bellack (Eds.), *The clinical psychology handbook* (pp. 35-56). New York: Pergamon.

Gannaway, T. W., Sink, J. M., & Becket, W. C. (1980). A predictive validity study of a job sample program with handicapped and disadvantaged individuals. *Vocational Guidance Quarterly, 29*(1), 4-11.

Gans, J. S. (1981). Depression diagnosis in a rehabilitation hospital. *Archives of Physical Medicine and Rehabilitation, 62,* 386-389.

Garraway, W. M., Akhtar, A. J., Hockey, L., & Prescott, R. J. (1980). Management of acute stroke in the elderly: Follow-up of a controlled trial. *British Medical Journal, 281,* 827-829.

Garraway, W. M., Akhtar, A. J., Prescott, R. J., & Hockey, L. (1980). Management of acute stroke in the elderly: Preliminary results of a controlled trial. *British Medical Journal, 281,* 1040-1043.

Gartner, A., & Joe, T. (Eds.). (1987). *Images of the disabled, disabling images.* New York: Praeger.

Gasparrini, B., & Satz, P. (1979). Treatment for memory problems in left hemisphere CVA patients. *Journal of Clinical Neuropsychology, 1,* 137-150.

Gay, E. G., Weiss, D. J., Hendel, D. D., Da ،ris, R. V., & Lofquist, L. H. (1971). *Manual for the Minnesota Importance Questionnaire.* Minneapolis: University of Minnesota, Vocational Psychology Research.

Gellman, W., Stern, D., & Soloff, A. (1963). *A scale of employability for handicapped persons.* Chicago: Jewish Vocational Services.

Genskow, J. K. (1980). Evaluation: A multi-purpose proposition. In B. Bolton & D. W. Cook (Eds.), *Rehabilitation client assessment* (pp. 204-212). Baltimore: University Park Press.

Gibson, D. L., Weiss, D. J., Hendel, D. D., Dawis, R. V., & Lofquist, L. H. (1970). *Manual for the Minnesota Satisfactoriness Scales.* Minneapolis: University of Minnesota, Vocational Psychology Research.

Gilberstadt, H. (1968). Relationship among scores of tests suitable for assessment of adjustment and intellectual functioning. *Journal of Gerontology, 23,* 483-487.

Gill, W. S. (1972). The psychologist and rehabilitation. In J. G. Cull & R. E. Hardy (Eds.), *Vocational rehabilitation: Profession and process* (pp. 470-483). Springfield, IL: Charles C Thomas.

Glaser, E. M., Abelson, H. H., & Garrison, K. N. (1983). *Putting knowledge to use: Facilitating the diffusion of knowledge and the implementation of planned change.* San Francisco: Jossey-Bass.

Glick, I. D., & Sternberg, D. (1969). Performance I.Q. as predictor of hospital treatment outcome. *Comprehensive Psychiatry, 10,* 365-368.

Glickman, N. (1986). Cultural identity and deafness and mental health. *Journal of Rehabilitation of the Deaf, 20,* 1-10.

Glueckauf, R. L. (1990). Program evaluation guidelines for the rehabilitation professional. In M. G. Eisenberg & R. Grzesiak (Eds.), *Advances in clinical rehabilitation* (Vol. 3, pp. 250-266). New York: Springer.

Glueckauf, R. L., Webb, P. M., Papandria-Long, M., Rasmussen, J. L., Markand, O., & Farlow, M. (in press). The Family and Disability Assessment System: Consistency and accuracy of judgments across coders and measures. *Rehabilitation Psychology, 37*(4).

Goffman, E. (1963). *Stigma: Notes on the management of spoiled identity.* Englewood Cliffs, NJ: Prentice-Hall.

Goldberg, L. R. (1968). Simple models or simple processes? Some research on clinical judgments. *American Psychologist, 23,* 483-496.

Goldberg, L. R. (1991). Human mind versus regression equation: Five contrasts. In D. Cicchetti & W. M. Grove (Eds.), *Thinking clearly about psychology: Vol. 1. Matters of public interest. Essays in honor of Paul E. Meehl* (pp. 173-184). Minneapolis: University of Minnesota Press.

Golden, C. J., Purisch, A. D., & Hammeke, T. A. (1985). *Luria-Nebraska Neuropsychological Battery: Forms I and II, manual.* Los Angeles: Western Psychological Services.

Goldenson, R., Dunham, J., & Dunham, C. (Eds.). (1978). *Disability and rehabilitation handbook.* New York: McGraw-Hill.

Goldfried, M. R., & D'Zurilla, T. J. (1969). A behavioral-analytic model for assessing competence. In C. D. Spielberger (Ed.), *Current topics in clinical and community psychology* (Vol. 1, pp. 151-196). New York: Academic Press.

Goldfried, M. R., & Kent, R. N. (1972). Traditional vs. behavioral assessment: A comparison of methodological assumptions. *Psychological Bulletin, 77,* 409-420.

Goldman, L. (1990). Qualitative assessment. *Counseling Psychologist, 18,* 205-213.

Goldsmith, J. B., & McFall, R. M. (1975). Development and evaluation of an interpersonal skill-training program for psychiatric inpatients. *Journal of Abnormal Psychology, 84,* 51-58.

Goldstein, A. P., Heller, K., & Sechrest, L. B. (1966). *Psychotherapy and the psychology of behavior change.* New York: John Wiley.

Gorsuch, R. L. (1983). *Factor analysis* (2nd ed.). Hillsdale, NJ: Lawrence Erlbaum.

Gorsuch, R. L. (1988). Exploratory factor analysis. In J. R. Nesselroade & R. B. Cattell (Eds.), *Handbook of multivariate experimental psychology* (2nd ed., pp. 231-258). New York: Plenum.

Gottlieb, H., Alperson, B. L., Schwartz, A. H., Beck, C., & Kee, S. (1988). Self-management for medication reduction in chronic low back pain. *Archives of Physical Medicine and Rehabilitation, 69,* 442-448.

Granger, C., Albrecht, G., & Hamilton, B. (1979). Outcome of comprehensive medical rehabilitation: Measurement by PULSES and the Barthel Index. *Archives of Physical Medicine and Rehabilitation, 60,* 145-154.

Granger, C. V. (1984). A conceptual model of functional assessment. In C. V. Granger & G. E. Gresham (Eds.), *Functional assessment in rehabilitation medicine* (pp. 14-25). Baltimore: Williams & Wilkins.

Granger, C. V., Dewis, L. S., Peters, N. C., Sherwood, C. C., & Barrett, J. E. (1979). Stroke rehabilitation: Analysis of repeated Barthel Index measures. *Archives of Physical Medicine and Rehabilitation, 60,* 14-17.

Granger, C. V., & Gresham, G. E. (Eds.). (1984). *Functional assessment in rehabilitation medicine.* Baltimore: Williams & Wilkins.

Granger, C. V., & Hamilton, B. B. (1992). The uniform data system for medical rehabilitation report of first admissions for 1990. *American Journal of Physical Medicine and Rehabilitation, 71,* 108-113.

Granger, C. V., Hamilton, B. B., Keith, R. A., Zielezny, M., & Sherwin, F. S. (1986). Advances in functional assessment for medical rehabilitation. *Topics in Geriatric Rehabilitation, 1*(3), 59-74.

Gresham, G. E., Fitzpatrick, T. E., Wolf, P. A., McNamara, P. M., Kannel, W. B., & Dawber, T. R. (1975). Residual disability in survivors of stroke: The Framingham study. *New England Journal of Medicine, 293,* 954-956.

Griggins, C. (1982). The disabled face a schizophrenic society. In M. Eisenberg, C. Griggins, & R. Duval (Eds.), *Disabled people as second-class citizens.* New York: Springer.

Grosjean, F. (1982). *Life with two languages.* Cambridge, MA: Harvard University Press.

Grzesiak, R. (1979). Psychological services in rehabilitation medicine: Clinical aspects of rehabilitation psychology. *Professional Psychology, 10,* 511-520.

Grzesiak, R. (1981). Rehabilitation psychology, medical psychology, health psychology, and behavioral medicine. *Professional Psychology, 12,* 411-413.

Guilmette, T. J., Faust, D., Hart, K., & Arkes, H. R. (1990). A national survey of psychologists who offer neuropsychological services. *Archives of Clinical Neuropsychology, 5,* 373-392.

Haffey, W. J., & Johnston, M. V. (1989). An information system to assess the effectiveness of brain injury rehabilitation. In R. L. Wood & P. Eames (Eds.), *Models of brain injury rehabilitation* (pp. 205-233). Baltimore: Johns Hopkins University Press.

Hagen, C., Malkmus, D., & Durham, P. (1979). *Levels of cognitive functioning in rehabilitation of the head injured adult: Comprehensive physical management.* Downey, CA: Rancho Los Amigos Hospital.

Halpern, A. S., & Fuhrer, M. J. (Eds.). (1984). *Functional assessment in rehabilitation.* Baltimore: Paul H. Brookes.

Halpern, A. S., Irwin, L. K., & Mundres, A. W. (1986). *Social and Prevocational Information Battery-Revised: Examiner's manual.* Monterey, CA: CTB/McGraw-Hill.

Halstead, L. S. (1976). Team care in chronic illness: A critical review of the literature of the past 25 years. *Archives of Physical Medicine and Rehabilitation, 57,* 507-511.

Hamilton, B. B., Granger, C. V., Sherwin, F. S., Zielezny, M., & Tashman, J. S. (1987). A uniform national data system for medical rehabilitation. In M. J. Fuhrer (Ed.), *Rehabilitation outcomes: Analysis and measurement* (pp. 137-147). Baltimore: Paul H. Brookes.

Hammill, D. D., Brown, L., & Bryant, B. R. (1989). *A consumer's guide to tests in print.* Austin, TX: Pro-Ed.

Harmon, L. W., Sharma, V., & Trotter, A. B. (1976). Vocational inventories. In B. Bolton (Ed.), *Handbook of measurement and evaluation* (pp. 133-158). Baltimore: University Park Press.

Hathaway, S. R., & McKinley, J. C. (1989). *MMPI-2: Manual for administration and scoring.* Minneapolis: University of Minnesota Press.

Haworth, R. J., & Hollings, E. M. (1979). Are hospital assessments of daily living activities valid? *International Rehabilitation Medicine, 1,* 59-62.

Hayes, S. C. (1987). The gathering storm. *Behavior Analysis, 22*(2), 41-45.

Healy, C. (1990). Reforming career appraisals to meet the needs of clients in the 1990's. *Counseling Psychologist, 18,* 214-226.

Heaton, R. K., Grant, I., Anthony, W. Z., & Lehman, A. W. (1981). A comparison of clinical and automated interpretation of the Halstead-Reitan Battery. *Journal of Clinical Neuropsychology, 3,* 122-141.

Heaton, R. K., & Pendleton, M. G. (1981). Use of neuropsychological tests to predict adult patients' every day functioning. *Journal of Consulting and Clinical Psychology, 49,* 807-821.

Heinemann, A. W., Goranson, N., Ginsburg, K., & Schnoll, S. (1989). Alcohol use and activity patterns following spinal cord injury. *Rehabilitation Psychology, 34,* 191-206.

Heinemann, A. W., Mamott, B., & Schnoll, S. (1990). Substance use by persons with recent spinal cord injuries. *Rehabilitation Psychology, 35,* 217-228.

Hertzog, C. (1989). Using confirmatory factor analysis for scale development and validation. In M. P. Lawton & A. R. Herzog (Eds.), *Special research methods for gerontology* (pp. 281-306). New York: Bayward.

Hickling, E. J., Sison, G. F., & Holtz, J. L. (1985). Role of psychologists in multidisciplinary pain clinics: A national survey. *Professional Psychology: Research and Practice, 16,* 868-880.

Higgins, P. (1980). *Outsiders in a hearing world: A sociology of deafness.* Beverly Hills CA: Sage.

Higgins, P. (1985). *Rehabilitation detectives: Doing human service work.* Beverly Hills, CA: Sage.

Hiskey, M. (1966). *Manual for the Hiskey-Nebraska Test of Learning Aptitude.* Lincoln, NE: Union College Press.

Holland, J. L. (1984). *Making vocational choices: A theory of vocational personalities and work environments* (2nd ed.). Englewood Cliffs, NJ: Prentice-Hall.

Hollin, C. R., & Trower, P. (1986). *Handbook of social skills training* (Vols. 1, 2). Oxford, UK: Pergamon.

House, A. (1988). Mood disorders in the physically ill: Problems of definition and measurement. *Journal of Psychosomatic Research, 32,* 345-353.

Hsu, T. C., & Shermis, M. D. (1989). The development and evaluation of a microcomputerized adaptive placement testing system for college mathematics. *Journal of Educational Computing Research, 5,* 473-485.

Hunter, J. E. (1980). *The dimensionality of the General Aptitude Test Battery (GATB) and the dominance of general over specific factors in the prediction of job performance* (USES Test Research Report No. 44). Washington, DC: U.S. Department of Labor.

Hunter, J. E., & Hunter, R. F. (1984). Validity and utility of alternative predictors of job performance. *Psychological Bulletin, 96,* 72-98.

Hursh, N. C., Rogers, E. S., & Anthony, W. A. (1988). Vocational evaluation with people who are psychiatrically disabled: Results of a national survey. *Vocational Evaluation and Work Adjustment Bulletin, 21*(4), 149-155.

Hyman, M. D. (1972). Social psychological determinants of patients' performance in stroke rehabilitation. *Archives of Physical Medicine and Rehabilitation, 53,* 217-226.

Hyman, R. (1977). "Cold reading": How to convince strangers that you know all about them. *Zetetic, 1,* 18-37.

In-home measurements for epidemiologic research. (1988, Spring). *Network,* pp. 1-2 (Watertown, MA: New England Research Institute).

Institute for Personality and Ability Testing. (1985). *Manual for Form E of the 16 PF.* Champaign, IL: IPAT.

Institute of Medicine. (1991). *Disability in America.* Washington, DC: National Academy Press.

International Association for Psychosocial Rehabilitation Services. (1985). *Organizations providing psychosocial rehabilitation and related community support services in the United States: A national directory.* McLean, VA: Author.

Jacobs, H. E. (1988). The Los Angeles Head Injury Survey: Procedures and initial findings. *Archives of Physical Medicine and Rehabilitation, 69,* 425-431.

Jacobsen, N. S., & Margolin, G. (1979). *Marital therapy: Strategies based on social learning and behavior exchange principles.* New York: Brunner/Mazel.

Jansen, M. A., & Eisenberg, M. (1982). Editorial. *Rehabilitation Psychology, 27,* 3.

Jansen, M. A., & Fulcher, R. (1982). Rehabilitation psychologists: Characteristics and scope of practice. *American Psychologist, 37,* 1282-1283.

Jastak, J. E., & Jastak, S. (1987). *Wide Range Interest-Opinion Test.* (Available from Jastak Associates, 1526 Gilpin Ave., Wilmington, DE)

Jette, A. M. (1980). Health status indicators: Their utility in chronic-disease evaluation research. *Journal of Chronic Diseases, 33,* 567-579.

Johnson, M. (1987). Emotion and pride: Search for a disability culture. *Disability Rag, 8,* 1, 4-10.

Johnston, M. V. (1987). Cost-Benefit methodologies in rehabilitation. In M. J. Fuhrer (Ed.), *Rehabilitation outcomes: Analysis and measurement* (pp. 99-113). Baltimore: Paul H. Brookes.

Johnston, M. V., Findley, T. W., DeLuca, J., & Katz, R. T. (1991). Research in physical medicine and rehabilitation. XII. Measurement tools with application to brain injury. *American Journal of Physical Medicine and Rehabilitation, 70*(Suppl.), S114-S130.

Johnston, M. V., & Keith, R. A. (1983). Cost-benefits of medical rehabilitation: Review and critique. *Archives of Physical Medicine and Rehabilitation, 64,* 147-154.

Jones, W. P. (1983). Measurement of personality traits of the visually limited. *Education of the Visually Handicapped, 15,* 12-19.

Jongbloed, J. (1986). Prediction of function after stroke: A critical review. *Stroke, 17,* 765-776.

Jöreskog, K. G., & Sörbom, D. (1984). *LISREL VI: Analysis of linear structural relationships by the method of maximum likelihood.* Mooresville, IN: Scientific Software, Inc.

Ju, J., & Thomas, K. (1987). Accuracy of counselor perception of client work values and client satisfaction. *Rehabilitation Counseling Bulletin, 30,* 157-166.

Kagitcibasi, C., & Berry, J. (1989). Cross cultural psychology: Current research and trends. In M. Rosenzweig & L. Porter (Eds.), *Annual review of psychology* (Vol. 40, pp. 493-531). Palo Alto, CA: Annual Reviews.

Kalsbeek, W. D., McLaurin, R. L., Harris, B. S. H., & Miller, J. D. (1980). National Head and Spinal Cord Injury Survey: Major findings. *Journal of Neurosurgery, 53,* S19-S31.

Kanfer, F. H., & Saslow, G. (1967). Behavioral diagnosis. In C. M. Frank (Ed.), *Behavior therapy: Appraisal and status.* New York: McGraw-Hill.

Kashani, J., Frank, R., Kashani, S., Wonderlich, S., & Reid, J. (1983). Depression among amputees. *Journal of Clinical Psychiatry, 44,* 256-258.

Kathol, R. (1985). Depression associated with physical disease. In E. E. Beckham & W. R. Leber (Eds.), *Handbook of depression: Treatment, assessment, and research* (pp. 745-762). Homewood, IL: Dorsey.

Kay, T., & Silver, S. M. (1989). Closed head trauma: Assessment for rehabilitation. In M. D. Lezak (Ed.), *Assessment of the behavioral consequences of head trauma* (pp. 145-170). New York: Alan R. Liss.

Keith, R. A. (1984). Functional assessment measures in medical rehabilitation: Current status. *Archives of Physical Medicine and Rehabilitation, 65,* 74-78.

Keith, R. A. (1986). Organizational effectiveness in the rehabilitation hospital: A cross-national comparison. *Rehabilitation Psychology, 31,* 131-141.

Keith, R. A. (1988). Observations in the rehabilitation hospital: Twenty years of research. *Archives of Physical Medicine and Rehabilitation, 69,* 625-631.

Keith, R. A. (in press). Comprehensive rehabilitation: Themes, models, and issues. In M. G. Eisenberg, R. L. Glueckauf, & H. Zaretsky (Eds.),

Medical aspects of disability: A handbook for the rehabilitation professional. New York: Springer.

Keith, R. A., & Breckenridge, K. (1985). Characteristics of patients from the Hospital Utilization Project data system: 1980-1982. *Archives of Physical Medicine and Rehabilitation, 66,* 768-772.

Keith, R. A., & Cowell, K. S. (1987). Time use of stroke patients in three rehabilitation hospitals. *Social Science and Medicine, 24,* 529-533.

Kelly-Hayes, M., Wolf, P. A., Kase, C. S., Gresham, G. E., Kannel, W. B., & D'Agostino, R. B. (1989). Time-course of functional recovery after stroke: The Framingham Study. *Journal of Neurological Rehabilitation, 3,* 65-70.

Kemp, B. (1985). Rehabilitation and the older adult. In J. E. Birren & K. W. Schaie (Eds.), *Handbook of the psychology of aging* (2nd ed., pp. 647-663). New York: Van Nostrand Reinhold.

Kemp, B. J., & Vash, C. L. (1971). Productivity after injury in a sample of spinal cord injured persons. *Journal of Chronic Disease, 27,* 337-343.

Kendall, P. C., Edinger, J., & Eberly, C. (1978). Taylor's MMPI correction factor for spinal cord injury: Empirical endorsement. *Journal of Consulting and Clinical Psychology, 46,* 370-371.

Kettner, P. M., Moroney, R. M., & Martin, L. L. (1990). *Designing and managing programs.* Newbury Park, CA: Sage.

Kirchner, C. (1984). *Assessing effects of VR on disadvantaged persons: Theoretical perspectives and issues for research.* Unpublished manuscript.

Klauber, M. R., Marshall, L. F., Toole, B. M., Knowlton, S. L., & Bowers, S. A. (1985). Cause of decline in head injury mortality rate in San Diego County, California. *Journal of Neurosurgery, 62,* 528-531.

Klippel, J., & DeJoy, D. (1984). Counseling psychology in behavioral medicine and health psychology. *Journal of Counseling Psychology, 31,* 219-227.

Klonoff, H., Fibiger, C. H., & Hutton, G. H. (1970). Neuropsychological patterns in chronic schizophrenia. *Journal of Nervous and Mental Disease, 50,* 291-300.

Konarski, E. A., Jr. (1985). The use of response deprivation to increase the academic performance of EMR students. *The Behavior Therapist, 8,* 61.

Koren, P. E., DeChillo, N., & Friesen, B. J. (in press). A brief questionnaire to assess empowerment in families who have members with disabilities. *Rehabilitation Psychology, 37*(4).

Kotila, M., Waltimo, O., Niemi, M. L., Laaksonen, R., & Lempinen, M. (1984). The profile of recovery from stroke and factors that influence outcomes. *Stroke, 15,* 1039-1044.

Kozak, M. J., & Miller, G. A. (1982). Hypothetical constructs versus intervening variables: A re-appraisal of the three-systems model of anxiety assessment. *Behavioral Assessment, 4,* 347-358.

Kravetz, S., Florian, V., & Wright, G. N. (1985). The development of a multifaceted measure of rehabilitation effectiveness: Theoretical rationale and scale construction. *Rehabilitation Psychology, 30,* 195-208.

Kreutzer, J. S., Leininger, B. E., & Harris, J. A. (1990). The evolving role of neuropsychology in community integration. In J. S. Kreutzer & P. Wehman (Eds.), *Community integration following traumatic brain injury* (pp. 49-66). Baltimore: Paul H. Brooks.

Kyle, J. (1987). *Adjustment to acquired hearing loss: Analysis, change, and learning* (Proceedings of conference at University of Bristol). Bristol: Center for Deaf Studies.

Laird, M., & Krown, S. (1991). Evaluation of a transitional employment program. *Psychosocial Rehabilitation Journal, 15*(1), 3-8.

Lang, P. J. (1968). Fear reduction and fear behavior: Problems in treating a construct. In J. M. Schlein (Ed.), *Research in psychotherapy* (Vol. 3, pp. 91-102). Washington, DC: American Psychological Association.

Lang, P. J., & Cuthbert, B. N. (1984). Affective information processing and the assessment of anxiety. *Journal of Behavioral Assessment, 6,* 369-395.

Lanyon, R., & Goodstein, L. (1982). *Personality assessment* (2nd ed.). New York: J. Wiley.

Lehman, A., & Cordray, D. S. (1991). *Prevalence of alcohol, drug, and mental health disorders among the homeless: A quantitative synthesis.* Prepared for the National Institute of Mental Health, under revision for publication.

Lehmann, J. F., De Lateur, B. J., Fowler, R. S., Warren, C. G., Arnold, R., Schertzer, G., Hurka, R., Whitmore, J. J., Masock, A. J., & Chambers, K. H. (1975). Stroke rehabilitation: Outcome and prediction. *Archives of Physical Medicine and Rehabilitation, 56,* 383-389.

Leli, D. A., & Filskov, S. B. (1984). Clinical detection of intellectual deterioration associated with brain damage. *Journal of Clinical Psychology, 40,* 1435-1441.

Lemke, S., & Moos, R. H. (1990). Measuring the social climate of congregate residences for older people. *Psychology and Aging, 2,* 20-29.

Lerner, M. (1986). *Surplus powerlessness: Psychodynamics of everyday life and the psychology of individual and social transformation.* Oakland, CA: Institute for Labor and Mental Health.

Leung, P. (1984). Training in rehabilitation psychology. In C. Golden (Ed.), *Current topics in rehabilitation psychology* (pp. 17-27). Orlando, FL: Grune & Stratton.

Leung, P., Sakata, R., & Ostby, S. (1990). Rehabilitation psychology professional training: A survey of APA accredited programs. *Rehabilitation Education, 4,* 177-183.

Levin, H. S., Benton, A. L., & Grossman, R. G. (1982). *Neurobehavioral consequences of closed head injury.* New York: Oxford University Press.

Levine, E. (1981). *Ecology of early deafness.* New York: Columbia University Press.

Lewis, F., & Bolton, B. (1986). Latent structure modeling of VR clients' occupational attainment. *Rehabilitation Counseling Bulletin, 29,* 166-172.

Lezak, M. D. (1983). *Neuropsychological assessment* (2nd ed.). New York: Oxford University Press.

Lezak, M. D. (1987). Assessment for rehabilitation planning. In M. J. Meier, A. L. Benton, & L. Diller (Eds.), *Neuropsychological rehabilitation* (pp. 41-58). New York: Guilford.

Lezak, M. D. (1988). Brain damage is a family affair. *Journal of Clinical and Experimental Neuropsychology, 10,* 111-123.

Lezak, M. D. (1989). Assessment of psychosocial dysfunctions resulting from head trauma. In M. D. Lezak (Ed.), *Assessment of the behavioral consequences of head trauma* (pp. 113-143). New York: Alan R. Liss.

Lichtenstein, S., Fischhoff, B., & Phillips, L. D. (1982). Calibration of probabilities: The state of the art to 1980. In D. Kahneman, P. Slovic, & A. Tversky (Eds.), *Judgment under uncertainty: Heuristics and biases* (pp. 306-334). Cambridge, UK: Cambridge University Press.

Linkowski, D. C. (1987). *The Acceptance of Disability Scale.* Washington, DC: George Washington University, Rehabilitation Research and Training Center.

Lipsey, M. W. (1990, May). Theory as method: Small theories of treatment. In L. Sechrest, E. Perrin, & J. Bunker (Eds.), *Research methodology: Strengthening causal interpretations of nonexperimental data* (pp. 33-51). Washington, DC: Agency for Health Care Policy and Research, Public Health Service, U.S. Department of Health and Human Services.

Lipsey, M. W. (1991). *Design sensitivity: Statistical power for experimental research.* Newbury Park, CA: Sage.

Lipsey, M. W., Crosse, S., Dunkle, J., Pollard, J., & Stobart, G. (1985). Evaluation: The state of the art and the sorry state of the science. *New Directions for Program Evaluation, 27,* 7-28.

Lipsey, M. W., & Pollard, J. A. (1989). Driving toward theory in program evaluation: More models to choose from. *Evaluation and Program Planning, 12,* 317-328.

Lister, M. J. (1987). Clinical measurement. *Physical Therapy, 67,* 1829.

Loehlin, J. C. (1987). *Latent variable models: An introduction to factor, path, and structural analysis.* Hillsdale, NJ: Lawrence Erlbaum.

Loevinger, J. (1966). The meaning and measurement of ego development. *American Psychologist, 21,* 195-206.

Lofquist, L. H. (1960). *Conference on research in the psychological aspects of rehabilitation.* Washington, DC: American Psychological Association.

Long, J. S. (1983). *Confirmatory factor analysis: A preface to LISREL.* Beverly Hills, CA: Sage.

Lorenze, E. J., & Cancro, R. (1962). Dysfunction in visual perception in hemiplegia: Its relation to activities of daily living. *Archives of Physical Medicine and Rehabilitation, 43,* 514-517.

Lowe, J. B., Windsor, R. A., Adams, B., Morris, J., et al. (1986). Use of a *bogus pipeline* method to increase accuracy of self-reported alcohol consumption among pregnant women. *Journal of Studies on Alcohol, 47,* 173-175.

Lubin, B., Larsen, R. M., & Matarrazzo, J. D. (1984). Patterns of psychological test usage in the United States: 1935-1982. *American Psychologist, 39,* 451-454.

Ludlow, L. H., et al. (1983, April 11-15). *Measuring change with the Rating Scale Model.* Paper presented at the annual meeting of the American Educational Research Association, Montreal.

Luey, H. (1980). Between worlds: The problem of deafened adults. *Social Work in Health Care, 5,* 253-265.

Luria, A. R. (1963). *Restoration of function after brain injury.* London: Pergamon.

Luria, A. R. (1980). *Higher cortical functions in man* (rev. ed.; B. Haigh, Trans.). New York: Basic Books.

Luria, A. R., Naydin, V. L., Tsvetkova, L. S., & Vinarskaya, E. N. (1969). Restoration of higher cortical function following local brain damage. In P. J. Vinken & G. W. Bruyn (Eds.), *Handbook of clinical neurology* (Vol. 3, pp. 368-433). Amsterdam, the Netherlands: North-Holland.

MacCorquodale, K., & Meehl, P. E. (1948). On the distinction between hypothetical constructs and intervening variables. *Psychological Review, 55,* 95-107.

MacGuffie, R. A., Misener, B. B., & Reichart, D. A. (1989). Present and ideal roles and functions of the medical rehabilitation counselor. *Journal of Applied Rehabilitation Counseling, 20,* 33-40.

Magistro, C. M. (1989). Clinical decision making in physical therapy: A practitioner's perspective. *Physical Therapy, 69,* 525-534.

Malec, J., & Neimeyer, R. (1983). Psychologic prediction of duration of inpatient spinal cord injury rehabilitation and performance of self-care. *Archives of Physical Medicine and Rehabilitation, 64,* 359-363.

Mariano, A. J. (1992). Chronic pain and spinal cord injury. *Clinical Journal of Pain, 8,* 87-92.

Marrone, J., Horgan, J., Scripture, D., & Grossman, M. (1984). Serving the severely psychiatrically disabled client within the VR system. *Psychosocial Rehabilitation Journal, 8*(2), 5-23.

Marsh, H. W. (1987). The hierarchical structure of self-concept and the application of hierarchical confirmatory factor analysis. *Journal of Educational Measurement, 24,* 17-39.

Marsh, H. W., Balla, J. R., & McDonald, R. P. (1988). Goodness-of-fit indexes in confirmatory factor analysis: The effect of sample size. *Psychological Bulletin, 103,* 391-410.

Marsh, H. W., & Hocevar, D. (1985). Application of confirmatory factor analysis to the study of self-concept: First- and higher order factor models and their invariance across groups. *Psychological Bulletin, 97,* 562-582.

Marsh, H. W., & Hocevar, D. (1988). A new, more powerful approach to multitrait-multimethod analyses: Application of second-order confirmatory factor analysis. *Journal of Applied Psychology, 73,* 107-117.

Mason, L., & Muhlenkamp, A. (1976). Patients' self-reported affective states following loss and caregivers' expectations of patients' affective states. *Rehabilitation Psychology, 59,* 573-579.

Massel, H. K., Liberman, R. P., Mintz, J., Jacobs, H. E., Rush, T. V., Giannini, C. A., & Zarate, R. (1990). Evaluating the capacity to work of the mentally ill. *Psychiatry, 53,* 31-43.

Matarazzo, J. D. (1990). Psychological assessment versus psychological testing: Validation from Binet to the school, clinic, and courtroom. *American Psychologist, 45,* 999-1017.

Matt, G. E., Vazquez, C., & Campbell, W. K. (1992). Mood-congruent recall of affectively toned stimuli: A meta-analytic review. *Clinical Psychology Review, 12,* 227-255.

McCaffrey, R. J., Malloy, P. F., & Brief, D. J. (1985). Internship opportunities in clinical neuropsychology emphasizing recent INS training certificate. *Professional Psychology: Research and Practice, 16,* 236-252.

McCarron, L., & Dial, J. (1986). *McCarron-Dial Work Evaluation System: A systematic approach to vocational, educational, and neuropsychological assessment.* Dallas, TX: Common Market Press.

McDowell, I., & Newell, C. (1987). *Measuring health.* New York: Oxford University Press.

McEwan, K. L., & Devins, G. M. (1983). Is increased arousal in social anxiety noticed by others? *Journal of Abnormal Psychology, 92,* 417-421.

McFall, R. M. (1991). Manifesto for a science of clinical psychology. *The Clinical Psychologist, 44,* 75-88.

McFall, R. M., & McDonel, E. C. (1986). The continuing search for units of analysis in psychology: Beyond persons, situations, and their interactions. In R. O. Nelson & S. C. Hayes (Eds.), *Conceptual foundations of behavioral assessment* (pp. 201-241). New York: Guilford.

McFarlane, W. R. (1991). Family psychoeducational treatment. In A. S. Gurman & D. P. Kniskern (Eds.), *Handbook of family therapy* (Vol. 2, pp. 363-395). New York: Brunner/Mazel.

McGlynn, S. M., & Kaszniak, A. W. (1991a). Unawareness of deficits in dementia and schizophrenia. In G. P. Prigatano & D. Schacter (Eds.), *Awareness of deficit after brain injury: Clinical and theoretical issues* (pp. 84-110). New York: Oxford University Press.

McGlynn, S. M., & Kaszniak, A. W. (1991b). When metacognition fails: Impaired awareness of deficit in Alzheimer's disease. *Journal of Cognitive Neuroscience, 3,* 184-189.

McGlynn, S. M., & Schacter, D. L. (1989). Unawareness of deficits in neuropsychological syndromes. *Journal of Clinical and Experimental Neuropsychology, 11,* 143-205.

McGrew, J. H., & McFall, R. M. (1990). A scientific inquiry into the validity of astrology. *Journal of Scientific Exploration, 4,* 75-83.

McKinlay, J. B., McKinlay, S. M., & Beaglehole, R. (1989). A review of the evidence concerning the impact of medical measures on recent mortality and morbidity in the United States. *International Journal of Health Services, 19,* 181-208.

McKinley, W. W., Brooks, D. N., Bond, M. R., Martinage, D. P., & Marshall, M. M. (1981). The short-term outcome of severe blunt head injury as reported by the relatives of the injured persons. *Journal of Neurology, Neurosurgery, and Psychiatry, 44,* 527-533.

McSweeney, A. J. (1990). Quality of life assessment in neuropsychology. In D. E. Tupper & K. D. Cicerone (Eds.), *The neuropsychology of everyday life: Assessment and basic competencies* (pp. 185-217). Boston: Kluwer Academic.

McSweeney, A. J., Grant, I., Heaton, R. K., Prigatano, G. P., & Adams, K. M. (1985). Relationship of neuropsychological status to everyday functioning in healthy and chronically ill persons. *Journal of Clinical and Experimental Neuropsychology, 7,* 281-291.

Meehl, P. E. (1950). On the circularity of the law of effect. *Psychological Bulletin, 47,* 52-75.

Meehl, P. E. (1954). *Clinical versus statistical prediction: A theoretical analysis and a review of the evidence.* Minneapolis: University of Minnesota Press.

Meehl, P. E. (1971). High school yearbooks: A reply to Schwarz. *Journal of Abnormal Psychology, 77,* 143-148.

Meehl, P. E. (1973). *Psychodiagnosis: Selected papers.* Minneapolis: University of Minnesota Press.

Meehl, P. E. (1984). Foreword. In D. Faust, *The limits of scientific reasoning.* Minneapolis: University of Minnesota Press.

Meehl, P. E. (1986). Causes and effects of my disturbing little book. *Journal of Personality Assessment, 50,* 370-375.

Meenan, R. F., Gertman, P. M., Mason, J. H., & Dunaif, R. (1982). The Arthritis Impact Measurement Scales: Further investigations of a health status measure. *Arthritis and Rheumatism, 24,* 544-549.

Meier, M. J., Strauman, S., & Thompson, W. G. (1987). Individual differences in neuropsychological recovery: An overview. In M. Meier, A. Benton, & L. Diller (Eds.), *Neuropsychological rehabilitation* (pp. 71-110). New York: Guilford.

Melvin, J. L. (1989). Status report on interdisciplinary medical rehabilitation. *Archives of Physical Medicine and Rehabilitation, 70,* 273-276.

Menchetti, B. M., & Flynn, C. C. (1990). Vocational evaluation. In F. R. Rusch (Ed.), *Supported employment: Models, methods, and issues* (pp. 111-130). Sycamore, IL: Sycamore.

Menchetti, B. M., & Rusch, F. R. (1988). Vocational evaluation and eligibility for rehabilitation services. In P. Wehman & M. S. Moon (Eds.), *Vocational rehabilitation and supported employment* (pp. 79-90). Baltimore: Paul H. Brookes.

Meyerson, L. (1955). Somatopsychology of physical disability. In W. M. Cruickshank (Ed.), *Psychology of exceptional children and youth.* Englewood Cliffs, NJ: Prentice-Hall.

Milberg, W. P., Hebben, N., & Kaplan, E. (1986). The Boston process approach to neuropsychological assessment. In I. Grant & K. M. Adams (Eds.), *Neuropsychological assessment of neuropsychiatric disorders* (pp. 65-86). New York: Oxford University Press.

Miller, E. (1984). *Recovery and management of neuropsychological impairments.* New York: John Wiley.

Millon, T. (1982). *Millon Clinical Multiaxial Inventory Manual.* Minneapolis: Interpretive Scoring Systems.

Millon, T., Green, C., & Meagher, R. (1982). *Millon Behavioral Health Inventory manual.* Minneapolis: National Computer Systems, Inc.

Minuchin, S. (1978). *Psychosomatic families.* Cambridge, MA: Harvard University Press.

Mischel, W. (1968). *Personality and assessment.* New York: John Wiley.

Moore, R. Y. (1974). Central regeneration and recovery of function: The problem of collateral reinnervation. In D. G. Stein, J. J. Rosen, & N. Butters (Eds.), *Plasticity and recovery of function in the central nervous system* (pp. 111-128). New York: Academic Press.

Moos, R. H. (1974). *The social climate scales: An overview.* Palo Alto, CA: Consulting Psychologist Press.

Moriarty, J. B. (1981). *Preliminary Diagnostic Questionnaire.* Dunbar: West Virginia Rehabilitation Research and Training Center.

Moryl, A. M. (1991). *A comparison of job performance ratings in two training sites for persons with serious mental illness.* Unpublished master's thesis, Indiana University-Purdue University, Department of Psychology, Indianapolis.

Mowbray, C. T., & Herman, S. E. (1991). Using multiple sites in mental health evaluations: Focus on program theory and implementation issues. *New Directions in Program Evaluation, 50,* 45-58.

Mulvey, E. P., Linney, J. A., & Rosenberg, M. S. (1987). Organizational control and treatment program design as dimensions of institutionalization in settings for juvenile offenders. *American Journal of Community Psychology, 15,* 321-335.

Murphy, S. T., & Hagner, D. C. (1988). Evaluating assessment settings: Ecological influences on vocational evaluation. *Journal of Rehabilitation, 54*(1), 53-59.

Murray, D. M., O'Connell, C. M., Schmid, L. A., & Perry, C. L. (1987). The validity of smoking self-reports by adolescents: A reexamination of the "bogus pipeline" procedure. *Addictive Behaviors, 12,* 7-15.

Muthard, J., & Salomone, P. (1969). The roles and functions of the rehabilitation counselor. *Rehabilitation Counseling Bulletin, 13,* 81-168.

Muthén, B. (1987). *LISCOMP: Analysis of linear structural relations with a comprehensive measurement model.* Mooresville, IN: Scientific Software, Inc.

Myers, B. A., Friedman, S. B., & Weiner, I. B. (1970). Coping with a chronic disability: Psychosocial observations of girls with scoliosis. *American Journal of Diseases of Children, 120,* 175-181.

Nagi, S. Z. (1976). An epidemiology of disability among adults in the United States. *Milbank Memorial Fund Quarterly/Health and Society, 54,* 439-467.

Nagi, S. Z. (1991). Disability concepts revisited: Implications for prevention. In Institute of Medicine, *Disability in America* (pp. 309-327). Washington, DC: National Academy Press.

National Association of Rehabilitation Facilities. (1988, November). *Medical rehabilitation. What it is and where it is: A discussion* (NARF Monograph Series). Washington, DC: NARF.

National Institute on Alcohol Abuse and Alcoholism. (1991). *Synopses of cooperative agreements for research demonstration projects on alcohol and other drug abuse treatment for homeless persons* (Contract No. ADM 281-89-0006). Rockville, MD: Author.

National Strategic Research Plan Task Force. (1989). *Report.* Bethesda, MD: National Institute on Deafness and Other Communication Disorders (NIDCD).

Neff, W. (1971). *Rehabilitation psychology.* Washington, DC: American Psychological Association.

Neff, W. S. (1977). *Work and human behavior* (2nd ed.). Chicago: Aldine.

Neff, W. S. (1980). Vocational assessment: Theory and models. In B. Bolton & D. W. Cook (Eds.), *Rehabilitation client assessment* (pp. 19-26). Baltimore: University Park Press.

Nemiah, J. C. (1957). The psychiatrist and rehabilitation. *Archives of Physical Medicine and Rehabilitation, 38,* 143-147.

Newman, L. (1970). Instant placement: A new model for providing rehabilitation services within a community mental health program. *Community Mental Health Journal, 6,* 401-410.

Newnan, O. S., Heaton, R. K., & Lehman, R. A. W. (1978). Neuropsychological and MMPI correlates of patients' future employment characteristics. *Perceptual and Motor Skills, 46,* 635-642.

Olshansky, S., & Hart, W. (1967). Psychologists in vocational rehabilitation or vocational rehabilitation counselors? *Journal of Rehabilitation, 33*(2), 28-29.

Orlans, H. (1985). *Adjustment to adult hearing loss.* San Diego, CA: College Hill Press.

Osmon, D. C. (1983). The use of test batteries in clinical neuropsychology. In C. J. Golden & P. J. Vicente (Eds.), *Foundations of clinical neuropsychology* (pp. 113-141). New York: Plenum.

Pacsofar, E. L. (1986). Assessing work behavior. In F. R. Rusch (Ed.), *Competitive employment: Issues and strategies* (pp. 93-102). Baltimore: Paul H. Brookes.

Padden, C. (1980). Deaf community and culture of deaf people. In C. Baker & K. Battison (Eds.), *Sign language and the deaf community: Essays in honor of William C. Stokoe.* Silver Spring, MD: National Association of the Deaf.

Paralyzed Veterans of America. (1988). *Final report: The PVA needs assessment survey.* Washington, DC: Author.

Parker, H. J., & Chan, F. (1990). Psychologists in rehabilitation: Preparation and experience. *Rehabilitation Psychology, 35,* 239-248.

Parker, R. M., & Hansen, C. E. (1976). Aptitude and achievement tests. In B. Bolton (Ed.), *Handbook of measurement and evaluation* (pp. 77-100). Baltimore: University Park Press.

Patrick, D. L., & Bergner, M. (1990). Measurement of health status in the 1990s. *Annual Review of Public Health, 11,* 165-183.

Patrick, D. L., & Peach, H. (Eds.). (1989). *Disablement in the community.* New York: Oxford University Press.

Patrick, D. L., Stein, J., Porta, M., Porter, C. Q., & Ricketts, T. C. (1988). Poverty, health services, and health statistics in rural America. *Milbank Memorial Fund Quarterly, 66,* 105-136.

Patton, M. Q. (1986). *Utilization-focused evaluation* (2nd ed.). Beverly Hills, CA: Sage.

Paul, G. L. (1987). Rational operations in residential treatment settings through ongoing assessment of client and staff functioning. In D. R. Peterson & D. B. Fishman (Eds.), *Assessment for decision* (pp. 145-203). New Brunswick, NJ: Rutgers University Press.

Peck, J., Smith, T. W., Ward, J., & Milano, R. (1989). Disability and depression in rheumatoid arthritis. *Arthritis and Rheumatism, 32,* 1100-1106.

Perlman, L. (Ed.). (1983). *Rehabilitation in the public mind.* Alexandria, VA: National Rehabilitation Association.

Peterson, D. R. (1968). *The clinical study of social behavior.* New York: Appleton-Century-Crofts.

Peterson, D. R. (1987). The role of assessment in professional psychology. In D. R. Peterson & D. B. Fishman (Eds.), *Assessment for decision* (pp. 5-43). New Brunswick, NJ: Rutgers University Press.

Pincus, T., Callahan, L., Bradley, L. A., Vaughn, W., & Wolfe, F. (1986). Elevated MMPI scores for hypochondriasis, depression, and hysteria in patients with rheumatoid arthritis reflect disease rather than psychological status. *Arthritis and Rheumatism, 29,* 1456-1466.

Piotrowski, C., & Keller, J. W. (1984). Attitudes toward clinical assessment by members of the AABT. *Psychological Reports, 55,* 831-838.

Piotrowski, C., & Lubin, B. (1990). Assessment practices of health psychologists: Survey of APA Division 38 clinicians. *Professional Psychology: Research and Practice, 21,* 99-106.

Piper, M. C., Darrah, J., & Byrne, P. (1989). Impact of gestational ages on preterm motor development at 4 months chronological and adjusted ages. *Child-Care, Health, and Development, 15,* 105-115.

Pollack, M., Levenstein, D. S. W., & Klein, D. F. (1968). A three-year posthospital follow up of adolescent and adult schizophrenics. *American Journal of Orthopsychiatry, 38,* 94-110.

Popper, K. (1962). *Conjectures & refutations.* New York: Basic Books.

Potsubay, R. T., & Fredrickson, R. H. (1985). The impact of vocational assessment on occupational consistency and employment stability of rehabilitation clients. *Vocational Evaluation and Work Adjustment Bulletin, 18*(1), 21-28.

Power, P. W. (1991). *A guide to vocational assessment* (2nd ed.). Austin, TX: PRO-ED.

Prediger, D. J. (1976). A World of Work Map for career exploration. *Vocational Guidance Quarterly, 24,* 198-208.

Premack, D. (1959). Toward empirical behavior laws: I. Positive reinforcement. *Psychological Review, 66,* 219-233.

Premack, D. (1965). Reinforcement theory. In D. Levine (Ed.), *Nebraska Symposium on Motivation, 1965* (pp. 123-180). Lincoln: University of Nebraska Press.

Pribram, K. H. (Ed.). (1969). *Brain and behavior 1: Mood states and mind.* Middlesex, England: Penguin.

Prigatano, G. P., Fordyce, D. J., Zeiner, H. K., Roueche, J. R., Pepping, M., & Wood, B. C. (1983). Neuropsychological rehabilitation after closed head injury in young adults. *Journal of Neurology, Neurosurgery, and Psychiatry, 47,* 505-513.

Prigatano, G. P., & Schacter, D. L. (Eds.). (1991). *Awareness of deficit after brain injury: Clinical and theoretical issues.* New York: Oxford University Press.

Pullin, D., & Zirkel, P. A. (1988, March 31). Testing the handicapped: Legislation, regulations and litigation. *West's Education Law Reporter, 44,* 1-18.

Putnam, S. H., & DeLuca, J. W. (1990). The TCN Professional Practice Survey: Part I: General practices of neuropsychologists in primary employment and private practice settings. *The Clinical Neuropsychologist, 4,* 199-244.

Quittner, A. L., Glueckauf, R. L., & Jackson, D. N. (1990). Chronic parenting stress: Moderating versus mediating effects of social support. *Journal of Personality and Social Psychology, 59,* 1266-1278.

Ragosta, M. (1988). *Issues in testing individuals with disabilities.* Unpublished manuscript, American Psychological Association, Committee on Disabilities and Handicaps, Washington, DC.

Rappaport, M., Herrero-Backe, C., Rappaport, M. L., & Winterfield, K. M. (1989). Head injury outcome up to ten years later. *Archives of Physical Medicine and Rehabilitation, 70,* 885-892.

Reding, M. J., & Potes, E. (1988). Rehabilitation outcome following initial unilateral hemispheric stroke. *Stroke, 19,* 1354-1358.

Reitan, R. M. (1988). Integration of neuropsychological theory, assessment, and clinical applications. *The Clinical Neuropsychologist, 2,* 331-349.

Reitan, R. M., & Wolfson, D. (1985). *The Halstead-Reitan Neuropsychological Test Battery: Theory and clinical interpretation.* Tucson, AZ: Neuropsychology Press.

Revell, W. G., Wehman, P., & Arnold, S. (1984). Supported work model of competitive employment for persons with mental retardation: Implications for rehabilitative services. *Journal of Rehabilitation, 50,* 30-38.

Richards, J. S. (1981). Pressure ulcers in spinal cord injury: Psychosocial correlates. *Model System's SCI Digest, 3,* 11-18.

Roberts-Gray, C., & Scheirer, M. A. (1988). Checking the congruence between a program and its organizational environment. *New Directions in Program Evaluation, 40,* 63-82.

Robertson, C., Gatchel, R. J., & Fowler, C. (1991). Effectiveness of a videotaped behavioral intervention in reducing anxiety in emergency oral surgery patients. *Behavioral Medicine, 17,* 77-85.

Rock, D. A., Bennett, R. E., & Jirele, T. (1988). Factor structure of the Graduate Record Examinations general test in handicapped and nonhandicapped groups. *Journal of Applied Psychology, 73,* 383-392.

Roe, A. (1956). *The psychology of occupations.* New York: John Wiley.

Roe, A. (1985). Career and life. *Counseling Psychologist, 13,* 311-326.

Roessler, R., & Bolton, B. (1978). *Psychosocial adjustment to disability.* Baltimore: University Park Press.

Roessler, R. T., & Boone, S. E. (1982). Evaluation diagnoses as indicators of employment potential. *Vocational Evaluation and Work Adjustment Bulletin, 15*(3), 103-106.

Rogan, P., & Hagner, D. (1990). Vocational evaluation in supported employment. *Journal of Rehabilitation, 56*(1), 45-51.

Rohe, D. E., & Basford, J. (1989). Traumatic spinal cord injury, alcohol, and the Minnesota Multiphasic Personality Inventory. *Rehabilitation Psychology, 34,* 25-32.

Romano, J. M., & Turner, J. (1985). Chronic pain and depression: Does the evidence support a relationship? *Psychological Bulletin, 97,* 18-34.

Rosenthal, R. (1963). On the social psychology of the psychological experiment: The experimenter's hypothesis as an unintended determinant of experimental results. *American Scientist, 51,* 268-283.

Rossi, P. H. (1978). Issues in the evaluation of human services delivery. *Evaluation Quarterly, 2,* 573-599.

Rossi, P. H., & Freeman, H. E. (1989). *Evaluation: A systematic approach.* Newbury Park, CA: Sage.

Rothenberg, R. B., & Koplan, J. P. (1990). Chronic disease in the 1990s. *Annual Review of Public Health, 11,* 267-296.

Rothstein, J. M. (Ed.). (1985). *Measurement in physical therapy: Clinics in physical therapy* (Vol. 7). New York: Churchill Livingstone.

Rourke, B. P. (1982). Central processing deficiencies in children: Toward a developmental neuropsychological model. *Journal of Clinical Neuropsychology, 4*, 1-18.

Ruddy, L. (1987). *Washington State DVR/U.S. Department of Labor "pilot project" for "community-based time-limited vocational assessment.* Unpublished manuscript, Washington State-DSHS/DVR, Olympia, WA.

Rudrud, E. H., Wendelgass, P., Markve, R. A., Ferrara, J. A., & Decker, D. S. (1982). Community referenced assessment of vocational knowledge and preference. *Vocational Evaluation and Work Adjustment Bulletin, 15*(1), 19-21.

Rudrud, E. H., Ziarnik, J., Bernstein, G., & Ferrara, J. (1984). *Proactive vocational rehabilitation.* Baltimore: Paul H. Brookes.

Russell, E. W. (1984). Theory and development of pattern analysis methods related to the Halstead-Reitan Battery. In P. E. Logue & J. M. Schear (Eds.), *Clinical neuropsychology: A multidisciplinary approach* (pp. 50-98). Springfield, IL: Charles C Thomas.

Rutman, L. (1980). *Planning useful evaluations: Evaluability assessment.* Beverly Hills, CA: Sage.

Sampaio, E., Bril, B., & Breniere, Y. (1989). Is vision necessary for learning to walk? Preliminary study and methodological approach. *Psychologie Francaise, 34*, 71-78.

Sather, W. S. (1985). Planning for improvement in counselor performance in the state/federal vocational rehabilitation program. *Journal of Rehabilitation Administration, 9*, 4-14.

Sawyer, J. (1966). Measurement *and* prediction, clinical *and* statistical. *Psychological Bulletin, 66*, 178-200.

Schalock, R. L. (1988). Critical performance evaluation indicators in supported employment. In P. Wehman & M. S. Moon (Eds.), *Vocational rehabilitation and supported employment* (pp. 163-174). Baltimore: Paul H. Brookes.

Scheff, S. W. (Ed.). (1984). *Aging and recovery of function in the central nervous system.* New York: Plenum.

Scherer, M. (1989). Differing perspectives of the use of assistive devices by people with physical disabilities. In *Computer technology/special education/rehabilitation proceedings of the Fourth Annual Conference.* Northridge: California State University.

Scherer, M., & McKee, B. (1989). *Assistive technology device predisposition assessment (ATDPA).* Rochester, NY: National Technical Institute for the Deaf, Rochester Institute of Technology.

Scherer, M., McKee, B., & Young, M. (1990). *Educational technology predisposition assessment (ETPA)*. Rochester, NY: National Technical Institute for the Deaf, Rochester Institute of Technology.

Schneider, C., & Anderson, W. (1980). Attitudes toward the stigmatized: Some insights from recent research. *Rehabilitation Counseling Bulletin, 23,* 299-313.

Schoenfeld, T. A., & Hamilton, L. W. (1977). Secondary brain changes following lesions: A new paradigm for lesion experimentation. *Physiology and Behavior, 18,* 951-967.

Schulz, R., & Decker, S. (1985). Long-term adjustment to physical disability: The role of social support, perceived control, and self-blame. *Journal of Personality and Social Psychology, 48,* 1162-1172.

Scott, A., & Sechrest, L. (1992). The role of theory in guiding cost-benefit analysis. In H. T. Chen & P. Rossi (Eds.), *Policy studies organization*. Westport, CT: Greenwood.

Seale, C., & Davies, P. (1987). Outcome measurement in stroke rehabilitation research. *International Disability Studies, 9,* 155-160.

Sechrest, L., & Figueredo, A. J. (in press). Approaches used in conducting outcomes and effectiveness research. In P. Budetti (Ed.), *A research agenda for outcomes and effectiveness research*. Alexandria, VA: Health Administration Press.

Sechrest, L., & Pitz, D. (1987). Commentary: Measuring the effectiveness of heart transplant programs. *Journal of Chronic Diseases, 40*(Suppl. 1), 155-158.

Sechrest, L. B., West, S. G., Phillips, M. A., et al. (1979). Some neglected problems in evaluation research: Strength and integrity of treatments. In L. Sechrest et al., *Evaluation studies review annual* (Vol. 4). Beverly Hills, CA: Sage.

Selleck, V. (1991, March). *Rehabilita ion in the real world*. Presentation at Indiana University-Purdue University, Indianapolis, Department of Psychology.

Selvini Palazzoli, M., Boscolo, L., Cecchin, G., & Prata, G. (1978). *Paradox and counterparadox*. New York: Jason Aronson.

Shannon, C. E., & Weaver, W. (1949). *The mathematical theory of communication*. Urbana: University of Illinois Press.

Shavelson, R. J., & Webb, N. M. (1991). *Generalizability theory: A primer*. Newbury Park, CA: Sage.

Shavelson, R. J., Webb, N. M., & Rowley, G. L. (1989). Generalizability theory. *American Psychologist, 44,* 922-932.

Shontz, F., & Wright, B. (1980). The distinctiveness of rehabilitation psychology. *Professional Psychology, 11,* 919-924.

Shurrager, H. C. (1961). *A haptic intelligence scale for adult blind*. Chicago: Illinois Institute of Technology.

Sigafoos, J., Cole, D. A., & McQuarter, R. J. (1987). Current practices in the assessment of students with severe handicaps. *Journal of the Association for Persons with Severe Handicap, 12,* 264-273.

Siller, J. (1969a). Psychological situation of the disabled with spinal cord injuries. *Rehabilitation Literature, 30,* 290-296.

Siller, J. (1969b). *The general form of the Disability Factor Scales series (DFS-G).* New York: New York University, Department of Educational Psychology.

Silverstein, B., Kilgore, K. M., Fisher, W. P., Harley, J. P., & Harvey, R. F. (1991). Applying psychometric criteria to functional assessment in medical rehabilitation: I. Exploring unidimensionality. *Archives of Physical Medicine and Rehabilitation, 72,* 631-637.

Smelt, H. R. (1989). Effect of an inhibitive weight-bearing mitt on tone reduction and functional performance in a child with cerebral palsy. *Physical and Occupational Therapy in Pediatrics, 9,* 53-80.

Smith, B. H., & Sechrest, L. (1991). The treatment of aptitude-treatment interactions. *Journal of Consulting and Clinical Psychology, 59,* 233-244.

Smith, D. S., Goldenberg, E., Ashburn, A., Kinsella, G., Sheikh, K., Brennan, P. J., Meade, P. W., Zutshi, D. W., Perry, J. D., & Reeback, J. S. (1981). Remedial therapy after stroke: A randomized controlled trial. *British Medical Journal, 282,* 517-520.

Snow, W. G. (1987). Standardization of test administration and scoring criteria: Some shortcomings of current practice with the Halstead-Reitan Battery. *The Clinical Neuropsychologist, 1,* 250-262.

Snyder, C. R., Handelsman, M. M., & Endelman, J. R. (1978). Can clients provide valuable feedback to clinicians about their personality interpretations? A reply to Greene. *Journal of Consulting and Clinical Psychology, 46,* 1493-1495.

Society of Behavioral Medicine. (1988). *Directory of training opportunities in behavioral medicine.* Knoxville, TN: Author.

Sohlberg, M. M., & Mateer, C. A. (1987). Effectiveness of an attention training program. *Journal of Clinical and Experimental Neuropsychology, 9,* 117-130.

Sohlberg, M. M., & Mateer, C. A. (1989). *Introduction to cognitive rehabilitation: Theory and practice.* New York: Guilford.

Spear, J., & Schoepke, J. (1981). Psychologists and rehabilitation: Mandates and current training practices. *Professional Psychology, 12,* 606-612.

Spiegel, J. S., Spiegel, T. M., Ward, N. B., Paulus, H. E., Leake, B., & Kane, R. L. (1986). Rehabilitation for rheumatoid arthritis patients: A controlled trial. *Arthritis and Rheumatism, 29,* 628-637.

Stein, D. G., Rosen, J. J., & Butters, N. (Eds.). (1974). *Plasticity and recovery of function in the central nervous system.* New York: Academic Press.

Stewart, L. (Ed.). (1986). *Clinical rehabilitation assessment and hearing impairment.* Fayetteville: University of Arkansas.

Stolov, W. (1982). Evaluation of the patient. In F. J. Kottke, G. K. Stillwell, & J. F. Lehmann (Eds.), *Krusen's handbook of physical medicine and rehabilitation* (3rd ed., pp. 1-18). Philadelphia: W. B. Saunders.

Stolov, W., & Clowers, M. (1981). *Handbook of severe disability.* Washington, DC: U.S. Department of Education.

Stubbins, J. (1984). Rehabilitation services as ideology. *Rehab Psych, 29,* 197-203.

Stubbins, J. (1988). Politics of disability. In E. Yuker (Ed.), *Attitudes toward persons with disabilities.* Westport, CT: Greenwood.

Sussman, A. (1986, May). Mentally healthy deaf person. In *Program on approaches in counseling and psychotherapy with deaf clients.* Fremont, CA: Ohlone College/Gallaudet Extension.

Sutcliffe, J. P. (1980). On the relationship of reliability to statistical power. *Psychological Bulletin, 88,* 509-515.

Sweet, J. J., & Moberg, P. J. (1990). A survey of practices and beliefs among ABPP and non-ABPP clinical neuropsychologists. *The Clinical Neuropsychologist, 4,* 101-120.

Tanaka, J. S., & Huba, G. J. (1984). Confirmatory hierarchical factor analyses of psychological distress measures. *Journal of Personality and Social Psychology, 46,* 621-635.

Taylor, G. P. (1970). Moderator-variable effects on personality-test-item endorsements of physically disabled patients. *Journal of Consulting and Clinical Psychology, 35,* 183-188.

Thomas, J. P. (1979). Rehabilitation of the spinal cord injured: The model systems approach. *SCI Digest, 1,* 3-6, 33.

Thompson, M. S. (1980). *Benefit-cost analysis for program evaluation.* Beverly Hills, CA: Sage.

Timberlake, W. (1980). A molar equilibrium theory of learned performance. In G. H. Bower (Ed.), *The psychology of learning and motivation* (Vol. 14, pp. 1-58). New York: Academic Press.

Timberlake, W., & Allison, J. (1974). Response deprivation: An empirical approach to instrumental performance. *Psychological Review, 81,* 146-164.

Timberlake, W., & Farmer-Dougan, V. A. (1991). Reinforcement in applied settings: Figuring out ahead of time what will work. *Psychological Bulletin, 110,* 379-391.

Timko, C., & Moos, R. H. (1991). A typology of social climates in group residential facilities for older people. *Journal of Gerontology, 46,* S160-S169.

Torkelson, R. M., Jellinek, H. M., Malec, J. F., & Harvey, R. F. (1983). Traumatic brain injury: Psychological and medical factors related to rehabilitation outcome. *Rehabilitation Psychology, 28,* 169-176.

Trexler, L. (1987). Neuropsychological rehabilitation in the United States. In M. Meier, A. Benton, & L. Diller (Eds.), *Neuropsychological rehabilitation* (pp. 437-460). New York: Guilford.

Trieschmann, R. B. (1988). *Spinal cord injuries: Psychological, social, and vocational rehabilitation.* New York: Demos.

Tucker, L. R., & Lewis, C. (1973). The reliability coefficient for maximum likelihood factor analysis. *Psychometrika, 38,* 1-10.

Tuma, J. M., & Pratt, J. M. (1982). Clinical child psychology practice and training: A survey. *Journal of Clinical Child Psychology, 11,* 27-34.

Tupper, D. E., & Cicerone, K. D. (1990a). Introduction to the neuropsychology of everyday life. In D. E. Tupper & K. D. Cicerone (Eds.), *The neuropsychology of everyday life: Assessment and basic competencies* (pp. 3-18). Boston: Kluwer Academic.

Tupper, D. E., & Cicerone, K. D. (Eds.). (1990b). *The neuropsychology of everyday life: Assessment and basic competencies.* Boston: Kluwer Academic.

Turk, D. C., & Rudy, T. (1987). Towards a comprehensive assessment of chronic pain patients. *Behaviour Research and Therapy, 25,* 237-249.

Turner, J. A., Clancy, S., & Vitaliano, P. (1987). Relationships of stress, appraisal and coping to chronic low back pain. *Behaviour Research and Therapy, 25,* 281-288.

Turner, R. J., & McLean, P. D. (1989). Physical disability and psychological distress. *Rehabilitation Psychology, 34,* 225-242.

Ugland, R. P. (1982). The Mankato Productivity Ratio: A method for measuring individual productivity and work adjustment. *Vocational Evaluation and Work Adjustment Bulletin, 15,* 131-135.

Umlauf, R., & Frank, R. G. (1983). A cluster-analytic description of patient subgroups in the rehabilitation setting. *Rehabilitation Psychology, 28,* 157-167.

Ungerstedt, U. (1971). Post synaptic supersensitivity after 6-hydroxydopamine induced degeneration of nigro-striatal dopamine system. *Acta Physiologica Scandinavica* (Suppl. 367), pp. 69-93.

Ursprung, A. W. (1986). Incidence and correlates of burnout in residential service settings. *Rehabilitation-Counseling Bulletin, 29,* 225-239.

U.S. Commission on Civil Rights. (1983). *Accommodating the spectrum of individual abilities.* Washington, DC: U.S. Commission on Civil Rights.

U.S. Department of Labor. (1970). *Manual for the USES General Aptitude Test Battery*. Washington, DC: Government Printing Office.

U.S. Department of Labor. (1979). *Guide for occupational exploration*. Washington, DC: Government Printing Office.

U.S. Department of Labor. (1982a). *Manual for the General Aptitude Test Battery, section I: Administration and scoring*. Minneapolis, MN: Intran Corporation.

U.S. Department of Labor. (1982b). *Manual for the USES Interest Inventory*. Minneapolis, MN: Intran Corporation.

Vandergoot, D. (1986). *Review of placement research literature: Implications for research and practice* (Rehabilitation Research Review). Washington, DC: D:ATA Institute.

Van Fossen, B. (1988, February). *Structural and cultural context of violence*. Paper presented at the conference on Violence and Relationships, Rochester, NY.

Vash, C. (1982). Women and employment. In L. Perlman & K. Arenson (Eds.), *Women and rehabilitation of disabled persons*. Alexandria, VA: National Rehabilitation Association.

Vernon, M., & Andrews, J. (1989). *Psychology of deafness*. New York: Longman.

Vineberg, S., & Willems, E. (1971). Observation and analysis of patient behavior in the rehabilitation hospital. *Archives of Physical Medicine and Rehabilitation, 52*, 8-14.

von Monakow, C. (1914). *Die lokalisation im grosshirn und der abbau der funktion durch kortikale herde*. Wiesbaden, Germany: J. F. Bergmann.

Wade, T. C., & Baker, T. B. (1977). Opinions and use of psychological tests: A survey of clinical psychologists. *American Psychologist, 32*, 517-521.

Walls, R. T., Zane, T., & Thvedt, J. E. (1979). *The Independent Living Behavior Checklist* (experimental edition). Morgantown: West Virginia Rehabilitation Research and Training Center.

Wang, M. C., & Walberg, H. J. (1983). Evaluating educational programs: An integrative, causal-modeling approach. *Educational Evaluation and Policy Analysis, 5*, 347-366.

Ware, J. E., Brook, R. H., Davies-Avery, A. R., et al. (1980). *Conceptualization and measurement of health for adults in the Health Insurance Study: Vol. 1. Model of health and methodology* (Publication No. LR-1987/I-HEW). Santa Monica, CA: RAND Corporation.

Wasylenki, D. A., Goering, P. N., Lancee, W. J., Ballantyne, R., & Farkas, M. D. (1985). Impact of a case manager program on psychiatric aftercare. *Journal of Nervous and Mental Disease, 173*, 303-308.

Wax, T. (1990). Deaf community leaders as liaisons between mental health and deaf cultures. *Journal of American Deafness and Rehabilitation Association, 24,* 33-40.

Webb, E. J., Campbell, D. T., Schwartz, R. D., & Sechrest, L. (1966). *Unobtrusive measures: Nonreactive research in the social sciences.* Chicago: Rand McNally.

Webb, E., Campbell, D. T., Schwartz, R. D., Sechrest, L., & Grove, J. B. (1981). *Nonreactive measures in the social sciences.* Boston: Houghton Mifflin.

Watzlawick, P., Weakland, J., & Fisch, R. (1974). *Change: Principles of problem formation and resolution.* New York: Norton.

Wechsler, D. (1945). A standardized memory scale for clinical use. *Journal of Psychology, 19,* 87-95.

Wechsler, D. (1981). *WAIS-R manual: Wechsler Adult Intelligence Scale-Revised.* New York: Psychological Corporation.

Wechsler, D. (1987). *WMS-R manual: Wechsler Memory Scale—Revised.* New York: Psychological Corporation.

Wedding, D., & Faust, D. (1989). Clinical judgment and decision making in neuropsychology. *Archives of Clinical Neuropsychology, 4,* 233-265.

Wedding, D., & Gudeman, H. (1980, February). Implications of computerized axial tomography for clinical neuropsychology. *Professional Psychology,* pp. 31-35.

Wegener, S., & Elliott, T. (1992). Pain assessment of persons with spinal cord injury. *Clinical Journal of Pain, 8,* 93-101.

Wehman, P. (1986). Supported competitive employment for persons with severe disabilities. *Journal of Applied Rehabilitation Counseling, 17,* 24-29.

Wehman, P. (1988). Supported employment: Toward zero exclusion of persons with severe disabilities. In P. Wehman & M. S. Moon (Eds.), *Vocational rehabilitation and supported employment* (pp. 3-14). Baltimore: Paul H. Brookes.

Weick, K. E. (1980). *Social psychology of organizing* (2nd ed.). New York: Random House.

Weinberg, N., & Williams, J. (1978). How the physically disabled perceive their disabilities. *Journal of Rehabilitation, 44,* 31-33.

Weiss, D. J., Dawis, R. V., England, G. W., & Lofquist, L. H. (1967). *Manual for the Minnesota Satisfaction Questionnaire.* Minneapolis: University of Minnesota, Vocational Psychology Research.

Westbrook, M. T., & Nordholm, L. (1986). Effects of diagnosis on reactions to patient optimism and depression. *Rehabilitation Psychology, 31,* 79-94.

Westerheide, W. J., Lenhart, L., & Miller, M. C. (1975). *Field test of a services outcome measurement form: Client change.* Oklahoma City: Department of Institutions, Social and Rehabilitation Services.

Whisnat, J. P. (1984). The decline of stroke. *Stroke, 15,* 160-168.

Wholey, J. (1977). Evaluability assessment. In L. Rutman (Ed.), *Evaluation research methods.* Beverly Hills, CA: Sage.

Widaman, K. F. (1985). Hierarchically nested covariance structure models for multitrait-multimethod data. *Applied Psychological Measurement, 9,* 1-26.

Wiggins, J. S. (1973). *Personality and prediction: Principles of personality assessment.* Reading, MA: Addison-Wesley.

Williams, D. E., Thompson, J. K., Haber, J. D., & Raczynski, J. M. (1986). MMPI and headache: A special focus on differential diagnosis, prediction of treatment outcome, and patient-treatment matching. *Pain, 24,* 143-158.

Williams, G., & Mourer, S. (1990). Psychological assessment of newly injured SCI patients: Survey results. *SCI Psychosocial Process, 3*(3), 12-15.

Winter, P. L., & Keith, R. A. (1988). A model of outpatient satisfaction in rehabilitation. *Rehabilitation Psychology, 33,* 131-142.

Wolfensberger, W. (1972). *Principle of normalization in human services.* Toronto, Canada: National Institute on Mental Retardation.

Wood, P. H. N., & Badley, E. M. (1980). *People with disabilities: Toward acquiring information which reflects more sensitively their problems and needs.* New York: World Rehabilitation Fund.

Wood-Dauphinee, S., Shapiro, S., Bass, E., Fletcher, C., Georges, P., Hensby, V., & Mendelsohn, B. (1984). A randomized trial of team care following stroke. *Stroke, 15,* 864-872.

World Health Organization. (1980). *International classification of impairments, disabilities, and handicaps.* Geneva, Switzerland: Author

Wortman, P. M. (1983). Evaluation research: A methodological perspective. *Annual Review of Psychology, 34,* 246-260.

Wright, B. (1959). *Psychology and rehabilitation.* Washington, DC: American Psychological Association.

Wright, B. (1960). *Physical disability: A psychological approach.* New York: Harper & Row.

Wright, B. (1972). Value-laden beliefs and principles for rehabilitation psychology. *Rehabilitation Psychology, 19,* 38-45.

Wright, B. (1983). *Physical disability: A psychosocial approach* (2nd ed.). New York: Harper & Row.

Wright, B. (1988). Attitudes and the fundamental negative bias: Conditions and corrections. In H. Yuker (Ed.), *Attitudes toward persons with disabilities.* Westport, CT: Greenwood.

Wright, B., & Fletcher, B. (1982). Uncovering hidden resources: A challenge in assessment. *Professional Psychology, 13,* 229-235.

Wright, G. N., & Remmers, H. H. (1960). *Manual for the Handicap Problems Inventory.* Lafayette, IN: Purdue Research Foundation.

Wright, J. D. (1991). Methodological issues in evaluating the National Health Care for the Homeless Program. *New Directions for Program Evaluation, 52,* 61-74.

Yates, B. T. (1985). Cost-effectiveness analysis and cost-benefit analysis: An introduction. *Behavioral Assessment, 7,* 207-234.

Yeaton, W. H., & Sechrest, L. (1981). Critical dimensions in the choice and maintenance of successful treatments: Strength, integrity, and effectiveness. *Journal of Consulting and Clinical Psychology, 29,* 156-167.

Yuker, H. E., Block, J. R., & Young, J. H. (1970). *The measurement of attitudes toward disabled persons.* Albertson, NY: Human Resources Center.

Zieziula, F. (Ed.). (1983). *Assessment of hearing impaired people.* Washington, DC: Gallaudet University.

Index

About the Editors

Robert L. Glueckauf (Ph.D.) is Assistant Professor and Clinical Training Coordinator of the clinical rehabilitation psychology doctoral program in the Department of Psychology at Indiana University—Purdue University at Indianapolis. He obtained his M.S. and Ph.D. degrees in clinical psychology at Florida State University. He is President-Elect of the American Psychological Association's Division of Rehabilitation Psychology. He serves as Book Review Editor and Consulting Editor for *Rehabilitation Psychology*. He has written several empirical articles and chapters and edited books in the field of rehabilitation. As a scientist and educator, he is deeply committed to improving the quality of life of persons with disabilities through the promotion of rehabilitation research and education. His current research interests lie primarily in the development and evaluation of counseling interventions for persons with disabilities and their families.

Lee B. Sechrest (Ph.D.) is Professor of Psychology at the University of Arizona, having held previous positions at Pennsylvania State University, Northwestern University, Florida State University, and the University of Michigan. He was Head of the Department of Research on the Utilization of Scientific Knowledge at Michigan from 1980 to 1984. He has been President of the Divisions of Clinical Psychology and Evaluation, Measurement, and Statistics of the American Psychological Association and of the American Evaluation Association. He is also the founder and President of the Evaluation Group for Analysis of Data, a nonprofit organization devoted to research and consultation in program evaluation research methods and data analysis. He has directed more than 100 doctoral dissertations and has served as both a member and chair of research review panels for the National Center for Health Services Research (now AHCPR) and the Veterans Administration Health Services Research and Development service.

Gary R. Bond (Ph.D.) is Professor of Psychology and Director of the Doctoral Program in Clinical Rehabilitation Psychology at Indiana University–Purdue University at Indianapolis, where he has been since 1983. He received his doctorate in psychology from the University of Chicago in 1975. His early work was on the evaluation of the processes and outcomes in therapy groups and self-help groups. From 1979 to 1983 he was the Director of Research at Thresholds, a psychiatric rehabilitation center in Chicago. Since that time his interests have focused primarily on the evaluation of community programs directed to the rehabilitation and treatment of persons with serious mental illness. In 1989 he received a 5-year Research Scientist Development Award from the National Institute of Mental Health. He also received research awards from the American Rehabilitation Counseling Association in 1987, the American Psychological Association (Division of Rehabilitation Psychology) in 1990, and the Purdue School of Science at Indianapolis in 1991. His publications include more than 30 articles in peer-reviewed journals and 15 book chapters. Consistent with his interest in developing a partnership between the university and the public mental health sector, he has collaborated with several state departments of mental health on a variety of federal grants. He has consulted and presented widely to mental health and rehabilitation organizations throughout the United States.

Elizabeth C. McDonel (Ph.D.) is currently on a 2-year Research Fellowship sponsored by the National Association of State Mental Health Program Directors. The fellowship focuses on mental health services and policy research and is organized as a public-academic partnership between the Department of Psychology at Indiana University-Purdue University at Indianaplois (IUPUI), and the Indiana State Department of Family and Social Services administration, Division of Mental Health. She recieved her Ph.D. in clinical psychology from Indiana University in 1986. She has published in the areas of psychological assessment, psychiatric rehabilitation, and sexual assault.

About the Contributors

Brian Bolton (Ph.D., Rehabilitation Psychology, University of Wisconsin—Madison) is University Professor and Director of Research at the Arkansas Research and Training Center in Vocational Rehabilitation, University of Arkansas, Fayetteville. He is a Fellow of the American Psychological Association (Evaluation, Measurement, and Statistics, and Rehabilitation Psychology), of the Society for Personality Assessment, and of the American Psychological Society and has received 10 research project awards from the American Rehabilitation Counseling Association. He received the Burlington Northern Foundation Faculty Achievement Award for scholarly research from the University of Arkansas in 1986, the Roger Barker Distinguished Research Award from the Division of Rehabilitation Psychology of the American Psychological Association in 1988, and the Distinguished Career in Rehabilitation Counseling Research Award from the American Rehabilitation Counseling Association in 1989. His publications include 10 edited or authored books, 40 chapters or reviews in books or reference volumes, and 100 articles in psychology and rehabilitation journals.

Jennifer J. Bortz (Ph.D.) is a postdoctoral fellow in neuropsychology and neurological rehabilitation at the Barrow Neurological Institute in Phoenix, Arizona. She received her Ph.D. in clinical psychology from the University of Arizona in 1992, with a specialization in clinical neuropsychology. She completed her internship in clinical psychology and neuropsychology at Brown University School of Medicine in 1992. Her prior research has investigated the role of depression in the sense of self-efficacy of Parkinson's disease patients and the processing of emotional stimuli in Alzheimer's disease. Current research interests extend her work on emotion to other neurological populations, with a focus upon implications for clinical management and rehabilitation.

Jeffrey B. Brookings (Ph.D.) is Professor and former Chair of the Department of Psychology at Wittenberg University, Springfield, Ohio. He has published more than 25 articles in psychology and rehabilitation journals, cowritten two books, and made more than 35 presentations at national and regional professional conferences. His current interests include rehabilitation psychology; personality, ability, and vocational interest measurement; and applications of covariance structure modeling techniques to construct validation research.

David S. Cordray (Ph.D.) is Professor of Public Policy and Psychology and Chair of the Department of Human Resources at Vanderbilt University. He also is Director of the Center for the Study of At-Risk Populations and Public Assistance Policy at the Vanderbilt Institute for Public Policy Studies. Prior to joining the faculty at Vanderbilt, he was Associate Professor in the Division of Methodology and Evaluation Research at Northwestern University and the Assistant Director of Federal Welfare and Statistical Policy in the Program and Evaluation Methodology Division of the U.S. General Accounting Office. He is currently involved in several major research projects, including a national evaluation of programs serving homeless substance abusers and a meta-analysis of the effectiveness of job training programs.

Laura L. Dietzen (M.S.) is a graduate of the master's program in Rehabilitation Psychology at Indiana University–Purdue University at Indianapolis (IUPUI). She is employed at IUPUI as a Research Associate and has collaborated with Dr. Gary Bond on a variety of projects concerning mental health services for persons with serious mental illness.

Timothy R. Elliott (Ph.D.) is Assistant Professor in the Department of Psychology at Virginia Commonwealth University/Medical College of Virginia in Richmond. His primary appointment is with the counseling psychology program, and he is an affiliate faculty member in the social psychology program and an adjunct faculty member with the Department of Rehabilitation Medicine. He earned his M.S. in Rehabilitation Counseling from Auburn University in 1981; he acquired his Ph.D. in Counseling Psychology from the University of Missouri in 1987. He holds memberships in Divisions 17 (Counseling Psychology) and 22 (Rehabilitation Psychology) in the American Psychological Association as well as in the American Association of Spinal Cord Injury Psychologists and Social Workers. In 1991, he received the Early Research Achievement Award from Division 22 of the APA. His research interests concern the adjustment and psychosocial aspects associated with chronic illness, injury, and stress.

David Faust received his Ph.D. in Clinical Psychology from Ohio University in 1979. He is currently Professor of Psychology, at the University of Rhode Island, and holds an affiliate appointment in the Department of Psychiatry and Human Behavior, Brown University Medical School. He was previously Director of Psychology at the Rhode Island Hospital and has been an active, practicing psychologist, with a focus on neuropsychology. He has published widely on such topics as neuropsychology, clinical judgment, psychology and law, and the philosophy of science and has been the recipient of various awards and honors in psychology.

Alfred W. Kaszniak (Ph.D., ABPP) is Professor and acting head of the Psychology Department at the University of Arizona. He received his Ph.D. in 1976 from the University of Illinois and interned in clinical neuropsychology at Rush-Presbyterian-St. Luke's Medical Center in Chicago. He holds Diplomate status in the specialty area of clinical neuropsychology of the American Board of Professional Psychology (ABPP) and is a Fellow of the American Psychological Association and American Psychological Society. His major research interest is in neuropsychological aspects of aging and age-related disorders of the central nervous system (e.g., Alzheimer's and Parkinson's diseases). Other research interests include cognitive and behavioral consequences of frontal lobe damage, brain systems in emotional expression and comprehension, and the neuropsychology of consciousness. His publications include two books (one coedited and one cowritten) and more than 70 scientific papers, chapters, and reviews.

Robert Allen Keith (Ph.D.) is Director of the Research and Planning Center at Casa Colina Hospital for Rehabilitative Medicine and Professor of Psychology Emeritus, Claremont Graduate School. He has a Ph.D. in clinical psychology from the University of California, Los Angeles, is a Diplomate in Clinical Psychology (American Board of Professional Psychology), and is a Fellow of the Division of Rehabilitation Psychology of the American Psychological Association. In his career, he has been a research fellow in the Department of Nutrition, School of Public Health, Harvard University; visiting scholar, Department of Child Development, University of London; and a fellow of the International Exchange of Experts and Information in Rehabilitation program of the World Rehabilitation Fund. Research and publication in rehabilitation medicine have been primarily in functional assessment, data systems, treatment delivery systems, program evaluation, and clinical research. A recent project has been to coauthor a set of measurement standards for medical rehabilitation.

Mark W. Lipsey (Ph.D.) is currently Professor in the Department of Human Resources, Vanderbilt University, on leave from the Department of Psychology, Claremont Graduate School. His Ph.D., in psychology, is from the Johns Hopkins University. He has been a visiting fellow at the U.S. General Accounting Office, Program Evaluation and Methodology Division, and a Fulbright Lecturer at University of Delhi, in India. Editorships have included Editor-in-Chief, *New Directions for Program Evaluation* and Associate Editor of *Evaluation Review.* He is the author of *Design Sensitivity: Statistical Power for Experimental Research.* Areas of specialization include evaluation and treatment research on juvenile delinquency and juvenile justice, for which he has held numerous research grants and contracts. He has been a consultant on evaluation and research design for a wide variety of social agencies. His writings include treatment effectiveness, human service organizations, quality of life, and applied research methodology, particularly with meta-analysis and experimental and quasi-experimental designs and analysis.

Richard M. McFall received his Ph.D. in clinical psychology from Ohio State University in 1965, joined the faculty of the Psychology Department at the University of Wisconsin—Madison in 1965, and left Wisconsin in 1979 to join the psychology faculty at Indiana University—Bloomington, where he served as Director of Clinical Training from 1979 to 1985 and again from 1991 to the current time. His primary research focus has been on the assessment and prediction of interpersonal competence and on the relationship between competence and psychopathology. In pursuing these interests, he and his colleagues have investigated the competencies of a variety of clinical populations, including schizophrenics, depressed college students, adolescent delinquents, eating disordered college students, shy men, and sexually coercive men. In recent years, he has proposed and investigated a social information-processing model of social competence.

Georgine M. Pion (Ph.D.) is currently Research Associate Professor of Psychology and Human Development at Vanderbilt University and Fellow in the Center for the Study of At-Risk Populations and Public Assistance Policy at the Vanderbilt Institute for Public Policy Studies. Along with David Cordray, she is involved in a large-scale, national effort to examine the effectiveness of NIAAA-funded research demonstration projects aimed at homeless substance abusers. Her other research focuses on science policy including strategies for assessing the effectiveness of federal research training policies and issues surrounding the sharing of research data.

Teena M. Wax (Ph.D.) is Assistant Professor and Staff Chair of Psychological Services at the National Technical Institute for the Deaf, Rochester Institute of Technology. Previously, she was Washington State's Coordinator of Statewide Mental Health Services for Hearing Impaired Persons and also taught at Gallaudet University's Department of Counseling in Washington, D.C. She received her Ph.D. in psychology from the University of Delaware, Newark, in 1975, and her M.S.W. from the University of Maryland, Baltimore, in 1980. Her initial research and practice interests were in gerontology, with studies in biorhythms and addictions. She has approximately 15 years of clinical, research, practice, and administrative experience in psychosocial, developmental, mental health, and rehabilitation issues with deaf and hearing individuals and their families and special interests in cross-cultural mental health, addictions, and use of animals in mental health therapy. Deaf herself, she currently resides in Rochester, New York, and owns a Hearing Ear Dog.